Measuring Caring

International Research on
Caritas as Healing

JOHN NELSON, RN, MS, PhDc, is currently the President of Healthcare Environment, Inc., an international data management and consultation company. His experience includes 14 years of clinical experience and 10 years of data management and consultation for health care organizations. Nelson specializes in statistical analysis of clinical, financial, and labor indicators that assist executives in understanding the strengths and vulnerabilities of their organizations. He integrates multiple methods of mathematics to establish understanding of data, including Gaussian, Parato, non-Euclidean, pattern analysis, and qualitative analysis. He is a facilitator for the Caring International Research Collaborative, the largest research community within Sigma Theta Tau International, and has conducted or participated in approximately 80 studies within 15 different constructs that relate to health care, including caring, relationship-based care, primary nursing, self-care, workload (faculty of nursing and staff nurses), and complexity science. He has published in peer-reviewed nursing journals and spoken at several conferences throughout the world. He is a doctoral candidate at the University of Minnesota and is a member of several professional health care organizations.

JEAN WATSON, PhD, RN, AHN-BC, FAAN, is Distinguished Professor of Nursing and holds an endowed Chair in Caring Science at the University of Colorado, Denver, and Anschutz Medical Center Campus. She is founder of the original Center for Human Caring in Colorado and is a Fellow of the American Academy of Nursing. She previously served as Dean of Nursing at the University Health Sciences Center and is a past President of the National League for Nursing. Her latest activities include Founder and Director of a new, nonprofit foundation: Watson Caring Science Institute (http://www.watsoncaringscience.org).

Dr. Watson has earned undergraduate and graduate degrees in nursing and psychiatric–mental health nursing and holds her PhD in educational psychology and counseling. She is a widely published author and recipient of several awards and honors, including the Fetzer Institute Norman Cousins Award in recognition of her commitment to developing, maintaining, and exemplifying relationship-centered care practices; an international Kellogg Fellowship in Australia; and a Fulbright Research Award in Sweden. She holds eight honorary doctoral degrees, including five international honorary doctorates (Sweden, the United Kingdom, Spain, British Columbia and Quebec, Canada).

Clinical nurses and academic programs throughout the world use her published works on the philosophy and theory of human caring and the art and science of caring in nursing. Dr. Watson's caring philosophy is used to guide transformative models of caring and healing practices for nurses and patients alike, in diverse settings worldwide

At the University of Colorado, Dr. Watson holds the title of Distinguished Professor of Nursing, the highest honor accorded a faculty member for scholarly work. In 1999 she assumed the Murchinson-Scoville Chair in Caring Science, the nation's first endowed chair in Caring Science, based at the University of Colorado, Denver, & Health Sciences Center.

She is author or coauthor of over 16 books on caring; her latest books range from empirical measurements of caring to new, postmodern philosophies of caring and healing, philosophy and science of caring, and caring science as sacred science. Her books have earned *American Journal of Nursing* books-of-the-year awards and seek to bridge paradigms as well as point toward transformative models for this 21st century.

Measuring Caring
International Research on
Caritas as Healing

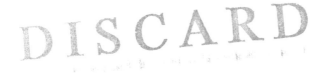

John Nelson, RN, MS, PhDc
Jean Watson, PhD, RN, AHN-BC, FAAN

Editors

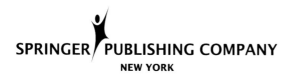

SPRINGER PUBLISHING COMPANY
NEW YORK

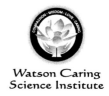

Watson Caring
Science Institute

Springer Publishing Company, LLC
11 West 42nd Street
New York, NY 10036
www.springerpub.com

Acquisitions Editor: Allan Graubard
Project Manager: Lindsay Claire
Composition: S4Carlisle Publishing Services

ISBN 978-0-8261-6351-6
E-book ISBN: 978-0-8261-6352-3
Caring Factor Surveys ISBN: 978-0-8261-9344-5

11 12 13 14/ 5 4 3 2 1

The author and the publisher of this Work have made every effort to use sources believed to be reliable to provide information that is accurate and compatible with the standards generally accepted at the time of publication. Because medical science is continually advancing, our knowledge base continues to expand. Therefore, as new information becomes available, changes in procedures become necessary. We recommend that the reader always consult current research and specific institutional policies before performing any clinical procedure. The author and publisher shall not be liable for any special, consequential, or exemplary damages resulting, in whole or in part, from the readers' use of, or reliance on, the information contained in this book. The publisher has no responsibility for the persistence or accuracy of URLs for external or third-party Internet Web sites referred to in this publication and does not guarantee that any content on such Web sites is, or will remain, accurate or appropriate.

The Caring Factor Surveys, the primary tools used for the major studies in this book, are available to download at www.springerpub.com/NelsonCaring

Library of Congress Cataloging-in-Publication Data
Measuring caring : international research on caritas as healing/edited by John Nelson, Jean Watson.
    p.; cm.
  Includes bibliographical references and index.
  ISBN 978-0-8261-6351-6 (alk. paper) — ISBN 978-0-8261-6352-3 (e-book)
  1. Nurse and patient. 2. Nursing—Philosophy. 3. Nursing. 4. Medical care.
  I. Nelson, John, R.N. II. Watson, Jean, 1940–
  [DNLM: 1. Nursing Theory. 2. Empathy. 3. Nurse's Role. 4. Nurse-Patient Relations.
  5. Nursing Care—methods. 6. Philosophy, Nursing. WY 86]
  RT86.3.M44 2012
  610.73—dc23
                                                                              2011020541

Special discounts on bulk quantities of our books are available to corporations, professional associations, pharmaceutical companies, health care organization, and other qualifying groups.

If you are interested in a custom book, including chapters from more than one of our titles, we can provide that service as well.

For details, please contact:
Special Sales Department, Springer Publishing Company, LLC
11 West 42nd Street, 15th Floor, New York, NY 10036-8002
Phone: 877-687-7476 or 212-431-4370; Fax: 212-941-7842
Email: sales@springerpub.com

Printed in the United States of America by Gasch Printing.

This book is dedicated to all the practitioners, educators, and scholars in caring science around the world who are interested in and committed to pursuing research and innovative approaches to assess and measure Caritas (caring and love), as well as theory validation.

To those who paved the way for this research and ventured into new models of experimentation and collaboration to make this happen.

Finally, to Springer Publishing for its support and encouragement in pursuing the publication of this international research.

Contents

Contributors

Gino Angelo S. Aloc, BSN, Remedios T. Romualdez Mem. Schools, Makati Medical Center, College of Nursing, Makati, Philippines

Gernalyn M. Antonio, BSN, Remedios T. Romualdez Mem. Schools, Makati Medical Center, College of Nursing, Makati, Philippines

Diana Marie Avecilla-Millare, BSN, Remedios T. Romualdez Mem. Schools, Makati Medical Center, College of Nursing, Makati, Philippines

Maritess M. Bedona, BSN, Remedios T. Romualdez Mem. Schools, Makati Medical Center, College of Nursing, Makati, Philippines

Gail Franka C. Beligrado, BSN, Remedios T. Romualdez Mem. Schools, Makati Medical Center, College of Nursing, Makati, Philippines

Kate Bent, PhD, National institutes of Health, Bethesda, Maryland

Marjorie Bott, PhD, University of Kansas School of Nursing, Kansas City, Kansas

Maria Brennan, MSN, St. Joseph's Healthcare System, Paterson, New Jersey

Rea Anna Buenaventura, BSN, Remedios T. Romualdez Mem. Schools, Makati Medical Center, College of Nursing NA Makati

Christelle Jolie O. Bulala, BSN, Remedios T. Romualdez Mem. Schools, Makati Medical Center, College of Nursing, Makati, Philippines

Kristal Capalungan, BSN, Remedios T. Romualdez Mem. Schools, Makati Medical Center, College of Nursing, Makati, Philippines

Joe Pak Leng Cheong, BSc, Kiang Wu Hospital of Macau, China

Selwynne Wan Cheong, BSc, MPHC, Kiang Wu Nursing College of Macau, China

Elizabeth Clerico, MSN, BSN, Roper Saint Francis Healthcare, Charleston, South Carolina

Gerri Clubb, BSN, MS, Indiana Wesleyan University, Marion, Indiana

Sandra Conklin, MSN, Wyoming Medical Center, Casper, Wyoming

Mae Shela S. Cruz, BSN, Remedios T. Romualdez Mem. Schools, Makati Medical Center, College of Nursing, Makati, Philippines

Maria Cutrera, BNS, Hospital "Piccole Figlie," Parma, Italy

Vickie Diamond, MS, Wyoming Medical Center, Casper, Wyoming

Pam DiNapoli, BSN, MSN, PhD, University of New Hampshire and Catholic Medical Center, Manchester, New Hampshire

Karen Drenkard, PhD, American Nurses Credentialing Center, Silver Spring, Maryland

Mally Ehrenfeld, PhD, Tel Aviv University, Tel Aviv, Israel

Nancy L. Fahrenwald, PhD, South Dakota State University, College of Nursing Brookings, South Dakota

Jayne Felgen, BS, MPA, Creative Health Care Management, Minneapolis, Minnesota

Margaret May A. Ga, MAN, Remedios T. Romualdez Mem. Schools, Makati Medical Center, College of Nursing, Makati, Philippines

Penelope Glynn, PhD, Regis College, School of Nursing, Weston, Massachucetts

Karen Gutierrez, BA, MS, PhD, Metro State University, St. Paul, Minnesota

Katherine R. Gutierrez, BSN, Remedios T. Romualdez Mem. Schools, Makati Medical Center, College of Nursing, Makati, Philippines

Sydrick D. G. Gutierrez, BSN, Remedios T. Romualdez Mem. Schools, Makati Medical Center, College of Nursing, Makati, Philippines

Christi Harley, BS, BSN, Roper Saint Francis Healthcare, Charleston, South Carolina

Winnie Hennessy, BSN, MSN, PhD, Roper Saint Francis Healthcare, Charleston, South Carolina

Anna Herbst, BSN, MSN, Inova Health System, Falls Church, Virginia

MaryAnn Hozak, MSN, St. Joseph's Healthcare System, Paterson, New Jersey

Shannon S. Spies Ingersoll, DNP, Olmsted Medical Center, Rochester, Minnesota

Michal Itzhaki, PhD, Tel Aviv University, Tel Aviv

Raffiel Jacinto, MAN, Remedios T. Romualdez Mem. Schools, Makati Medical Center, College of Nursing, Makati, Philippines

Jennifer Johnson, ADN, BA, MA, MSNEd, Our Lady of Lourdes Memorial Hospital, Binghamton, New York

Sandy Johnson, BA, San Joaquin Community Hospital, San Joaquin, California

Dawn Julian, BA, MS, DNP, Geary Community Hospital - Rural Health Clinic, Junction City, Kansas

Mavra Kear, PhD, Polk State College, Winter Haven, Florida

Erin Kosak, BSN, Bon Secour St. Francis Hospital, Charleston, South Carolina

Sara Sio Wa Lao, BSc, Kiang Wu Nursing College of Macau, China

Iris Lawrence, BS, Winter Haven Hospital, Winter Haven, Florida

Patti Leger, BSN, Wyoming Medical Center, Casper, Wyoming

Iris Kate R. Llorca, BSN, Remedios T. Romualdez Mem. Schools, Makati Medical Center, College of Nursing, Makati, Philippines

Grace Ka In Lok, BSc, MNS, Kiang Wu Nursing College of Macau, China

Tanya Lott, BSN, MSN, Roper Saint Francis Healthcare, Charleston, South Carolina

Giuliana Masera, MS, MBA, PhD, Univerisity of Parma, Parma, Italy

Peggy McCartt, PhD, Baptist Health, Jacksonville, Florida

Cheryl McDavitt, BSN, Norwood Hospital, Norwood, Massachucetts

Yvonne Michel, BS, PhD, Statistical Consulting (self employed), Daniel Island, South Carolina

John Nelson, AD, BSN, MS, PhDc, Healthcare Environment, St. Paul, Minnesota

Lynda Olender, AD, BSN, MA, PhDc, James J. Peters, Veterans Affairs Medical Center, New York, New York

Dax Andrew Parcells, BS, MA, PhDc, Florida Atlantic Univsersity, Boca Raton, Florida

Georgia Persky, BSN, MBA, DNSc, New York-Presbyterian Hospital/Columbia University Medical Center, New York, New York

Sheri Phifer, BSN, Duke University Hospital, Durham, North Carolina

Melinda M. Phillips, ASN, BSN, MSN, Galen College of Nursing, Louisville, Kentucky

Diane Raines, MSN, RN, Baptist Health, Jacksonville, Florida

Princess M. Ramos, BSN, Remedios T. Romualdez Mem. Schools, Makati Medical Center, College of Nursing, Makati, Philippines

Patricia Clarisse V. Reyes, BSN, Remedios T. Romualdez Memorial Schools, Makati Medical Center, College of Nursing, Makati, Philippines

Linda S. Rieg, BSN, MBA, MSN, PhD, Indiana Wesleyan University, Marion, Indiana

Maria Romana, MSN, New York-Presbyterian Hospital, New York, New York

Elena O. Rubis, BSN, Remedios T. Romualdez Mem. Schools, Makati Medical Center, College of Nursing, Makati, Philippines

Jill Rye, MA, Avera McKennan Hospital, Sioux Falls, South Dakota

Ana M. Schaper, BSN, MS, PhD, Gundersen Lutheran Health System, La Crosse, Wisconsin

Darcy Sherman-Justice, MS, Avera McKennan Hospital & University Health Center, Sioux Falls, South Dakota

Alfonso Sollami, PhD, Azienda Ospedaliero University of Parma, Parma, Italy

Deanne Sramek, BSN, DNP, Wyoming Medical Center, Casper, Wyoming

Janina Sweetenham, M.A. (Ed. Psych), Dip. N. Ed (London), Dip. Ed., Dip N. Ed, Rotherham Foundation Trust, Rotherham, South Yorkshire, England

Robin L. Testerman, MSN, MBA, Lakeland, Florida

Allison Tinker, BA, Hons CHCN, PG Dip HCE, Rotherham Foundation Trust, Rotherham, South Yorkshire, England

Linda Toomer, MSN, Grady Health System, Atlanta, Georgia

Marian Turkel, BSN, MSN, PhD, Albert Einstien Healthcare Network, Philadelphia, Pennsylvania

Joyce Turner, ADN, BSN, MSN, Grady Health System, Atlanta, Georgia

Pamela Turner, PhD, Wolfson Children's Hospital, Jacksonville, Florida

Jeff Vasquez, BSN, MN, Rotorua Hospital, Rotorua, New Zealand

John Carlo G. Villamero, BSN, Remedios T. Romualdez Mem. Schools, Makati Medical Center, College of Nursing, Makati, Philippines

Jean Watson, PhD, University of Colorado, Denver, Watson Caring Science Institute, Boulder, Colorado

Michelle Ming Xia Zhu, MSN, PhD, Kiang Wu Nursing College of Macau, China

Foreword

Caritas Consciousness Through
an Integral Lens

This book is the first collection of research that tests the construct of Caritas (caring and love) within the context of caring science and the theory of human caring assembled over the last 30 years by Dr. Jean Watson and her colleagues. This book represents the efforts of a community of practice—a group of people who share a passion for something they know how to do and who interact regularly in order to learn how to do it better (Wegner, 2005).

The collection of chapters in this volume supports and extends the evidence of measuring the impact of caring consciousness and the role Caritas plays in healing and value-driven philosophy health. The fact that this book is bringing *Caritas consciousness* to other nurses and health care professionals around the world illustrates the wisdom and power of a value-driven philosophy—theory and the importance of good science. Reading this book is likely to support personal and professional transformation and to support development of nurses' *collective consciousness*.

I think Dr. Jean Watson and her colleagues are integral philosopher–scientists. The word *integral* means "to include, to bring together, to join, to link, to embrace." Ken Wilber (2007) has advanced an integral theory based on internal-external, inside-outside, individual and collective perspectives related to experience in the world. Integral philosophy attempts to include and coordinate the many faces of the Good (the "we"), the True (the "it"), and the Beautiful (the "I"), as all of them evolve across a spectrum, from sensory forms (seen with the eye of flesh) to mental forms (seen with the eye of mind), to spiritual forms (seen with the eye of contemplation).

To be integral involves adoption of three integrative principles (Wilber, 2007): nonexclusion (acceptance of truth claims that pass the validity tests for their own paradigms in respective fields), enfoldment (sets of practices that are more inclusive, holistic, and comprehensive than others), and enactment (various types of inquiry that disclose different phenomena, depending on the quadrants—self, relationship, body–mind, systems—levels, lines, states, and types of the inquiry).

Within integral theory there are lines of development. Predictably, people develop from preconventional to conventional to postconventional ways of thinking, being, and doing. I believe *Caritas consciousness* is a cognitive-ethical-moral-spiritual line of development enhanced through practice and verified through multiple forms of inquiry and evidence. The works described in this book are establishing the foundations of good science in the discipline.

Good science from an integral perspective involves instrumental injunctions, direct apprehensions, communal confirmations, or rejections. As explained by Sean Esbjorn-Hargens and Ken Wilber (2006):

> Instrumental injunction refers to an actual practice, an exemplar, a paradigm, an experiment or an ordinance. It is always of the form "If you want to know this, do this." Direct apprehension refers to an immediate experience of the domain brought forth by the injunction: that is, a direct experience or apprehension of data (even if those data are mediated, at the moment of experience they are immediately apprehended). Communal confirmation or rejection is a checking of the results, the data, the evidence with others who have completed the injunction and apprehensive strands adequately. Thus all kinds of science are in fact empirical in the broadest sense of experiential. This is a much broader definition of science than the narrow definition of sensory experience usually associated with it. (p. 534)

This text contains many examples about the application and use of pluralistic inquiry methods. Integral Methodological Pluralism (IMP) proposes that different types of inquiry have their own methods and validity claims (Esbjorn-Hargens, 2006). For example, phenomenological inquiry includes mindful practices such as reflection, journaling, prayer, and shadow work. The validity claims associated with these inquiry methods include truthfulness, honesty, sincerity, integrity, and the identification and acknowledgment of bias and assumptions. Hermeneutical interpretive methods include storytelling, collective reflection, and textual analysis. Validity claims for these methods include issues of intersubjective justness. Empirical inquiries include surveys, field observations, the development of measures and metrics and include validity claims of propositional objective truth through repeatable, controlled, empirical, logical conditions. Finally, when inquiry is focused on systems, direct experience with the system(s) through mapping, statistical analysis, and study can gain validity claims of functional fit as data and evidence from multiple and reputable sources converge. Examples of phenomenological, hermeneutic, empirical, and systems inquiry are represented in the chapters contained in this volume. Each study examines self, relationships, body, mind, and systems in the context of caring theory and practices.

This book brings the theory, practice, and evidence of *Caritas consciousness* to other nurses and health care professionals around the world. The efforts of the community of practice involved in this work illustrate the purpose and power of a value-driven philosophy—theory with the influence of good science to enable the appreciation of the wisdom of caring and love in health and healing. A careful read of this book will support personal and professional transformation through the development and evolution of our *collective consciousness*. Personal and professional transformation is hard work that takes time and intention.

Robert Kegan (1994) notes that personal and professional transformation takes place when we develop fifth-order consciousness. Kegan describes the development of consciousness this way: As we grow and develop we realize differences between self and other—the "me" and "not me." We evolve from self-consciousness to "self-other" consciousness. We then progress to a second level of consciousness that he calls the "we" or "socialized mind." Most people's growth and development become arrested at this conventional level of consciousness. With critical experiences and time, some of us master the *hidden curriculum of daily life*. We transcend our third level of consciousness and develop a fourth-order consciousness that Kegan calls "self-authoring mind." Self-authoring individuals view work, school, parenting, therapy, intimate relationships, and citizenship differently than those who operate at the level of socialized mind. At work, fourth-order consciousness manifests itself in the following ways. A person is:

- the inventor or owner of one's own work and distinguishes work from job.
- self-initiating, self-correcting, self-evaluating rather than being dependent on others to frame the problems, initiate adjustments, or determine whether things are going acceptably well.
- guided by one's own visions at work rather than being without vision or being captive of the authority's agenda.
- responsible for what happens to oneself at work externally and internally (rather than seeing present internal circumstances and future external possibilities as caused by someone else).

- an accomplished master of one's particular work roles, jobs, or careers (rather than having an apprentice or imitating relationship to what one does).
- conceiving the organization from "outside in" as a whole, seeing one's relation to the whole and seeing the relation of the parts to the whole, rather than seeing the rest of the organization and its parts only from the perspective of one's own part, from the "inside out" (Kegan, 1994, p. 302).

In educational settings, those with a "self-authoring mind"

- exercise critical, creative, and systems thinking.
- examine self, culture, and milieu in order to understand what we feel from what we should feel, what we value from what we should value, and what we want from what we should want.
- are self-directed learners (they take initiative, set their own goals and standards, use experts, institutions, and other resources to pursue these goals, take responsibility for their own direction and productivity in learning).
- see themselves as cocreators of the culture (rather than shaped by the culture).
- read actively (rather than receptively) with a purpose in mind.
- write to themselves and bring their teachers into their self-reflection (rather than write mainly to the teachers or for the teachers).
- take charge of the concepts, theories of a course or discipline and marshal on behalf of themselves an independently chosen topic and its internal procedures for formulating and validating knowledge (Kegan, 1994, p. 303).

Kegan argues that continual, professional growth and development in a postmodern society may require a "fifth order of consciousness, or the growth and creation of a 'self-transforming mind.'" At this level people integrate polarities and contradictions in their own behavior as they develop and appreciate complexity thinking and engage in the really hard work of psychological and spiritual integration. I believe this book challenges all nurses to aspire to fifth-order consciousness of a self-transforming mind.

As you read this book, I hope you appreciate and value the integral nature of the work and the evidence gathered. May your exploration and analysis of these ideas and methods stimulate the development of your own personal and professional *Caritas consciousness* in support of your own healing work and the healing care of others.

REFERENCES

Esbjorn-Hargens, S. (2006). Integral research: A multimethod approach to investigating phenomena. *Constructivism in the Human Sciences, 11*(2), 79–107.

Esbjorn-Hargens, S., & Wilber, K. (2006). Toward a comprehensive integration of science and religion: A postmetaphysical approach. In P. Clayton & Z. Simpson (Eds.), *The Oxford handbook of religion and science* (pp. 523–546). Oxford: Oxford University Press.

Kegan, R. (1994*). In over our heads: The mental demands of modern life.* Cambridge, MA: Harvard University Press.

Wegner, E. (2005). *Cultivating communities of practice: A quick start-up guide.* Retrieved, from http://www.ewenger.com/theory/start-up_guide_PDF.pdf

Wilber, K. (2007). *The integral vision.* Boston: Shambala.

Daniel J. Pesut, PhD, RN, PMHCNS-BC, FAAN

Preface

The intent of this book is to build a scientific–theoretical argument that Caritas (caring and love) is an intervention for healing. There is much evidence that pharmacotherapy and technology heal, but we lack evidence on the healing power of caring and love.

Skeptics will state, "You can't measure the impact of caring and love." If that is true, then we must negate the science regarding stress, quality of life, coping, and all the other abstract dimensions of the human experience. The body of science relating to the power of love follows the same trajectory as these other abstract/latent dimensions of life and human experiences associated with all the vicissitudes of living and dying. As such, this book is the first collection of research that tests the construct of Caritas (caring and love) within the context of Caring Science and the Theory of Human Caring assembled over the last 30 years by Dr. Jean Watson.

Here our focus is for nurses engaged in the theory-guided practices of the Caritas processes within the context of health provision as well as for all health providers. The book focuses on nurses because nursing and health care are in need of new methods of human caring and healing that are low cost, can be used by all, and can influence outcomes. Simply, we propose that Caritas interventions will influence practitioner/patient, organizational, and financial outcomes in a positive direction.

Caring interventions begin with self. Research within this book reveals that caring for self relates to caring for others, specifically, coworkers and patients. Caring, according to Watson, includes 10 Caritas processes. When applied within the appropriate time, using the appropriate method, caring and love will be perceived and healing will follow. Behaviors include treating oneself with loving kindness, taking time for relationships, tending to one's basic needs of life, embracing both positive and negative aspects of oneself, honoring spiritual aspects of life, taking time to acquire knowledge, having belief and hope, allowing oneself to believe in the impossible, creative problem solving, and creating a healing environment. Theoretically, if these behaviors are enacted toward self, there will be greater access to one's inner healing processes for wholeness.

This book has initiated a mass collaboration of researchers worldwide who are testing these theories. There is already enough research, prompted by the completion of this book, to write a second volume on how we have built the scientific argument, including how we are correlating nurse and patient reports of caring with their respective biophysical, physiological markers. Once we are able to show how caring behaviors toward self and others decrease the prevalence and incidence of illness, we may be able to initiate training and reimbursement for effective caring. Thus, this work has practical and empirical implications as well as theoretical validation for Caring Science as a growing field.

This book has several applications, including those for educators who teach nursing theories, for research professors who are building the scientific argument, and for teachers who focus on professional leadership and clinical scholar roles. The book is organized in sections, with several chapters relating to that topic or dimension of caring. The first section reviews the theory of caring and possibilities for the use of Watson's concept of Caritas. The second section reviews research that connects caring to the care provider who, in this case, is the nurse. The third section provides exemplars of interventions aimed at the enhancement of Caritas toward self and others. The fourth section presents international perspectives from cross-sectional studies across the globe. Finally, the fifth section, along with the appendices, includes several studies that examine caring in specific contexts such as addiction, electroconvulsive therapy (ECT), and other particular populations. All the tools described within this book that are derived from the Caring Factor Survey (CFS), the primary tool used for the majority of the studies in this book, can be downloaded at the Springer Publishing website at www. springerpub.com/nelsoncaring.

The authors of this book readily participated in what could be called a mass collaboration. The networking occurred mostly through the Caring International Research Collaborative (CIRC) and Watson's Caring Science Institute (WCSI). The CIRC group is a research community within Sigma Theta Tau International and WCSI is a nonprofit foundation created by Dr. Jean Watson. Together, participants are all learning from each other, and thus this work furthers that goal of clinical scholarship.

John Nelson

Acknowledgments

I thank John for his leadership and vision for this book and all the intense international communication and follow-up required for this research. I appreciate the many researchers who were willing to take chances and engage in further developing and validating concepts of caring, love, and Caritas as empirical variables worthy of researching. My continuing appreciation goes to the collaborating organizations, the contributing authors, and colleagues who participated in the birthing of this work, and to Allan Graubard at Springer for his support, encouragement, and guidance for this book. I am grateful also for his creation of Springer Publishing's Watson Caring Science Library in conjunction with Watson Caring Science Institute (WCSI).

As founder of the WCSI, I am pleased and delighted to endorse this work as part of the Watson Caring Science Library. It is an exemplar of the nature of caring-science research and the assessment and measurement of caring and healing, the foundations of authentic nursing care and caring in our world. May it serve as a foundation for further research in Caritas—Caring and Love, the ultimate source of healing and true health.

Jean Watson

First, I thank my family for their love and support. Deb has been the best wife/friend/partner I could ask for. I am so grateful for my four children, Jared, Bryce, Isaac, and Grace, who all bring such meaning and love to my life. I am deeply grateful for my coeditor, Jean Watson, who has provided the content of philosophy and theory in caring science. Theory is the foundation and guide for scientific inquiry, and her years of work in the caring science has helped guide the conversations and thought in developing the studies contained within this book. I am also grateful for all those in the Caritas Consortium, which is based in the Watson Caring Science Institute. This work would not have been possible without the vision of my wonderful friends and colleagues who colead the Caring International Research Collaborative (CIRC) with me. Jayne Felgen's exuberance and knowledge in operations and relationship-based care provide the inspiration to show continued progress in the mass collaboration of research. Geraldine Murray, my Irish counterpart, is one of the most organized and authentic individuals I have ever met. Her ability to get so much done, as well as being so forthright yet kind, has made her collaboration nothing less than enjoyable. Thank you, Jayne and Geraldine. I am grateful for my fellow researchers, academicians, clinicians, and students in the CIRC. Without their inspiring theories (hunches) about where love occurs, this work would not be possible. Thanks to each of you who have contributed to the investigation of Caritas as an intervention of healing!

Finally, I would like to thank God for being the source of love, knowledge, wisdom, and guidance.

John Nelson

SECTION I

Theoretical Background of Caritas

1

Concepts of Caring as Construct of Caritas Hierarchy in Nursing Knowledge: Conceptual-Theoretical-Empirical (CTE)

John Nelson, Pam DiNapoli,
Marian Turkel, and Jean Watson

Contemporary nursing practice focuses on creating caring environments for nurses, patients, and families within today's complex health care organizations. With the emergence of the American Nurses Credentialing Center's (ANCC) Magnet Recognition Program® (Magnet), nursing theory has moved from its central place in academia and research to practice. The majority of Magnet hospitals have implemented a theoretical framework grounded in caring science. Indeed, the theme for the 2010 ANCC National Magnet Conference, "Magnet: A Culture of Caring," was characteristic here with Jean Watson giving the keynote address on caring and caring science to an audience of nearly 6,000 nurses (October 2010). Watson's (1979, 1985, 2005, 2008, 2011) theory of human caring has become the theory of choice as direct care registered nurses (RNs) return to caring values. Theory-guided practice advances both the discipline and profession of nursing. Practice outcomes demonstrate the creation of a caring-healing environment at all levels and facilitate both human and environmental well-being (DiNapoli, Nelson, Turkel, & Watson, 2010; Turkel & Ray, 2004; Watson, 2008).

Theories are part of the knowledge structure of any discipline (Parker & Smith, 2010). According to Parker and Smith (2010), the major reason for structuring and advancing nursing knowledge through nursing theory is clear: to develop, understand, and transform nursing practice. Nursing is a professional discipline, and nursing theory guides and informs practice. As the work of nursing scholars and theorists has transformed professional nursing practice, so has the everyday practice of nursing enriched and advanced nursing theory. According to Parker (2006), "creative nursing practice is the direct result of ongoing theory-based thinking, decision making, and action of nurses" (p. 15).

Various definitions of theory exist. According to Parson (1949), theories tell us what we already know and what we need to know. Dickoff and James (1968) defined theory as a "conceptual system or framework invented for some purpose" (p. 198), whereas Ellis (1968) termed it "a coherent set of hypothetical, conceptual and pragmatic principles for forming a general frame of reference for a field of inquiry" (p. 217). Watson (1985) defined theory as "an imaginative grouping of knowledge, ideas, and experience that are represented symbolically and seek to illuminate a given phenomena" (p. 1). Watson (2005, 2008, 2011) further related theory to the Latin origin *Theoria*, which means "to see"—acknowledging theory as another way to see phenomena that are right in front of us. Although definitions vary, they meet in one purpose: to give meaning and explanation to, and understanding of, nursing practice. Theory represents the intellectual life of nursing (Levine, 1995).

The conceptual-theoretical-empirical (CTE) system of nursing practice as described in Fawcett (2000) is the purposeful way that nurses can apply the hierarchy of nursing knowledge to predict quality patient outcomes. The structural components of the CTE are a conceptual model, or theory, that is made up of concepts and propositions. Although not tangible entities, scholars propose them to help clinicians better understand a phenomenon. These conceptual definitions can then be formalized through empirical research methods designed to test and confirm the linkages between the concepts in a theory. It is this knowledge—of the linkages between concepts in a theory—that practitioners can use to help predict quality patient outcomes (Fawcett, 1999). Examination of caring theory through the lens of the CTE clarifies for practitioners how to demonstrate that caring practices and professional models of care, grounded in the tenets of caring theory, make a difference in nursing, patient, or organizational outcomes.

Implementing the CTE system to understand caring theory must begin with clarification of the concept as it relates to the metaparadigm concepts of nursing. Let us recall that a paradigm, as defined by Kuhn (1970, 1977), serves as a basis for understanding nursing knowledge (Parker, 2001). According to Kuhn, a paradigm is a framework or worldview consisting of assumptions held by members of the discipline considered as essential in the development of the discipline. Traditionally, the metaparadigm of nursing includes these concepts: nursing, person, health, and environment (Fawcett, 1984). Nursing scholars continue to advance knowledge within the discipline, which has in turn generated new ideas—also from nursing scholars—that have shifted the focus of the traditional metaparadigm. "Caring is considered by many as one central feature within the meta-paradigm of nursing knowledge and practices" (p. 456). The notion of replacing the concept "nursing" with "caring" within the disciplinary metaparadigm was advanced by Watson (1979) and by a group of scholars at the Wingspread Conference (1989) on

Knowledge About Care and Caring: State of the Art and Future Developments (Stevenson & Tripp-Reimer, 1990).

Caring, as the essence of nursing practice, has evolved over time since Watson's conception in *Nursing: The Philosophy and Science of Caring* (Watson, 1979), and later in *Nursing: Human Science and Human Care* (1985). These original theory books developed the concepts of transpersonal caring relationships between the nurse and the patient, the caring occasion, phenomenal field, and caring moment, advancing the notion that caring should be considered a metaparadigm concept of nursing and not simply something that nurses do. Watson and Smith (2002) also have fostered an understanding of the concept of caring from a theoretical perspective of caring science, which seeks to unify and connect as an "evolving philosophical-ethical-epistemic field of study that is grounded in the discipline of nursing and informed by related fields" (p. 456).

Indeed, Jean Watson's seminal work offers justification for the conceptual-theoretical link between the essential aspects of caring in nursing and the core of professional nursing by identifying 10 Carative Factors that can be measured empirically. Nursing-sensitive quality patient outcomes guided by the Carative Factors and grounded in a humanistic value system are what differentiate professional nursing practice and nursing practice focused solely on mechanics or tasks. Watson's original work has continued to evolve and grow—the Carative Factors were redefined as the Caritas Processes, reflecting a deeper connection among nursing praxis, caring science, and the universal concept of love. In Latin, *caritas* means "Christian love" and has been further defined as love for humanity. Caritas nursing practice involves the integration of transpersonal caring and love within the context of the nurse-patient relationship and interactions, resulting in a caring, healing relationship (Watson, 2005, 2008).

NURSING THEORY: ADVANCING
THE DISCIPLINE AND TRANSFORMING PRACTICE

Watson's (1979, 1985, 2005, 2008, 2011) philosophy brought to light caring science as the essence of nursing and as the foundational core of the discipline. Caring is a dynamic, transpersonal relationship between the nurse and the patient that involves ethical choice and action within the present moment (past, future, and present all at once), which manifests the potential for harmony of body, mind, and soul (spirit) (Watson, 1985, 2005, 2008). Thus, the process of caring is a moral ideal committed to a specific end, "the protection, enhancement, and preservation of the person's humanity which helps to restore inner harmony and potential healing" (Watson, 1985, p. 58).

To further advance the discipline of nursing and transform nursing practice it is necessary to empirically measure caring. This opens another debate essential to the development of psychometrically sound instruments: how to articulate the place caring has within an increasingly pharmacologic and mechanistic health care environment. As such, is caring a single concept that can be measured or a construct requiring the creation of a series of subscales to measure the identity and nature of a human phenomenon? Clearly, this debate must include scholars and practitioners.

A careful examination of the concept of caring—through the theory of caring science as proposed by Watson—might suggest that to measure Caritas is to view the concept of caring as a construct (*Caritas*), which implies a composite of elements that, when taken together, creates a single structure/construct. This conceptualization assists with examining Caritas as a paradigm of healing while allowing flexibility in testing individual processes (as interventions of healing). The composite elements of the construct are individual concepts that, when taken separately, have their own definitions and empirical indicators. Conceptualizing each of the Caritas Processes separately allows for the classification of each as a middle-range theory.

CONCEPT ANALYSIS

Concepts represent meaning, experience, or ideas of the human experience (Chinn & Kramer, 1995). Concept analysis is used to determine the state of the science of the concept in relation to science. In order for a concept to progress from analysis to scientific analysis of relevance within the lived experience, the concept must be validated within the context in which it is being examined (Hupcey & Penrod, 2005). Thus each concept within Watson's theory is proposed to be valid as a part of the construct of Caritas within the contexts being studied. When the concept is challenged within contexts being examined, further concept analysis may need to be conducted as it relates to the use of the concept within the construct of Caritas. It is important to examine the concept within the consideration of the entire construct within which it is embedded. Isolation of the concept without consideration of the entire construct limits the application of the concept to the human experience (Hupcey & Penrod, 2005).

In the case of the Caritas Processes, it must be considered, when examining a concept separately, how it relates to healing within the construct of Caritas. For example, how does loving kindness as a concept relate, and potentially contribute, to healing within the construct of Caritas? How does nurses' teaching in a way patients can learn contribute to healing within the construct of Caritas? Without considering how each concept contributes to the construct of interest (Caritas), the concepts lose scientific meaning. How they each contribute to healing from a theoretical and empirical point of view grows opaque, which, in turn, inhibits our ability to interpret findings of science (Hupcey & Penrod, 2005).

Wilson's classic work (1963) provides a framework to examine a concept within various contexts, including social context, similar concepts, practical application, and language (Hupcey & Penrod, 2005). Because constructs are prone to evolve, their concepts are temporal entities as well (Walker & Avant, 1995). Thus concept analysis is not a one-time event but a recurring aspect of construct validation within various contexts and points of time. Notably, Rodgers (2000) also viewed concepts as dynamic within context and time.

The three primary types of concept analysis previously referred to include Wilsonian-derived, evolutionary, and pragmatic utility. In fact, Wilson (1963) proposed 11 techniques to isolate a concept for useful dialogue in science. This method was contemporized by Walker and Avant in 1983 by reducing the 11 techniques to 8 (Weaver & Mitcham, 2008). Although other revisions of the Wilsonian approach were conducted by Chinn and Jacobs (1983) and Schwartz-Barcott and Kim (2000), the Walker-Avant approach is the most widely used in graduate schools (Weaver & Mitcham, 2008). Rodgers's (2000) evolutionary method also considers context and time as well as application within practice (Weaver & Mitcham, 2008). The final method, the pragmatic utility approach developed by Morse (2000), advises researchers to consider concept within the critical appraisal, specifically as it relates to research perspective, questions, assumptions, and methods (Weaver & Mitcham, 2008).

In terms of developing middle-range theories, some authors proposed that concept analysis can be used in that regard (Bu & Jezewski, 2007). Once the concepts' defining attributes, antecedents, consequences, and context of concepts are defined, the concept is potentially ready for examination as a middle-range theory to test within practice. The authors provide a walkthrough of the process they used to examine the concept of patient advocacy and possible future work as a middle-range (Bu & Jezewski, 2007).

THE FUTURE OF NURSING KNOWLEDGE: CARITAS PROCESSES AS MIDDLE-RANGE THEORY CONCEPTS

The development of nursing knowledge is an ongoing process. Middle-range theory, whose development has increased over time, focuses on specific aspects of nursing practice and is often viewed as more relevant and applicable to nursing practice than grand theories. Middle-range theories present concepts and propositions at a lower level of abstraction and are useful for increasing theory-based research and evidence-based nursing practice initiatives (Smith & Leiher, 2008). Certainly, future advances in nursing knowledge can be made by considering the development of middle-range theories based on caring science.

A place to start may be examination of each of the Caritas Processes as a specific phenomenon in middle-range theory. The conceptual analysis of several of the Caritas Processes has already been completed by Watson and others. Following are the 10 Caritas Processes and concept analyses found in the literature to address each concept.

Caritas Process 1: Cultivating the Practice of Loving Kindness and Equanimity Toward Self and Others (layman's terms: loving kindness, compassion, and forgiveness for self and others). This process involves listening and respecting others, honoring human dignity, treating self and others with loving kindness, recognizing vulnerabilities in self and others, and accepting self and others as they are. Upon examination of the literature, no concept analyses were found that were specific to loving kindness. However, the literature did reveal that this concept is being considered. Carson et al. (2005) tested a century-old practice of meditation of loving kindness practiced by the Buddhist tradition ($n = 43$). It was their desire to understand if meditation on loving kindness would decrease perception of pain for patients suffering from chronic low back pain. The 8-week study revealed a statistically significant decline in perception of pain for the loving kindness group, whereas no change occurred for the control group. Deeper examination of the loving kindness group revealed that the pain was lowest on the days that loving kindness meditation was practiced (Carson et al., 2005). Another study in meditation on loving kindness showed that only a few minutes of loving kindness increased perception of social connection (Hutcherson, Seppala, & Gross, 2008). Meanwhile, the control group showed no increase in perception of social connection (Hutcherson et al., 2008). These two studies suggest that loving kindness has potential to be examined further as a concept of healing physically, mentally, and/or spiritually.

Caritas Process 2: Being Authentically Present: Enabling, Sustaining, and Honoring Faith and Hope (layman's terms: faith and hope). The concept analysis of authenticity addressed self-discovery, which may include faith and hope (Starr, 2008). Search strategies to identify the concept of faith and hope revealed that they were analyzed as separate concepts. Benzein and Saveman (1998) used the Walker and Avant (1995) method of concept analysis to examine hope. Hope is future oriented, includes positive expectations, requires intentionality and action, involves interconnectedness, and includes a realistic goal (Benzein & Saveman, 1998). Others have conducted concept analysis in specific populations, including in the pediatric oncology population (Hendricks-Ferguson, 1997). The concept of hope as a subconcept of caring is reviewed in much more detail in Chapter 3 by Giuliana Masera and Karen Gutierrez of this book as an example of how health care professionals, academicians, and/or researchers can examine hope at a more extensive level.

One challenge in the identification of literature related to a specific concept is the verbiage used to label concepts that use different words but hold very similar, if not the same, meaning. According to Dyess

(2008), faith is related to spiritual belief rather than a more broad examination as a concept of believing in or for an outcome. Further discussion in supporting one's belief and hope as a process of healing is warranted.

Caritas Process 3: Cultivation of One's Own Spiritual Practices and Transpersonal Self, Going Beyond Ego-Self (layman's terms: spiritual support, growth and development, and evolution of higher consciousness). It is important to identify that the concept of spirituality, like other concepts in the construct of Caritas, uses different terms to identify the same or very similar concepts. For the concept of spirituality, there is some overlap in the terms *religiosity* and *spirituality*. These are not the same, but the concepts and overlap must be addressed within this discussion.

Bjarnason (2007) used the concept-analysis method espoused by Rodgers to examine religiosity, which has to do with traditions, practices, and affiliation. According to Bjarnason (2007), religiosity includes external behaviors such as attending a place of worship like a temple, mosque, church, or other formal gathering place for people of similar religiosity. It can also include internal behaviors such as reading religious text or private prayer (Bjarnason, 2007). The terms *spirituality, coping, belief,* and *hope* serve as surrogates for this concept in some literature (Bjarnason, 2007). Religiosity has been shown to have protective qualities for patients from conditions such as depression, hypertension, suicide, and drug involvement (Bjarnason, 2007). It also has been reported to aid in coping for stressful life events and chronic joint pain (Bjarnason, 2007).

Spirituality, as a concept, was analyzed by McBrien (2006) using the method of Walker and Avant (1995). Spirituality goes beyond the traditions and practices of religiosity to an individual's search for meaning and connection (McBrien, 2006). Spirituality includes the attributes of belief in God or a higher power; inner strength and peace derived from acceptance of one's situation; and connectedness to self, others, and God, which leads to deeper meaning in life (McBrien, 2006). Spirituality then may or may not include religiosity, per se, but allows the exploration of the individual in to deeper connectedness and meaning.

Caritas Process 4: Developing and Sustaining a Helping-Trusting Caring Relationship (layman's terms: helping–trusting relationship). Search terms used to identify concept analysis included *helping, help, trusting, trust,* and *helping-trusting*. Using the databases CINAHL and Medline, 31 articles were identified and three were selected to review for this chapter: Bell and Duffy (2009) analyzed the concept of nurse-patient trust; Hams (1997) conducted a concept analysis of trust from the perspective of coronary care; and Johns (1996) also conducted a concept analysis of trust. No concept analysis was found that examined helping-trusting or helping. However, within the concept of trust, help was reported to be an important attribute of trust (Bell & Duffy, 2009). Johns (1996) stated that trust includes the reliance on another to meet an unmet need. This could be referred to as being "helped" by another.

Caritas Process 5: Being Present to, and Supportive of, the Expression of Positive and Negative Feelings (layman's terms: promote feelings, both positive and negative). Concept analysis of listening was the closest concept found to "promotion of feelings, both positive and negative." According to Shiley (2010), listening is a skill and concept that has not received warranted attention as it relates to outcomes in health care. Attributes of listening include use of empathy and silence while maintaining a nonjudgmental and accepting attitude of what is being said both verbally and nonverbally (Shiley, 2010). No tools were found by Shiley to measure the patient's perception of listening skills of nurses. Therefore, the empirical data regarding the impact of listening as perceived by the patient and associated outcomes were also missing. This provides a future opportunity to examine the skill of listening as it relates to healing.

Caritas Process 6: Creative Use of Self and All Ways of Knowing as Part of the Caring Process; Engage in the Artistry of Caritas (layman's terms: creative problem solving). When looking for a concept analysis for creative problem solving or use of all ways of knowing, the closest terms found were *problem solving* and *intuition*. Zander (2007) examined the concept of ways of knowing from an historical perspective and how it has evolved as a concept over time. Rodgers's (2000) process of concept analysis was used because it includes the dynamics of a concept over time and possible evolution. Epistemology (Carper, 1978) and ontology (Jacobs-Kramer & Chinn, 1988), as resources for making decisions, were reviewed (Zander, 2007). Intuition was also identified as one "other" way of knowing (Zander, 2007).

Based on the historical review of Zander (2007), it is plausible that creative problem solving as a Caritas Process could be broken down and examined as a number of concepts, including aesthetic knowing, empirical knowing, ethical knowing, and personal knowing. Zander (2007) also identified other aspects of knowledge, including experience (Benner, Tanner, & Chesla, 1992; Burnard, 1987) and intuition (Agan, 1987; Rew & Barrow, 1987; Young, 1987). Simmons (2010) conducted a concept analysis of intuition as an aspect of knowing. It is proposed that knowing contains several concepts in itself as a separate construct. Further inquiry is needed to understand which aspects of knowing relate most strongly to problem solving as a Caritas Process that in turn relates to healing.

Caritas Process 7: Engage in Genuine Teaching-Learning Experience That Attends to Unity of Being and Subjective Meaning—Attempting to Stay Within Others' Frame of Reference (layman's terms: effective teaching). Two concept analyses were found that are central to teaching patients: health literacy (Speros, 2004) and information needs (Timmins, 2006).

Health literacy relates to the patients' ability to comprehend the necessary information to promote their own health (Speros, 2004). Speros used the Walker and Avant method to examine health literacy. Attributes of health literacy included both cognitive and social skills (Speros, 2004). Cognitive skills included the patients' ability to read and use numbers as well as comprehend either or both (Speros, 2004). Social aspects included the patients' ability to function as health care consumers and past experiences in health care (Speros, 2004). Speros did identify health outcomes of health literacy, including perceived health status and lower health care costs. Lower costs included decreased length of stay, less frequent use of health care services, and better health-promotion knowledge that resulted in better health status (Speros, 2004).

Timmins (2006) used Rodgers's (2000) evolutionary approach to examine the concept of information needs. Timmins identified that humans have individual learning needs and motivations. This fact requires health care professionals to understand the concept of information needs to be successful in teaching patients what they need to know (Timmins, 2006). Information-needs attributes include individual coping, problem-solving approach, perception of illness or health, and perception of health care professionals' competence in educating them (Timmins, 2006). The dynamics of measuring the impact of teaching are complicated by the constant change of demographics of society, advancement of technology, and increased access by consumers to electronic information (Timmins, 2006). These challenges prevent patients' information needs from being met, despite multiple methods and instruments to measure patient information needs (Timmins, 2006). No matter what method or instrument is used, each patient must be asked specifically what his or her information needs are, rather than assuming that each individual's information needs match those of the population that shares the individual's respective diagnosis (Timmins, 2006).

Qualitative research conducted by Turkel (1997) revealed that both patients and registered nurses valued patient education or patient teaching as a caring behavior or caring practice. An outcome of this caring was enchantment of learning when the teaching was done by a caring nurse. Patient participants talked about being able to ask questions and wanting to learn when they had a caring nurse. They believed they "could remember better" with a caring nurse. In terms of economic outcomes caring makes a difference. If patients are readmitted within 30 days after discharge with the same diagnosis because they do not understand how to care for themselves the hospital will not be reimbursed. Recidivism is costly to patients and hospitals: costly to patients in terms of increased time required for healing and recovery and costly to hospitals that will not be reimbursed for treatment.

Caritas Process 8: Creating a Healing Environment at All Levels (layman's terms: creates healing environment). No concept analysis was found for Caritas Process 8. Terms used to search for this concept analysis included *healing environment, optimal healing environment,* and *environment.* Articles related to each of these terms were identified, but no concept analysis. Although no specific content analysis was found in the nursing literature related to a healing environment, components of this Caritas Process have been found in the nursing literature from both a theoretical and research perspective. Nightingale (1859), in the seminal work *Notes on Nursing,* wrote that "unnecessary noise is the cruelest absence of care." Watson (2008) described noise reduction as a comfort measure that facilitates creation of a healing environment. As part of integration in practice, RNs have implemented quiet times in acute care settings where noise levels are intentionally reduced, lights are dimmed, and the patient is allowed to rest. Findings from Press Ganey indicated that patients complained about noise two times more often than about anything else in a hospital, including the food (Mazer, 2010). A recent study by Lawson et al. (2010) validated that high levels of sound in critical care result in poor sleep quality, which leads to slower healing, poorer immune response, and decreased cognitive function.

Additional healing modalities, including massage therapy, therapeutic touch, guided imagery, music, aromatherapy, and art therapy, are being used by RNs in practice to facilitate creation of a healing environment at all levels. Each of these modalities has empirical research validating its positive effect on healing. A few studies are presented. Therapeutic touch (TT) is an intervention that involves the intentional direction of energy for the purpose of healing. In an intervention study of 21 postoperative surgical patients, findings showed that participants who received TT had significantly lower level of pain, lower cortisol level, and higher natural killer cells (NKC) level.

The purpose of a study by Locsin, McCaffrey, and Purnell (2009) was to describe RN experiences of being cared for in a hospital healing-arts space in a southeast Florida hospital. Written narratives from 16 respondents to the question "What was your experience like, using the healing arts space?" were transcribed and analyzed following Colaizzi's (1978) phenomenological approach. Three themes were found to describe the nurses' experience of being cared for: freely appreciating oneness with the environment; "caring for self" as centering, relaxing, and knowing; and being physically present is living in a calm and gentle space all at once.

Twiss, Seaver, and McCaffrey (2006) studied the effect of music on anxiety and length of intubation time for 60 patients undergoing coronary artery bypass surgery. The researchers found that patients who listened to music had lower scores on anxiety measures and were able to be removed from the ventilator 3 hours earlier. McCaffrey (2008) reviewed numerous research articles, providing evidence that listening to music is a way to create and provide a healing environment for older adults and that music improves the healing environment from a physiologic and psychologic perspective.

Numerous research studies show the efficacy of aromatherapy and massage. One particular study (Lemon, 2004) examined the effect of massage with essential oils in 32 patients with psychiatric illness in an acute care setting. Findings indicated that the patients receiving massage with essential oils showed significantly more improvement in scores on depression, anxiety, and severity of emotional symptoms.

Caritas Process 9: Administering Sacred Acts of Caring-Healing by Tending to Basic Needs (layman's terms: holistic care). No concept analysis was found for holistic care. Although no specific concept analysis was found in the nursing literature, Watson (2008) invited RNs to assist with basic human needs with an intentional caring consciousness. An example of this is the evidence-based practice work of Sauer (2010) reducing bloodstream infections in the neonatal intensive care unit (NICU). The purpose of this evidence-based practice initiative was to change nursing practice in the NICU from clean to sterile technique for the tubing change of central venous catheters (CVCs). Bloodstream infections in the NICU patient population have the potential to be life threatening. Premature infants have a weakened immune system, and an infection compromises reserves and impacts the body system as a whole. Creating a healing environment by attending to safety and sterility potentiated comfort and healing. Changing CVC tubing is a sacred nursing act when the nurse practices with intentionality, will, and commitment. Realizing that it is a privilege to care for this patient population in all their vulnerability allows the "task" to become a caring interaction. The change from nursing task to Caritas practice has resulted in zero bloodstream infections in the past nine months.

From a theoretical perspective, Hektor and Touhy (1997) reflected, "Have we not thrown out the 'baby with the bath water' when we reduce bathing to a task to be accomplished, often without the expertise and involvement of the professional nurse?" Rather than being a healing and positive experience for older persons, bathing in institutions becomes routine, depersonalized, and often harmful. According to Hektor and Touhy, attention to the aesthetics of the bath could return bathing to its prior status as therapeutic healing intervention. From their perspective, examining the art of nursing as it was historically practiced helps us to rediscover the meaning of the skillful and artful therapeutic bath.

Disruptive behaviors, including physical and verbal aggression, often occur during bathing and are especially common among nursing home residents who are cognitively impaired. Research facilitated by Hoeffer, Rader, McKenzie, Lavelle, and Stewart (1997) aimed at changing the psychosocial environment in which bathing occurred and addressed the function, frequency, and form of bathing as well. Nursing practice emphasizing an individualized person-focused, rather than task-focused, approach reduced aggressive behavior during bathing and made it a more positive experience for nursing assistants and less stressful for residents.

Caritas Process 10: Opening and Attending to Spiritual/Mysterious and Existential Unknowns of Life-Death (layman's terms: allows belief in miracles). No concept analysis was found for miracles. However, the topic of miracles is described in many professional books and journals. For example, a book titled *Daily Miracles* (Briskin & Boller, 2006) captures stories and the practice of humanity, caring, and excellence in health care. Physicians and RNs from various practice settings reflected on and then shared stories of the human experience of caring and compassion.

CARING IN THE METAPARADIGM OF NURSING

Nightingale never explicitly defined caring in her seminal work, *Notes on Nursing* (1859, 1992); however, her professional and personal life exemplified an ethos of caring (Dunphy, 2006). In this regard, Watson (1992) has written: "Although Nightingale's feminine based caring healing model has transcended time and is prophetic for this century's healthcare reform, the model is yet to truly come of age in nursing or the healthcare system." Watson's (1979) work advanced the concept of caring within the discipline of nursing and, at that time, Watson called for caring to be included within the metaparadigm of nursing.

Numerous other scholars of caring have continued to advance it as a substantive area of study (Benner et al., 1992; Boykin & Schoenhofer, 1993; Duffy, 2005, 2007; Leininger, 1981; Ray, 1989, 2006, 2008, 2011; Roach, 1987; Smith, 1999, 2010; Sumner, 2010; Sumner & Fisher, 2008; Swanson, 1991, 1999). As concept, caring is broad enough to encompass the discipline of nursing and capture the nature of nursing (Ray, 2006). This transtheoretical identification recognizes the commonality of caring among the various theories, philosophies, and conceptual frameworks of the discipline. Nurses in practice are able to articulate caring as a philosophical and theoretical foundation for practice.

Qualitative research continues to advance the reflective, human nature of caring and captures the meaning and experience of giving and receiving caring. Quantitative research continues to show that caring can be measured and that it influences patient and nurse satisfaction and facilitates healing. Over 25 instruments with demonstrated reliability and validity have been developed to empirically assess and measure caring mindfully and intentionally (Watson, 2008).

Given this in-depth development of scholarly knowledge, and the ongoing advancement of caring in professional practice, the authors acknowledge caring as the unifying focus of the discipline. With respect to its historical development, and the influence of scholars who contributed to the original metaparadigm of nursing, the time has come to embrace caring as part of that same metaparadigm. Thus this book helps to explore the evolution of the concepts of caring within the construct of Caritas as emerging middle-range theories worthy of empirical validation and measurement.

REFERENCES

Agan, R. D. (1987). Intuitive knowing as a dimension of nursing. *Advances in Nursing Science, 10*(1), 63–70.

Bell, L., & Duffy, A. (2009). A concept analysis of nurse-patient trust. *British Journal of Nursing, 18*(1), 46–51.

Benner, P., Tanner, C., & Chesla, C. (1992). From beginner to expert: Gaining a differentiated clinical world in critical care nursing. *Advances in Nursing Science, 14*(3), 13–28.

Benzein, E., & Saveman, B. I. (1998). One step towards the understanding of hope: A concept analysis. *International Journal of Nursing Studies, 35*(6), 322–329.

Bjarnason, D. (2007). Concept analysis of religiosity. *Home Health Care Management & Practice, 19*(5), 350–355.

Boykin, A., & Schoenhofer, S. (1993). *Nursing as caring: A model for transforming practice.* New York, NY: National League for Nursing.

Briskin, A., & Boller, J. (2006). *Daily miracles: Stories and practices of humanity and excellence in health care.* Indianapolis, IN: Sigma Theta Tau International.

Bu, X., & Jezewski, M. A. (2007). Developing a mid-range theory of patient advocacy through concept analysis. *Journal of Advanced Nursing, 77*(1), 101–110.

Burnard, P. (1987). Towards an epistemological basis for experiential learning in nurse education. *Journal of Advanced Nursing, 12,* 189–193.

Carper, B. A. (1978). Practice oriented theory. Fundamental patterns of knowing in nursing . . . part 1 (2). *Advances in Nursing Science, 1,* 13–23.

Carson, J. W., Keefe, F. J., Lynch, T. R., Carson, K. M., Goli, V., Fras, A. M., Thorp, S. R. (2005). Loving-kindness meditation for chronic low back pain: Results from a pilot trial. *Journal of Holistic Nursing, 23*(3), 27–304.

Chinn P. L., & Jacobs, J. K. (1983). *Theory and nursing: A systematic approach.* St. Louis, MO: Mosby.

Chinn, P. L., & Kramer, M. K. (1995). *Theory and nursing, a systematic approach.* St. Louis, MO: Mosby.

Colaizzi, P. (1978). Psychological research as the phenomenologist views it. In R. Valle & M. King (Eds.), *Existential phenomenological alternative for psychology* (pp. 48–71). New York, NY: Oxford University Press.

Dickoff, J., & James. P. (1968). A theory of theories: A position paper. *Nursing Research, 17*(5), 415–435.

DiNapoli, P., Nelson, J., Turkel, M., & Watson, J. (2010). Measuring the caritas processes: Caring factor survey. *International Journal of Human Caring, 14*(3).

Duffy, J. R., Hoskins, L. M., & Dudley-Brown, S. (2005). Development and testing of a caring-based intervention for older adults with heart failure. *Journal of Cardiovascular Nursing, 20*(5), 325–333.

Duffy, J. R., Hoskins, L. M., & Seifert, R. F. (2007). Dimensions of caring: Psychometric evaluation of the caring assessment tool. *Advances in Nursing Science, 30*(3), 235–245.

Dunphy, L. (2006). Florence Nightingale's legacy of caring and its applications. In M. Parker (Ed.), *Nursing theories and nursing practice* (pp. 39–57). Philadelphia, PA: F. A. Davis.

Dyess, S. M. (2008). Faith: A concept analysis. *Southern Online Journal of Nursing Research, 8*(2), 2p.

Ellis, R. (1968). Characteristics of significant theories. *Nursing Research, 17*(3), 217–222.

Fawcett, J. (1984). The metaparadigm of nursing: Current status and future refinements. *Image: The Journal of Nursing Scholarship, 16*, 84–87.

Fawcett, J. (1999). *The relationship of theory and research* (2nd ed.). Philadelphia, PA: F. A. Davis.

Fawcett, J. (2000). *Analysis and evaluation of contemporary nursing knowledge; Nursing models and theories*. Philadelphia, PA: F. A. Davis.

Hams, S. P. (1997). Concept analysis of trust: A coronary care perspective. *Intensive and Critical Care Nursing, 13*, 351–356.

Hektor, L., & Touhy, T. (1997). The history of the bath: From art to task. *Journal of Gerontological Nursing, 23*(5), 7–16.

Hendricks-Ferguson, V. L. (1997). An analysis of the concept of hope in the adolescent with cancer. *Journal of Pediatric Oncology Nursing, 14*(2), 73–82.

Hoeffer, B., Rader, J., McKenzie, D., Lavelle, M., & Stewart, B. (1997). Reducing aggressive behavior during bathing cognitively impaired nursing home residents. *Journal of Gerontological Nursing, 23*(5), 16–23.

Hupcey, J. E., & Penrod, J. (2005). Concept analysis: Examining the state of the science. *Research and Theory for Nursing Practice: An International Journal, 19*(2), 197–208.

Hutcherson, C. A., Seppala, E. M., & Gross, J. J. (2008). Loving-kindness meditation increases social connectedness. *Emotion, 8*(5), 720–724.

Jacobs-Kramer, M. K., & Chinn, P. L. (1988). Perspectives on knowing: A model of nursing knowledge. *Scholarly Inquiry Nursing Practice, 2*(2), 129–139.

Johns, J. L. (1996). A concept analysis of trust. *Journal of Advanced Nursing, 24*, 76–83.

Kramer, M., & Chinn, P. L. (2007). *Integrated theory and knowledge development in nursing*. St. Louis, MO: Mosby.

Kuhn, T. (1970). *The structure of scientific revolutions* (2nd ed.). Chicago, IL: University of Chicago Press.

Kuhn, T. (1977). *The essential tension: Selected studies in scientific tradition and change* (2nd ed.). Chicago, IL: University of Chicago Press.

Lawson, N., Thompson, K., Saunders, G., Saiz, J., Richardson, J., Brown, D., . . . Pope, D. (2010). Sound intensity and noise evaluation in a critical care unit. *American Journal of Critical Care, 19*, 88–98.

Leininger, M. (Ed.). (1981). *Caring: An essential human need*. Thorofare, NJ: Slack.

Lemon, K. (2004). An assessment of treating depression and anxiety with aromatherapy. *International Journal of Aromatherapy, 14*(2), 63–69.

Levine, M. (1995). The rhetoric of nursing theory. *Image: Journal of Nursing Scholarship, 27*, 11–14.

Locsin, N., McCaffrey, R., & Purnell, M. (2009). Nurses describe their experience of being cared for in a hospital healing arts space. *Journal of Holistic Nursing, 5*(1), 16–25.

Mazer. S. (2010). *Hospital noise and the patient experience: Seven ways to create and maintain a quieter environment*. Reno, NV: Healing HealthCare Systems.

McBrien, B. (2006). A concept analysis of spirituality. *British Journal of Nursing, 15*(1), 42–45.

McCaffrey, R. (2008). Music listening: Its effects in creating a healing environment. *Journal of Psychosocial Nursing, 46*(10), 39–44.

Morse, J. M. (2000). Exploring pragmatic utility: Concept analysis by critically appraising the literature. In B. L. Rodgers & K. A. Knafl (Eds.), *Concept development in nursing: Foundations, techniques, and applications*. Philadelphia, PA: W. B. Saunders.

Nightingale, F. (1859/1992). *Notes on nursing: What it is and what it is not*. Philadelphia, PA: Lippincott.

Parker, M. (2001). *Nursing theories and nursing practice*. Philadelphia, PA: F. A. Davis.

Parker, M. (2006). *Nursing theories and nursing practice* (2nd ed.). Philadelphia, PA: F. A. Davis.

Parker, M., & Smith, M. (2010). *Nursing theories and nursing practice* (3rd ed.). Philadelphia, PA: F. A. Davis.

Parson, T. (1949). *Structure of social action*. Glencoe, IL: The Free Press.

Ray, M. (1989). The theory of bureaucratic caring for nursing practice in the organizational culture. *Nursing Administration Quarterly, 13*(2), 31–42.

Ray, M. (2006). Marilyn Anne Ray's theory of bureaucratic caring. In M. Parker (Ed.). *Nursing theories and nursing practice* (2nd ed.). Philadelphia, PA: F. A. Davis.

Ray, M. A. (2008). Caring scholar response to achieving compassionate excellence: A cooperative accelerated BSN program. *International Journal for Human Caring, 12*(2), 39–41.

Ray, M. A. (2011). A celebration of a life of commitment to transcultural nursing: Opening of the Madeleine M. Leininger Collection on Human Caring and Transcultural Nursing. *Journal of Transcultural Nursing, 22*(1), 97.

Rew, L., & Barrow, E. M. (1987). Intuition: A neglected hallmark of nursing knowledge. *Advances in Nursing Science, 10*(1), 49–62.

Roach, S. (1987). *Caring, the human mode of being: A blue-print for the health professions*. Ottawa, Ontario: Canadian Hospital Association.

Rodgers, B. (2000). Concept analysis: An evolutionary view. In B. L. Rodgers & K. A. Knafl (Eds.), *Concept development in nursing: Foundations, techniques, and applications* (2nd ed., pp. 77–102). Philadelphia, PA: Saunders. (Original work published 1993.)

Sauer, S. (2010). Watson's theory of human caring as a framework for practice in the neonatal intensive care unit. *International Journal for Human Caring, 14*(3), 76–77.

Schwartz-Barcott, D., & Kim, H. S. (2000). An expansion and elaboration of a hybrid model of concept development. In B. L. Rogers & K. A. Knafl (Eds.), *Concept developments in nursing: Foundations and applications*. Philadelphia, PA: W. B. Saunders.

Shiley, S. D. (2010). Listening: A concept analysis. *Nursing Forum, 45*(2), 125–134.

Simmons, B. (2010). Clinical reasoning: Concept analysis. *Journal of Advanced Nursing, 66*(5), 1151–1158.

Smith, M. C. (1999). Caring and the science of unitary human beings. *Advances in Nursing Science, 21*(4), 14–28.

Smith, M. C. (2010). Marlaine Smith's theory of unitary caring. In M. Parker & M. C. Smith (Eds.), *Nursing theories and nursing practice* (3rd ed.). Philadelphia, PA: F. A. Davis.

Smith, M. J., & Lieher, P. (2008). *Middle range theory for nursing*. New York, NY: Springer.

Speros, C. (2004). Health literacy: Concept analysis. *Journal of Advanced Nursing, 50*(6), 633–640.

Starr, S. (2008). Authenticity: A concept of analysis. *Nursing Forum, 43*(2), 55–62.

Stevenson, J., & Tripp-Reimer, T. (1990). Knowledge about care and caring: State of the art and future developments. *Proceedings of a Wingspread Conference.* Kansas City, MO: American Academy of Nursing.

Sumner, J. (2010). A moral framework for caring in nursing: Neo-Stoic Eudaemonism. *International Journal for Human Caring, 14*(1), 51–57.

Sumner, J. F., & Fisher, W. P., Jr. (2008). The moral construct of caring in nursing as communicative action: The theory and practice of a caring science. *Advances in Nursing Science, 31*(4), E19–36.

Swanson, K. (1991). Empirical development of a middle-range theory of caring. *Nursing Research, 40*, 161–166.

Swanson, K. M. (1999). Effects of caring, measurement, and time on miscarriage impact and women's well-being. *Nursing Research, 48*(6), 288–298.

Timmins, F. (2006). Exploring the concept of "information need." *International Journal of Nursing Practice, 12*, 375–381.

Turkel, M. (1997). *Struggling to find a balance: The paradox between caring and economics.* Doctoral dissertation, University of Miami.

Turkel, M., & Ray, M. (2004). Creating a caring practice environment through self-renewal. *Nursing Administration Quarterly, 28*(4), 249–254.

Twiss, E., Seaver, J., & McCaffrey, R. (2006). The effect of music listening on older adults undergoing cardiovascular surgery. *Nursing in Critical Care, 11*, 224–231.

Walker, L. O., & Avant, K. C. (1995). *Strategies for theory construction in nursing* (3rd ed.). Norwalk, CT: Appleton-Century-Crofts.

Watson, J. (1979). *Nursing: The philosophy and science of caring.* Boston, MA: Little, Brown.

Watson, J. (1985). *Nursing: Human science and human care.* Norwalk, CT: Appleton-Century-Crofts.

Watson, J. (1992). *Notes on nursing: Commemorative edition with commentaries by contemporary nursing leaders.* Philadelphia, PA: J. B. Lippincott.

Watson, J. (2005). *Caring science as sacred science.* Philadelphia, PA: F. A. Davis.

Watson, J. (Ed.). (2008). *Assessing and measuring caring in nursing and health science.* New York, NY: Springer.

Watson, J. (2011). *Human caring science.* Sudbury, MA: Jones & Bartlett.

Watson, J., & Smith, M. (2002). Caring science: The science of unitary human beings: A theoretical discourse for nursing knowledge development. *Journal of Advanced Nursing, 37*(5), 452–461.

Weaver, K., & Mitcham, C. (2008). Nursing concept analysis in North America: State of the art. *Nursing Philosophy, 9*, 180–194.

Wilson, J. (1963). *Thinking with concepts.* Cambridge, UK: Cambridge University Press.

Young, C. E. (1987). Intuition and nursing process. *Holistic Nursing, 7*(3), 52–62.

Zander, P. (2007). Ways of knowing in nursing: The historical evolution of a concept. *The Journal of Theory Construction & Testing, 11*(1), 7–11.

2

Caring Science as Metaparadigm

Jean Watson

*I*n considering the concepts of caring within the construct of Caritas, it is helpful to have the background and clarity of caring science itself. The broader model of human caring science provides the larger context for the emergence of this research. A paradigm of caring science makes explicit a deep ethic and philosophical worldview as the starting point, which unites caring and love as the basis for healing. *Caritas,* as the leading theoretical construct within caring science and the theory of human caring (Watson, 1985, 2008, 2011), is derived from the Latin word, which gives a deeper meaning for the concept of caring. It makes direct connections between caring and love, reminding us that human caring is delicate and fragile; it has to be honored, named, and cultivated to be sustained. Thus, human caring is very precious and more than a job. It is a lifelong mutual process of a giving-receiving gift to humanity. Caring-science approach has a covenant with humanity to sustain the dignity and deepest evolution of humankind (Watson, 2008):

> Caring Science has as its starting point in a relational ontology that honors the fact that we are all connected and Belong to Source—the universal spirit field of infinity/universal Love. A Caring Science orientation moves humanity closer to a moral community closer to peaceful relationships with self-other communities-nations, states, other worlds and time. (p. 17)

Caritas thinking invites a total transformation of self and systems. In this model, the changes come from the inner center of each person, opening the heart and a consciousness of humanity.

Basic assumptions and premises of caring science have been identified and named that provide a foundation for the construct of Caritas.

BASIC ASSUMPTIONS OF CARING SCIENCE

- Caring science is the essence of nursing and the foundational, disciplinary core of the profession.

- Caring can be most effectively demonstrated and practiced interpersonally; however, caring consciousness can transcend and be communicated beyond time, space, and physicality.
- The intersubjective human-to-human processes and connections keep alive a common sense of humanity; they teach us how to be human by identifying ourselves with others, whereby the humanity of one is reflected in the other.
- Caring consists of *Caritas Processes* that facilitate healing, honor wholeness, and contribute to the evolution of humanity.
- Effective caring promotes healing, health, and individual and family growth; a sense of wholeness, forgiveness, and evolved consciousness; an inner peace that transcends the crisis and fear of disease, diagnosis, illness, traumas, life changes, and so on.
- Caring responses accept a person not only as he or she is now but as what he or she may become and is becoming.
- A caring relationship is one that invites emergence of human spirit, opening to authentic potential, being authentically present, allowing the person to explore options—choosing the best action for self for "being in right relation" at any given point in time.
- Caring is more "healthogenic" than curing.
- Caring science is complementary to curing science.
- The practice (and research) of caring/Caritas is central to nursing. Its social, moral, and scientific contributions lie in its professional commitment to the values, ethics, and ideals of caring science in theory, practice (education), and research (Watson, 2008, pp. 17, 18).

PREMISES OF CARING SCIENCE

- Knowledge of caring cannot be assumed; it is an epistemic-ethical-theoretical endeavor that requires ongoing explication and development.
- Caring science is grounded in a relational, ethical ontology of unity within the universe that informs the epistemology, methodology, pedagogy, and praxis of nursing and related fields.
- Caring science embraces epistemological pluralism, seeking to understand the intersection and underdeveloped connections between the arts and humanities and the clinical sciences.
- Caring science embraces all ways of knowing, being, and doing: ethical, intuitive, personal, empirical, aesthetic, and even spiritual and metaphysical ways of knowing and Being.
- Caring-science inquiry encompasses methodological pluralism, whereby the method flows from the phenomenon of concern—diverse forms of inquiry seek to unify ontological, philosophical, ethical, and theoretical views while incorporating empirics and technology.

■ The culture of nursing—the discipline and profession of nursing—has a vital, social-scientific role in advancing, sustaining, and preserving human caring as a way of fulfilling its mission to society and broader humanity (Watson, 2005, pp. 218–219, in Watson, 2008, p. 18).

Caring science encompasses a humanitarian, human science orientation to human caring processes, phenomena, and experiences. Thus, Caritas as a construct for assessing and measuring authentic human caring is located within caring science and is a specific construct within the theory of human caring, identifying and naming the authentic caring process: the 10 Caritas Processes. The measurement of Caritas within the backdrop of caring science invites a total transformation of self and systems. In this model, changes occur not from an outer focus on systems but from that deep place within the creativity of the human spirit. Here is where humanity—the individual heart, consciousness, and actions of practitioners—evolves and connects with the ultimate source of all true transformation (Watson, 2008, p. 36).

MEASUREMENT OF CARITAS

To consider "measuring Caritas" involves another focus to both ground and expand the caring science model while empirically validating the deeper dimensions of caring, love, and healing. The caring assessment measures in this book strive to do just that from a variety of perspectives, populations, and countries. Although rhetorical questions remain about nursing's tendency to jump to methods and measurements before addressing the meaningful philosophical questions that inform knowledge, in this instance it is caring science that facilitates our measuring Caritas. Indeed, measuring Caritas with its origins in theoretical and philosophical beginnings helps to bridge opposing viewpoints, dualisms, and conflicting paradigms. Thus, these multiple approaches to measuring Caritas as a core element of caring lead us closer to putting caring in our clinical research formulas, further advancing caring-science scholarship, and informing and transforming practices (Watson, 2009).

Caritas, once glimpsed through empirical measurements in a variety of conditions, may help us to see what has long been hidden from the public as well as from our science models.

As this book unfolds, the reader can integrate a better understanding of the purpose and use of formal measurements of Caritas as evidence of caring-science scholarship and application. These include:

■ Continuous improvement of caring through the use of outcomes and more mindful, authentic Caritas interventions to improve practice;

- Benchmarking of structures and environments in which Caritas is more evident and overly manifest in patient and system outcomes;
- Tracking of levels and models of Caritas in care settings against routine-care, industrial practices;
- Evaluation of consequences of Caritas versus noncaring for both nurses and patients;
- Increased development of our knowledge and understanding of the relationship between Caritas practices and health and healing outcomes;
- Empirical validation of extant caring theory and caring science, as well as generation of new theories and understanding of caring and nursing practices;
- Stimulation of new directions for nursing and health-science educational programs, including interdisciplinary and transdisciplinary education and research (Watson, 2009, p. 7).

In summary, this chapter provides an overview of caring science and the foundation for the Caritas construct of caring with its theoretical origin in Watson's theory of human caring (Watson, 1979, 1985, 1999, 2008, 2011). Toward that end, ethical and philosophical premises are outlined, offering some reconciliation of paradigm and theoretical issues in the quest to measure caring through Caritas construct as embedded in the Caring Factor Survey (Nelson, Watson, & Inova Health, 2009).

Although this book traces similarities and differences in and across countries, with respect to measuring caring/Caritas, the basic ground of scholarship emerges from a different model of science: caring science. This work advances empirical research emerging from caring science and the specific theoretical construct of Caritas, bringing caring and love into our knowledge and practices of healing and patient outcomes for self and systems.

REFERENCES

Nelson, J., Watson, J., & Inova Health. (2009). Caring factor survey. In J. Watson, *Assessing and measuring caring in nursing and health sciences* (2nd ed., pp. 253–260). New York, NY: Springer.

Watson, J. (1979). *Nursing: The philosophy and science of caring.* Boston, MA: Little Brown.

Watson, J. (1985). *Nursing: Human science and human care. A theory of nursing.* New York, NY: National League for Nursing.

Watson, J. (1999). *Postmodern nursing and beyond.* Edinburgh, Scotland: Churchill Livingstone/New York, NY: Elsevier.

Watson, J. (2008). *Nursing: The philosophy and science of caring* (Rev. ed.). Boulder, CO: University Press of Colorado.

Watson, J. (2009). *Assessing and measuring caring in nursing and health sciences* (2nd ed.). New York, NY: Springer.

Watson, J. (2011). *Human caring science.* Sudbury, MA: Jones & Bartlett.

3

The Caritas Process of Hope as a Midrange Theory

Giuliana Masera and Karen Gutierrez

*H*ope is central to life and is an essential dimension for success-fully dealing with illness and preparing for death. Patient, family, and health care provider concerns regarding hope have been firmly established in the literature. Researchers have made significant strides in seeking to define hope, describe experiences of hope, and delineate factors that promote and diminish hope. Thus, we first review research on hope to clarify it in nursing practice before examining how the concept of hope is integrated into the construct of caring as proposed within Watson's theory of caring.

DEFINING THE CONCEPT OF HOPE

Researchers have analyzed the concept of hope in an effort to define it and delineate its many facets. Stephenson (1991) reviewed literature from multiple domains including theology, philosophy, psychology, psychiatry, and nursing in a concept analysis of hope. From this analysis, hope was described as a "positive feeling state," which includes a "feeling of confidence diluted by a degree of uncertainty" (p. 1458). In addition to the emotional aspect of hope, there was also a thinking component whereby an individual visualizes something meaningful to the person that is not yet in existence. Thus, hope had a strong association with personal meaning in life. It also incorporated a perception of needing help from something or someone outside of oneself, such as another person or a spiritual or religious entity. Antecedents to hope, according to Stephenson, were "anything that would be significant to the person since hope is uniquely related to the individual's life experiences" (p. 1459). The consequences of hope, identified in the analysis, included renewed energy, peace, and a new perspective. The culmination of the review and analysis was a definition of hope: Hope is "a process of anticipation that involves the interaction of thinking, acting, feeling, and relating, and is directed toward a future fulfillment that is personally meaningful" (p. 1459).

Dufault and Martocchio (1985) implemented research aimed at clarifying and expanding knowledge related to the concept of hope. These researchers observed 82 terminally ill patients and their providers in a variety of settings over a 2-year period, including in an acute care hospital and patients' homes. The researchers, who sought to define and describe hope's "spheres and dimensions," culminated their analysis with this definition: "a multidimensional dynamic life force characterized by a confident yet uncertain expectation of achieving a future good which, to the hoping person, is realistically possible and personally significant" (p. 380). This definition is similar to Stephenson's in many ways. Both definitions suggest hope is a feeling state that is positive (confidence), yet uncertain; is future oriented and meaningful to the individual; and has multiple dimensions.

Dufault and Martocchio (1985) expanded this definition of hope by describing two "spheres" of hope: "generalized hope" and "particularized hope." Generalized hope "is a sense of some future beneficial but indeterminate developments. It is broad in scope and not linked to any particular concrete or abstract object of hope" (p. 380). Conversely, particularized hope "is concerned with a particularly valued outcome, good, or state of being, in other words a hope object. Objects of hope, that which are hoped for, may be concrete or abstract" (p. 380). Generalized hope is described as promoting particular hope and providing support when particular hope is perceived as unrealistic. Dufault and Martocchio also described six dimensions for hope that frame both spheres of hope including affective, cognitive, behavioral, affiliative, temporal, and contextual dimensions.

Marcel (1995) differentiated the concept of hope as including two spheres as well. These spheres were described as "I hope that" and "I hope." The former described hope as focused on a specified object or condition to be achieved, whereas the latter described hope as more generalized and not goal directed. Thus, a significant contribution of both Marcel's and Dufault and Martocchio's work was the description of a second sphere of hope that is generalized and not focused on a particular goal.

Morse and Doberneck (1995) sought to describe hope by interviewing groups of chronically ill, but not "terminal," patients as well as individuals without current health issues. The four sample groups interviewed included patients undergoing heart transplant, patients with spinal cord injuries, breast cancer survivors, and breastfeeding mothers. Based on these interviews, the researchers identified seven components of hope:

1. A realistic initial assessment of the predicament or threat
2. The envisioning of alternatives and the setting of goals
3. A bracing for negative outcomes
4. A realistic assessment of personal resources and of external conditions and resources

5. The solution of mutually supportive relationships
6. The continuous evaluation for signs that reinforce the selected goals
7. A determination to endure (p. 277)

Based on these seven components as well as four patterns of "hoping" identified in the study, Morse and Doberneck (1995) defined hope as:

> Hope is a response to a threat that results in the setting of a desired goal, the awareness of the cost of not achieving the goal, the planning to make the goal a reality, the assessment, selection, and use of all internal and external resources and supports that will assist in achieving the goal, and the reevaluation and revision of the plan while enduring, working, and striving to reach the desired goal. (p. 284)

The meaning and significance of hope depends on an individual's life circumstance and personal philosophical stance regarding hope. Farran, Herth, and Popovich (1995) conceptualized hope as encompassing four key components:

1. The experiential process of accepting human "trials" as a part of being human while allowing imaginative possibilities to occur
2. A spiritual/transcendent process with hope being inseparable from faith
3. A rational thought process grounding hope in reality with goals and needed resources (physical, emotional, and social)
4. A relational process in that hope occurs between persons and it is influenced by another's hope, presence, communications, and strength

THE "LIVED EXPERIENCE" OF HOPE

Researchers have further expanded knowledge of the concept of hope by focusing on hope in relation to its "lived experience." Hall (1989), who focused on the experience of hope in patients with stage 2 (asymptomatic) HIV disease, interviewed 11 men. Based on their disclosure of how they live with this disease and her experience with previous HIV patients, as well as the researcher's own diagnosis of metastatic cancer, she surmised: "My experience, and those of my informants, have brought me to the conclusion that hope is something all people need until they take their last breath. I have seen very little evidence that most people accept death. Rather, they accept life. If they accept life well, then they die well" (p. 178).

Hall (1989) also examined and critiqued the commonly held medical notion that promoting and encouraging hope in individuals with a terminal illness encourages denial. Citing Kübler-Ross's work (1969), Hall pointed out that denial was presented as a healthy means of coping with a threat. Hall also reasoned that mortality is a known human reality. Thus, we are all dying yet we look to the future and are hopeful because this is human nature. If people not diagnosed as dying need hope, those who are dying need even more.

Herth (1990) conducted a longitudinal study focused on hope in patients diagnosed with terminal illness. Herth used interviews of patients, along with a tool she developed—the Herth Hope Index—to measure level and focus of hope over time. Study results identified that the focus of hope for the terminally ill patients in her sample changed over time from "tangible, time-focused expectations to a desire for serenity and inner peae as death approached" (p. 1258).

Another study by Herth (1993) focused solely on hope in caregivers of terminal patients. The results of this study demonstrated that time and the changing health status of the dying patient resulted in the focus of hope for caregivers changing from "doing" to "being" as death came nearer. Caregivers viewed hope as "continually unfolding and changing in response to life situations. . . . Hope enabled them to 'see beyond the present'" (p. 544).

Benzein (2001) interviewed 11 patients with cancer receiving palliative home care regarding their "lived experience of hope" after a cancer diagnosis. Her analysis revealed "a tension between hoping for something, that is a hope of getting cured, and living in hope, that is reconciliation and comfort with life and death" (p. 117). The patients described their experience of hope in the context of a terminal diagnosis as trying to live their lives as normally as possible and garnering hope from positive relationships, including relationships with self, significant others, their environment (e.g., the hope that resulted from living in their home), pets, and a spiritual relationship. A dual focus of hope existed for these patients: hope for a cure, with treatment representing hope, despite acknowledging that they knew they would not get better; and hope for being prepared for death. The balance in the level of hope placed on each of these foci shifted from day to day. Benzei concluded, "Living with an incurable illness does not mean living without hope. . . . The lived experience of hope for patients in palliative home care is not only hoping for something, but also living in hope" (pp. 123–124).

INFLUENCES ON HOPE

Many researchers have sought to identify influences that promote and discourage hope. Herth conducted multiple studies focused on hope using a variety of samples including terminally ill patients, family caregivers of terminally ill patients, and nurses in hospice and home health agencies. The results of these studies identified that caring relationships were associated with an increased level of hope, whereas uncaring relationships discouraged hope (Buckley & Herth, 2004; Herth, 1990, 1991,

1993). Caring relationships that promoted hope included relationships with family, friends, health care professionals, and/or God or a "higher being" (Herth, 1993). The "presence" of a caring person who was "fully there," physically and psychologically, listening to and attending to needs, was a significant source of hope for caregivers of terminally ill patients (Herth, 1993). Herth suggested that dying patients and their families need physical and emotional support; encouragement of patient-family physical closeness; facilitation of expression of spiritual beliefs; and an active, listening presence from care providers (Herth, 1990). In relationships, "the little things matter," such as asking what name the person prefers, willingness to answer questions, and showing respect (Buckley & Herth 2004). Communication of bad news in a "non caring" manner diminished hope (Buckley & Herth, 2004).

Herth's studies also identified specific methods to support hope. Strategies used by family caregivers to promote hope included participating in warm and caring relationships; cognitively reframing thoughts from negative to positive; praying and meditating; positive visualization; humor; and comparing the situation to that of others (Herth, 1993). Additional strategies included limiting the focus of time or measuring it based on upcoming meaningful events; focusing on and redefining attainable expectations; finding comfort in spiritual beliefs; and balancing energy with demands (Herth, 1993). Methods used by nurses to maintain hope were similar to those of family caregivers and included providing comfort; facilitating positive relationships; promoting meaningful spiritual beliefs and practices; positive thinking; redefining specific areas of hope in life; communicating one's own sense of hope; recalling joyous, meaningful events; recognizing, valuing, and accepting personhood and individuality; pointing out positive attributes such as courage and determination; focusing attention on attainable short-term, specific aims; and supporting the desire for inner peace and eternal rest (Buckley & Herth, 2004).

Kennedy and Lloyd-Williams (2006) conducted a review of the literature related to maintaining hope in communication in the context of palliative care. In this review, the authors identified that health care providers limited prognostic information communicated to patients and families to protect them from the pain of disclosure, but this, paradoxically, resulted in increased distress as a result of denying patients and families the opportunity to prepare for future outcomes. The review identified that patients' hope has multiple foci from cure, to relief of pain and a good death. The relationships between patient and family and provider influenced patients' and family members' responses to information provided as well as their level of hope. Provider behaviors that promoted hope included demonstrating empathy, trust, interest, and commitment; being receptive to questions; providing information compassionately; and "being there." Conversely, uncaring provider behaviors diminished hope, such as communicating in a harsh, disrespectful, or cold manner, as did receiving discrepant information from providers. Although balancing hope with truth was a central premise identified in the review, the authors stated that this does not mean that providing "false promises" is warranted; it means realizing hope can be garnered from providing caring relationships rather than viewing the situation solely as focused on hope for a cure. Thus, "information should be given in a way that is 'not unduly negative or falsely reassuring'. . . . This is believed to allow patients to put their affairs in order without feeling as if they are 'giving up'" (p. 53).

Findings from an ethnographic study of end of life in an intensive care unit (ICU) by Gutierrez (2010) expanded Kennedy and Lloyd-Williams's (2006) finding that providers attempt to "balance" hope with truth. In Gutierrez's study, ICU nurses and physicians attempted to identify the "appropriate" level of hope in accordance with a "realistic" picture of a specific patient situation in their own minds first, and then worked to "align" patients' and family members' prognostic "picture" and levels of hope with their own via communication processes. Alignment included either promoting or deterring hope, depending on whether family members' levels of hope were higher or lower than those of providers. This was described by providers as identifying whether family members and patients were "realistic" or "not realistic." If the nurses and physicians still had hope for patient recovery, they included positive aspects of the patient's condition in their communication with the patient and family (e.g., what was going "well"), including expressions of hope and a focus on treatment. If providers no longer had hope for recovery and perceived that it was time for withdrawing life support, they purposefully "keep the hope out of it," as one nurse described, by focusing on the negative aspects of the patient's condition (e.g., what is not going well) and excluding any statements of hope or further treatment options that represented hope. The purpose of deterring hope was viewed by providers as an attempt to "help" family members come to terms with the probability of impending patient death and enable them to make necessary end-of-life decisions. Although one ICU physician described attempting to transition the focus of hope to a peaceful death, a majority of providers viewed hope solely as goal oriented, and more specifically, focused on hope for patient "cure" or recovery (Gutierrez, 2010).

Clayton, Butow, Arnold, and Tattersall (2005) found similar findings when conducting interviews with focus groups and individuals—to foster coping and hope when discussing end-of-life issues and prognosis. They included in their interviews 19 patients with advanced cancer, 24 palliative care providers, and 22 health professionals. All groups described the need to maintain hope with only the health provider sample expressing concerns regarding not offering "unrealistic" hope in order to avoid harming the patient and family by preventing preparation for death. Influences on hope were delineated with all groups confirming the importance of sensitive communication of information that was not "too blunt" and not in more detail than desired by patients and/or families. Patients described perceiving hope when health care professionals treated them in a manner that made them feel "valuable and important" (p. 1972). Patients and palliative care providers most frequently described the hope perceived from good care. The uncertainty related to prognosis was a source of hope, because it suggested the possibility of living beyond what was expected. Health providers identified that goals for hope can change over time and that providers should assist patients in refocusing their goals for hope toward those that are more obtainable. There was general agreement regarding the importance of being "honest" without providing prognostic information when it was not desired, as well as providing hope by focusing on positive aspects without promoting "false hope."

Dufault and Martocchio (1985), in their study of the dimensions of hope, noted the affiliative dimension of hope that included treating others as "intelligent, worthwhile, and feeling persons." This promoted hope, as did the willingness of others to listen (p. 386). The researchers suggested means to promote hope by providing empathy, providing information, encouraging "courage, endurance, and patience," assisting in shifting the goal for hope, and providing knowledge of others' experiences for comparison purposes.

RELATIONSHIPS BETWEEN HOPE AND OTHER CONCEPTS

Marcel's (1995) philosophy of hope views it as the final guarantor of fidelity; that which shields a person from despair and provides strength to continue to create oneself in availability to the other. Although this might appear to be nothing more than optimism—frequently misplaced, as events too often reveal—that things will turn out for the best, Marcel insists that this is not the case. Following now familiar distinctions, he makes a differentiation between the realm of fear and desire on the one hand and the realm of despair and hope on the other.

Marcel (1995) views fear and desire as anticipatory and focused, respectively, on the object of fear or desire. To desire is "to desire that X" and to fear is "to fear that X." Optimism exists in the domain of fear and desire because it imagines and anticipates a favorable outcome. However, the essence of "I hope" is not "to hope that X," but merely "to hope. . . ." Thus, it is hope—which does not accept the current situation as final while at the same time resists imagining or anticipating specific circumstances—that can resolve the plight. In other words, hope is willing deliverance from the situation. The more hope transcends any anticipation of the form that deliverance might take, the less it is open to the objection that, in many cases, the hoped-for deliverance does not take place. If I desire that my disease be cured by a given surgical procedure, it is very possible that my desire might be thwarted. However, if I simply maintain myself in hope, no specific event (or absence of event) need shake me from this hope.

This does not mean, Marcel asserts, that hope is inert or passive, however, or even stoic. Stoicism is merely the resignation of a solitary consciousness. Hope is neither resigned, nor solitary. "Hope consists in asserting that there is, at the heart of being, beyond all data, beyond all inventories and all calculations, a mysterious principle which is in connivance with me" (p. 5). While hope is patient and expectant, it remains active and, as such, it might be characterized as an "active patience." The assertion contained in hope reveals a kinship with willing rather than desiring. Thus, "inert hope" would be an oxymoron.

> No doubt the solitary consciousness can achieve resignation [stoicism], but it may well be here that this word actually means nothing but spiritual fatigue. For hope, which is just the opposite of resignation, something more is required. There can be no hope that does not constitute itself through a "we" and for a "we". I would be tempted to say that all hope is at the bottom choral. (Marcel, 1973)

Finally, it should be no surprise that, "speaking metaphysically, the only genuine hope is hope in what does not depend on ourselves, hope springing from humility and not from pride" (Marcel, 1995). And here is found yet another aspect of the withering that takes place as a result of *indisponibilité,* in general, and pride in particular. The same arrogance that keeps the proud person from communion with fellows keeps her or him from hope. This example points to the dialectical engagement of despair and hope: where there is hope there is always the possibility of despair, and only where there is the possibility of despair might there be a response of hope. Despair, says Marcel, is equivalent to saying that there is nothing in the whole of reality to which I can extend credit, nothing worthwhile. "Despair is possible in any form, at any moment and to any degree, and this betrayal may seem to be counseled, if not forced upon us, by the very structure of the world we live in" (Marcel, 1995). Hope is the affirmation in response to this denial. Where despair denies that anything in reality is worthy of credit, hope affirms that reality will ultimately prove worthy of an infinite credit, the complete engagement and disposal of myself.

THE ROOT OF NURSING: CARING

In the new millennium, the crisis in modern medicine and nursing seems to lie in the lack of a meaningful philosophy for the nature of practice and the deeper dimensions of caring work. It seems that nursing's very survival is at stake at this moment in its history. Thus, it is a deeper level of nursing, its very source, that we must explore and excavate for the new era now upon us (Watson, 2002). Health care delivery systems around the world have intensified nurses' responsibilities and workloads. Nurses must now deal with patients' increased acuity and complexity in regard to health care situations. Despite such hardships, nurses must find ways to preserve their caring practice.

Watson's caring theory, which represents the archetype of an ideal nurse, is an indispensable guide to advance nursing practice. Its structure facilitates nursing's return to its professional roots and values. Not only does it guide nurses in the art of providing compassionate care to ease patients' and families' suffering and promote healing and dignity, but it also assists nurses' progression toward personal actualization. Applying caring values in nursing practice is essential to nurses' health because it is fundamentally tributary to providing meaning in nursing work (Chantal, 2003).

Caring theory and pain theory are congruent in their contemporary focus on subjective human experience, inner life processes, and meaning of the experience. Pain theory describes the pain experience as a dynamic interaction among biological, physiological, psychosocial, cultural, and spiritual influences. Thus, nurses must seek to know and recognize patients in all these dimensions in order to aid patients experiencing pain. The human caring process, too, requires knowledge of holistic personhood, including the unity of mind, body, and spirit; one's strengths, limitations, and responses; and knowledge of how to provide comfort, compassion, and empathy within the context of a caring relationship (Watson & Foster, 2003).

CARATIVE FACTORS

Developing her caring theory in 1979, and revising it in 1985, 1988, and 2008, Jean Watson views her caring theory and the "Carative Factors" (later transposed as Caritas Processes) as the foundation for her theory and the essence of nursing practice. She uses the term *carative* to contrast with conventional medicine's curative factors. Her Carative Factors attempt to "'honor' the human dimensions of nursing's work and the inner life world and subjective experiences of the people we serve" (Watson, 1997, p. 50). In all, the original Carative Factors comprise 10 elements:

1. Humanistic-altruistic system of value
2. Faith-hope
3. Sensitivity to self and others
4. Helping-trusting, human care relationship
5. Expressing positive and negative feelings

6. Creative problem-solving caring process
7. Transpersonal teaching-learning
8. Supportive, protective, and/or corrective mental, physical, societal, and spiritual environment
9. Human needs assistance
10. Existential-phenomenological-spiritual forces (Watson, 1988)

As her theory evolved, Watson introduced the concept of "clinical Caritas Processes," which have now replaced her Carative Factors. The word *caritas* originates from the Latin vocabulary, meaning "to cherish and to give special loving attention." The reader will be able to observe a greater spiritual dimension in these new processes. The following is Watson's translation of the Carative Factors into clinical Caritas Processes: the practice of loving kindness and equanimity within the context of caring consciousness.

1. Creative use of self and all ways of knowing as part of the caring process; to engage in artistry of caring-healing practices
2. Engaging in genuine teaching-learning experience that attends to unity of being and meaning, attempting to stay within others' frames of reference
3. Creating a healing environment at all levels (physical as well as non-physical), maintaining an environment of energy and consciousness whereby wholeness, beauty, comfort, dignity, and peace are potentiated
4. Opening and attending to spiritual, mysterious, and existential dimensions of one's own life-death; soul care for self and the one being cared for (Watson, 2001)

"TO CURE" OR "TO CARE"?

The distance between people and their worlds is particularly evident in health services, where the separation between health care professionals and users is distinct and markedly asymmetrical. The elements of separation between everyday life and institutional experiences and procedures also are easily recognizable in health-related situations.

The current task assumed by health providers seems to be providing care for "object-bodies," not "person-bodies." But can a nurse truly provide care for an anonymous body, viewed as a mechanism, a body-machine to repair, while ignoring the person subject? Curing without caring is the paradox that the division between science and person has caused, making the person in need of care ever more anonymous. This anonymity is marked by rules imposed by procedures (though understandable) that break rhythms of life and submit family relationships to emotional wounds: postponing a request, a meeting, or a word of comfort. Here, the relational need is not only of, and for, the patient but also of, and for, family members.

The impersonal nature of health care's communication systems makes it difficult for providers to move beyond their mask and role. This may be related to fear of burnout—a valid concern. Burnout is more prevalent, however, when there are few opportunities to develop emotionally and nurses present themselves poorly prepared to meet relational needs, especially in extreme situations. When suffering patients and families most need to receive care, there is a vacuum of knowledge and skills to meet their needs.

Cultivating knowledge of feelings and relational communication is essential to promote confidence and avoid being overwhelmed. Medical and nursing skills will not be diminished but rather enhanced by a psychological and human provision that providers bring into play in a relationship with the sick and suffering: viewing a patient as a whole person rather than discrete organs and systems (Iori, 2003).

CONCLUSION

Hope is a complex, multidimensional concept that has been studied from the perspectives of multiple disciplines. In nursing, promoting and sustaining hope in situations of distress, discomfort, inadequacy, and dependency is an important goal.

The value of promoting hope in nursing is related to its therapeutic healing power. Positive effects of hope are measurable and are the focus of nurse researchers seeking knowledge of the impact of nurse-patient caring interactions on patient healing. For these reasons, Watson's caring theory includes hope as a significant component in the Caritas Processes.

In caring, simple gestures of humanity, patience, and compassion are very important. Hope is the figure of the company. "I'm here beside you, do not be afraid." "Hope offers the prospect of a future, any future that life reserves for us, which may be death for a terminal patient. If the relationship between nurse and patient is the plot through which an achievement unfolds, it is here that hope can promote and support vitality and courage. Hope may return momentum even in times of life significantly affected" (Masera, 2008).

REFERENCES

Benzein, E., Norberg, A., & Saveman, B. (2001). The meaning of the lived experience of hope in patients with cancer in palliative home care. *Palliative Medicine, 15,* 117–126.

Buckley, J., & Herth, K. (2004). Fostering hope in terminally ill patients. *Nursing Standard, 19*(10), 33–41.

Chantal, C. (2003). Continuing education: A pragmatic view of Jean Watson's caring theory. *International Journal for Human Caring, 7*(3), 51–61.

Clayton, J. M., Butow, P. N., Arnold, R. M., & Tattersall, M. H. (2005). Fostering coping and nurturing hope when discussing the future with terminally ill cancer patients and their caregivers. *Cancer, 103*(9), 1965–1975.

Dufault, K. J., & Martocchio, K. B. (1985). Hope: Its spheres and dimensions. *Nursing Clinics of North America, 20*, 379–391.

Farran, C., Herth, K., & Popovich, J. (1995). *Hope and hopelessness: Critical clinical constructs.* Thousand Oaks, CA: Sage.

Gutierrez, K. (2010). *Communication of prognostic information in an ICU at end of life: Practices among and between nurses, physicians, and family members.* Unpublished dissertation, University of Minnesota.

Hall, B. (1989). The struggle of the diagnosed terminally ill person to maintain hope. *Nursing Science Quarterly,* 177–184.

Herth, K. (1990). Fostering hope in terminally-ill people. *Journal of Advanced Nursing, 15*, 1250–1259.

Herth, K. (1991). Development and refinement of an instrument to measure hope. *Scholarly Inquiry for Nursing Practice: An International Journal, 5*(1), 39–51.

Herth, K. (1993). Hope in the family caregiver of terminally ill people. *Journal of Advanced Nursing, 18*, 538–548.

Iori, V. (2003). Emozioni e sentimenti nel lavoro educativo e sociale, Il sapere dei sentimenti, in Strumenti n.9 [Emotions and feelings in the educational and social work, n. 9]. Milan: Guerini Studio.

Kennedy, V., & Lloyd-Williams, M. (2006). Maintaining hope: Communication in palliative care. *Recent Results in Cancer Research*, 47–60.

Kübler-Ross, E. (1969). *On death and dying.* New York, NY: Macmillan.

Marcel G. (1973). *Tragic wisdom and beyond* (S. Jolin & P. McCormick, Trans.). (Publication of the Northwestern University Studies in Phenomenology and Existential Philosophy, J. Wild, Ed.) Evanston, IL: Northwestern University Press.

Marcel, G. (1995). *The philosophy of existentialism* (pp. 26, 28, 31, M. Harari, Trans.). New York, NY: Carol.

Masera, G. (2008). *Educare alla speranza, quale significato nel lavoro di cura? Polikromie* [Educating for hope]. *III*(1), 3–8.

Morse, J., & Doberneck, B. (1995). Delineating the concept of hope. *Image: The Journal of Nursing Scholarship, 27*(4), 277–285.

Stephenson, C. (1991). The concept of hope revisited for nursing. *Journal of Advanced Nursing, 16*, 1456–1461.

Watson, J. (1988). *Nursing: Human science and human care. A theory of nursing.* New York, NY: National League for Nursing. (Original work published 1985.)

Watson, J. (1997). The theory of human caring: Retrospective and prospective. *Nursing Science Quarterly, 10*(1), 49–52.

Watson, J. (2001). Jean Watson: Theory of human caring. In M. E. Parker (Ed.), *Nursing theories and nursing practice* (pp. 343–354). Philadelphia, PA: F. A. Davis.

Watson, J. (2002, Spring). Guest editorial: Nursing: Seeking its source and survival. *ICUs and Nursing Web Journal,* (9), 1–7.

Watson, J. (2008). *Nursing: The philosophy and science of caring.* Denver, CO: University Press of Colorado.

Watson, J., & Foster, R. (2003) The attending nurse caring model: Integrating theory, evidence and advanced caring-healing therapeutics for transforming professional practice. *Journal of Clinical Nursing, 12*, 360–365.

4

Caring Factor Survey and Adaptations

*T*his chapter reviews seven different versions of the Caring Factor Survey (CFS). The CFS is based on Watsons's 10 Caritas Processes (Watson, 2008) and has been tested extensively and described elsewhere (DiNapoli, Nelson, Turkel, & Watson, 2010; Nelson, Watson, & Inova Health, 2009; Persky, Nelson, Watson, & Bent, 2008). Authors within this chapter all believe that the caring moment is important to all relationships that are directly or indirectly related to the care provider and patient relationship. Hypothetically, if caring is occurring all around the care provider and patient, this will potentiate the caring energy and interaction between care provider and patient. The most vital relationship outside of the care provider and patient relationship is relationship to self, which includes perceived competence of caring and caring behaviors toward self. Other important caring relationships include those with coworkers, nurse managers, patients' families, preceptors, and the organization itself. The original CFS was adapted to measure these important caring relationships. Use and refinement of these tools will help to continue to build the science of caring and test the authors' collective belief that Caritas is an intervention of healing.

REFERENCES

DiNapoli, P., Nelson, J., Turkel, M., & Watson, J. (2010). Measuring the caritas processes: Caring Factor Survey. *International Journal of Human Caring, 14*(3), 16–21.

Nelson, J., Watson, J., & Inova Health. (2009). Caring Factor Survey. In J. Watson (Ed.), *Assessing and measuring caring in nursing and health sciences* (2nd ed., pp. 253–260). New York, NY: Springer.

Persky, G. J., Nelson, J. W., Watson, J., & Bent, K. (2008). Creating a profile of a nurse effective in caring. *Nursing Administration Quarterly, 32*(1), 15–20.

Watson, J. (2008). *Nursing: The philosophy and science of caring* (Rev. ed.). Boulder, CO: University Press of Colorado.

The Practice of Loving Kindness to Self and Others as Perceived by Nurses and Patients in the Cardiac Interventional Unit (CIU)

Iris Lawrence and Mavra Kear

*I*n her theory of human caring, Jean Watson stresses the importance of the practice of loving kindness toward self and others. Caring and healing are rooted in the transpersonal caring relationship—the occasion when the one cared for and the one caring connect in a meaningful way. This connection cannot be attained fully if nurses do not attend to their own mind-body-spirit needs. In contemplating the full meaning of Caritas Process 1 ("Cultivating the Practice of Loving Kindness and Equanimity Toward Self and Others"), the nursing staff of the cardiac interventional unit (CIU) at Winter Haven Hospital, a 525-bed, not-for-profit, licensed, community hospital, began to wonder if nurses truly practice loving kindness toward self and coworkers. The staff decided to conduct a study and set out to adapt the psychometrically tested Caring Factor Survey (CFS) (Nelson, Watson, & Inova Health, 2009) to assess care of self and care of coworkers. A new instrument to measure self-care and care for coworkers could then be examined in a deeper analysis of how care for self and others relates to the patients' perception of caring. It was hypothesized that (1) patients give nurses higher average (mean) Caritas scores than nurses give themselves for self-care, and (2) nurses rate coworkers' practice of Caritas toward each other higher than Caritas toward oneself within self-care.

With the permission and assistance of John Nelson, one of the authors of the CFS, the CFS was modified to measure staff nurses' perceptions of self-care and was titled Caring Factor Survey–Caring for Self (CFS-CS). Similarly, the CFS was modified to measure nursing staffs' perceptions of Caritas of coworkers and the survey was titled Caring Factor Survey–Caring for Coworkers (CFS-CC). John Nelson then formatted the surveys for electronic data collection. After approval by the institutional review board at Winter Haven Hospital, CIU nurses were invited to complete the surveys. All 24 CIU nurses received invitations via e-mail, copies of the e-mail in their unit-based mailbox, and verbal invitations and reminders. Reminder e-mails were sent every 2–3 weeks over the 6-week data collection period. Each nurse was given two unique identifiers to use to access each of the online surveys: one identifier for CFS-CS and one identifier for CFS-CC. Once the nurse submitted the completed survey, the identifier could no longer be used. This log-in method helped ensure confidentiality of responses and prevented individuals from responding more than once. Space was provided on the electronic survey for staff to add comments about behaviors, attitudes, or events that prompted their responses. Participation in the study was voluntary and no incentives were offered.

The first hypothesis was measured by asking patients to complete the CFS during the same data-collection period as the staff surveys. The CIU averages 120 admissions per month and patient selection was randomized by every third admission. A target of 30 patients was set as an equivalent sample size to the number of staff nurses on the unit. For the purposes of this study, only patient responses were accepted and the survey was completed during the hospitalization instead of being mailed after discharge. Patients unable to complete the survey independently were assisted by the primary investigator. No patient identifiers were attached to the survey and voluntarily returning the completed CFS constituted implied consent to participate in the study. At the end of the data-collection period, all of the patient surveys were bundled and mailed to John Nelson, who entered the data into a data file for analysis.

Reliability for all instruments was established. Cronbach's alpha for the 30 patients who responded to the CFS was 0.92. Of the 24 CIU nurses invited to participate, 14 (58%) completed the CFS-CS and 13 (54%) completed the CFS-CC. Cronbach's alpha was 0.89 for the CFS-CS and 0.91 for the CFS-CC.

Patients ranked nurses highest for decision making (mean score 6.57) and lowest for spiritual beliefs and practices (mean score 5.36). The bar graph and rank order of all Caritas factors for patients are shown in Figure 4.1 and it is noted that the practice of loving kindness is ranked third with a mean score of 6.47. It was noted that all mean scores were above 4.0 (scale 1.0–7.0), indicating a generalized agreement that Caritas was conveyed by the care providers at Winter Haven Hospital (Figure 4.2).

The average (mean) score for the CFS-CS was 5.66. The mean score of 4.79 supports the hypothesis that nurses will give themselves low scores for the practice of loving kindness and it is also noted that it is the lowest score of any of the Caritas factors in this study.

The average (mean) score for the CFS-CC was 5.55. Similar to the CFS-CS, loving kindness was ranked as the lowest Caritas Process (mean 5.08). All scores were noted to be above 4.0 on the CFS-CC, indicating a generalized perception of coworker Caritas. However, it should be noted that the scores for loving kindness ranged from 1.0 to 7.0, so not all perceived Caritas from coworkers.

The total score (all 10 caring processes combined) of each scale was used to evaluate support of the proposed hypothesis. The preceding results support the first hypothesis that patients would rank caring higher than nurses reported self-care. The second hypothesis, that Caritas of coworkers would be ranked higher than Caritas for self, was not supported.

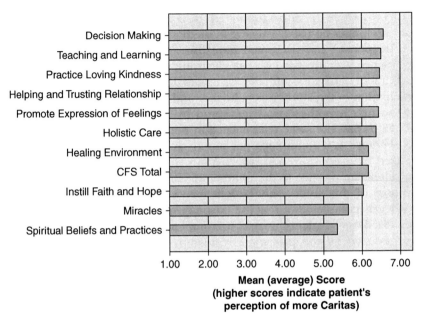

FIGURE 4.1 Mean scores for Caritas processes as measured by CFS, in rank order.

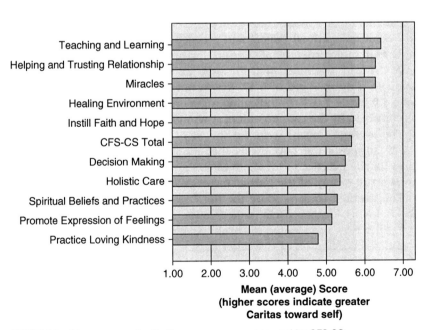

FIGURE 4.2 Mean scores for Caritas processes, measured by CFS-CS.

The results of this study suggest that nurses working in this nursing unit may not be tending to self-caring and mind-body-spirit renewal practices. If self-care is a concept that adds to the construct of Caritas, then these findings should be discussed and examined further. Authors of this study recognized the fact that this small study represented only a small proportion of nurses in the organization; however, the authors also hypothesized that similar results related to self-care and caring of coworkers would be found throughout the organization. This study offers an opportunity to investigate and develop interventions within the organization to help nurses attend to Caritas Process #1 of tending to self and others with loving kindness.

It is unclear from this small study if the lack of self-care is a global issue for registered nurses. Replication of this study with broader samples is needed. If it does become evident that nurses consistently fail to attend to the loving care needed to preserve the wholeness of self and others, then the authors assert that they have a professional obligation to make every effort to change the culture of nursing.

One place to start refinement of caring processes for coworkers is with Graduate Nurse Preceptor Training. A subcommittee is now focusing on revising the training to add emphasis on the importance of role-modeling self-care and care of others when serving as a mentor to new nurses. If this organization is to reach the goal of becoming a Caritas organization with Caritas nurses, there must be a culture in which the practice of loving kindness to self and coworkers is not merely a "theory" but the normative behavior of all nurses who practice within the organization.

REFERENCE

Nelson, J, Watson, J., & Inova Health. (2009). Caring factor survey. In J. Watson (Ed.), *Assessing and measuring caring in nursing and health sciences* (2nd ed., pp. 253–260). New York, NY: Springer.

Creation of the Caring Factor Survey–Care Provider Version (CFS-CPV)

Jennifer Johnson

*T*his section of the chapter reviews the development of an instrument that measures care providers' self-perception of demonstrating caring behaviors to patients within their care. The instrument was based on Watson's theory of Caritas (Watson, 2008). The instrument was developed during the implementation of relationship-based care (RBC), a professional model of care that uses the theory of Caritas.

The development of the instrument began with the discovery of the Caring Factor Survey (CFS) during a literature search for an instrument that measured care providers' self-perceptions of caring for patients. Due to no instrument being found that measured care provider perception of caring, it was decided to amend the CFS for this purpose. The CFS measures patients' perceptions of caring behaviors of those who are taking care of them, based on Watson's theory of Caritas. It was deemed the best instrument for amending to measure care providers' self-perceptions of delivering caring behaviors. The new tool was named the Caring Factor Survey–Care Provider Version (CFS-CPV). The original CFS was designed by John Nelson, Dr. Jean Watson, and Dr. Karen Drenkard and Gene Rigotti, who were employed at Inova Health. The CFS-CPV was designed to understand empirically how care was perceived by care providers.

The hospital where the instrument was targeted to be developed and tested within had recently subscribed to RBC as the professional practice model for its nurses. It was desired to measure caring as proposed by Watson because it was the central theory presented within RBC as well as the theory selected by the hospital of interest. This particular study was compelling because it has long been asserted historically by nurses that caring heals. However, caring is an elusive construct to measure. In order to measure caring, a tool that was consistent with Watson's theory of Caritas would need to be developed.

The first step was to perform a literature search and compile an annotated bibliography on appropriate journal articles that pertained to caring. Several journal articles on the topic of RBC and human caring were found, many of which referenced Jean Watson and her theory of human caring. Other resources were found that were written by John Nelson, Jayne Felgen, and Georgia Persky. The concept of RBC aligns with Watson's human caring theory and consists of three distinct elements that are interconnected: (a) the care provider's relationship with self, with patients and families, and with colleagues; (b) healing happens when therapeutic relationships are encouraged, developed, and nurtured; and (c) RBC must be introduced as a model of caregiving with an emphasis on the caring and healing environment in order to demonstrate excellence in this area of nursing practice.

It became clear during this project that human caring could be measured by using the unique CFS designed by the aforementioned Nelson et al., and based on Jean Watson's Carative Factors as it impacts healing. With the able assistance of John Nelson and the expertise of Jean Watson, the CFS was adapted in order to measure nurses' perceptions of care given rather than patients' perceptions of care received. The new tool was called the CFS-CPV.

After corresponding at length with John Nelson, the adapted survey was based on "I" statements from nurses', rather than patients', perspectives of care received. The survey in its adapted format worked well within the parameters of this project. Power analysis using G-Power 2.0 revealed that at least 60 respondents were needed for adequate power of the study.

Prior to data collection, a 1-hour in-service was conducted in the hospital as well as in the off-site physician office for the intended project. Each 1-hour in-service reviewed the topic of RBC and the theory of human caring. It was at the end of the in-service that attendees were given the CFS-CPV to complete. This time was used because it was deemed an efficient way to administer the CFS-CPV to a large group of nurses, nurse practitioners, and patient care assistants. Continuing education units (CEUs) were given to all who attended, which influenced attendance and procured the number of responses needed for an adequate sample size.

The in-services were held in December 2008 and consisted of the administration of the CFS-CPV; a PowerPoint presentation on Jean Watson's theory of human caring; a 2–3-minute clip of Nurse Ratchet from *One Flew Over the Cuckoo's Nest;* and a 2–3-minute clip of the nurse, Susie, from the movie *Wit.* The audience was encouraged to experience the contrast and discuss the comparison between a nontherapeutic and a therapeutic nurse-patient relationship as it pertained to caring. During the last five minutes, an audio of Jean Watson herself was played narrating her "caring moment," which was very moving spiritually and emotionally. Additionally, the participants received the CFS research studies time line in which Lourdes Hospital, site of the study, was included among approximately 60 other studies in caring science in John Nelson's research network.

By the end of the 4 in-services that occurred over a 2-month period, 76 nursing staff had responded to the CFS-CPV. There were 55 registered nurses (RNs) in the sample, 14 licensed practical nurses (LPNs), 2 advanced practice nurses (APNs), and 5 "other." There were no differences found using a *t* test to compare RNs and LPNs, using an alpha of

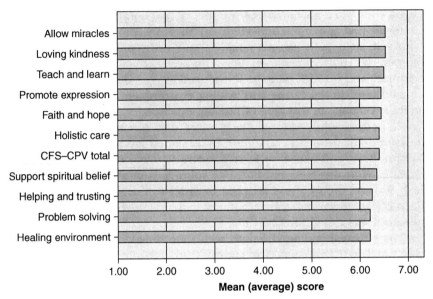

FIGURE 4.3   Rank order of all Caritas factors.

0.05. All respondents were included in the analysis. Psychometrics of the CFS-CPV revealed a Cronbach's alpha of 0.92. Descriptive statistics revealed that the highest scoring variable was perception of allowing patients to believe in a miracle (mean score 6.55, range 4.0–7.0), whereas the lowest scoring variable was creation of a healing environment (mean score 6.21, range 4.0–7.0). It was interesting to note that problem solving was second to last. The bar graph and rank order of all caring factors are noted in Figure 4.3.

This project was an excellent opportunity not only to develop a tool to measure nurses' perceptions of caring behaviors, but also to use data to reflect on delivery of caring behaviors. The in-services provided an opportunity to discuss the caring moment and how the concepts of RBC could be used to enhance the caring moment. The in-services provided opportunities outside of the in-service to carry on informal conversations of the impact of caring on patients as well as each other. Further research is needed to strengthen the validity and reliability of this new instrument to measure nurses' perceptions of caring. Continued research in understanding nurses' perceptions and competences in caring research may assist with documenting scientifically how caring is an intervention of healing.

REFERENCE

Watson, J. (2008). *Nursing: The philosophy and science of caring* (Rev. ed.). Boulder, CO: University Press of Colorado.

Family Used as Proxy to Measure Caring

*Patti Leger, Deanne Sramek,
Sandra Conklin, and Vickie Diamond*

*P*rior to the early 1900s, the question of the family's role in providing information, support, and care for the patient would not have been necessary because almost all care for the sick was provided at home by relatives. The ontological assumptions of objectivism, positivism, and reductionism that framed science and medicine during the industrial revolution led to an increase in hospitals, although initially they were considered only for the dying poor. A New York hospital superintendent in the early 1900s noted, "It can be put down as one of the advantages of a hospital that the relatives and friends do not take care of the patient. . . . It is much better for them [patients] not to be under the care of any one who is over-concerned for them" (Levine & Zuckerman, 2000, p. 4). The concept of family-centered care was introduced in health care settings in the 1960s when consumers, particularly parents of hospitalized children, insisted on health care information and the right to be present at the bedside. Health care professionals have made progress in the past four decades in researching and recognizing the importance of keeping the patient's family informed of health status, inviting family presence during invasive procedures and resuscitation, initiating liberal visiting policies, and involving the family in discharge planning decisions (Hodges, 2009; Li, 2005; Marco et al., 2006; Meyers et al., 2004). Most health care professionals recognize the many benefits of forming partnerships with families to provide excellent patient care and quality outcomes, yet families are often noted to be troublesome, distracting, and challenging in a variety of acute care settings and situations (Demir, 2008; Fisher et al., 2008; Levine & Zuckerman, 1999; Sjöblom, Pejlert, & Asplund, 2005; Yetman, 2009). With the ambivalence identified between health care professionals and the patient's family, the question of whether families can be used as proxy to measure patient caring becomes relevant.

LITERATURE REVIEW

Family-centered nursing literature acknowledges the importance of maintaining family unity in the acute care setting (Van Horn & Kautz, 2007). It is recognized that families are systems and when a family

43

member is ill and hospitalized, it affects the entire family (Benzein, Hagberg, & Saveman, 2008). Families experience vulnerability and helplessness (Eggenberger & Nelms, 2007). They worry about the patient's health and the patient's care received from health care providers (Li, 2005). Nursing research has demonstrated that the presence of family members enhances patient outcomes and adds to the strength of the family to endure difficulties (Marco et al., 2006). Families have commonly been used as proxy to assist in making health care decisions and goal planning for patients lacking decision-making capacity (Burkhardt & Nathaniel, 2008; Eicher & Johnson, 2003; Levack, Siegert, Dean, & McPherson, 2009). Qualitative nursing research has demonstrated strong feelings of connection between family members and the patient, particularly during critical illness and critical events (Eggenberger & Nelms, 2007; Meyers et al., 2004). Nursing research concerning the development of family partnerships during patient care is advancing the paradigm for the family as a system, yet there is a lack of literature concerning family perceptions of nurses' caring behaviors.

METHODS

A descriptive study using the 20-item Caring Factor Survey (CFS) was used to collect data from a convenience sample of 314 patients or their families over a 3-month time frame. Volunteers were recruited and trained to approach patients who met the inclusion criteria for the study. Inclusion criteria required that the patient be 18 years of age or older unless the parent or guardian consented to participation, the patient had to have been admitted to the hospital a minimum of 12 hours prior to being surveyed, and the patient had to be cognitively able to complete the survey or a family member could complete the survey for the patient. Descriptive statistics were used for the demographic variables. The t test was used to examine if there was a statistically significant difference using an alpha level of 0.05. A power analysis using G-Power 2.0 software revealed that a sample of 314 afforded an effect size of 0.30, power of 0.84, and alpha of 0.05. Data analysis was conducted using SPSS version 14.0 statistical software. The internal review board approved the study design.

RESULTS

The CFS dataset included responses from 137 family members due to the patient being too sick or too young to respond. The CFS data to date has revealed that there was no difference between the patient's and the family's CFS scores.

DISCUSSION

The results support the use of family as proxy to measure caring in one health care setting. The idea that a family member's perceptions of caring are similar to those of the patient's is supported by the transpersonal caring theory. Watson (2005) noted the connections between the tenets of transpersonal human caring theory and the science of unitary human beings: "Transpersonal caring resides within a field of caring consciousness and energy that transcends time, space, and physicality and is one with the universal field of consciousness (spirit)—the infinity" (p. 7). Invoking caring as part of our consciousness and intention affects the holographic universal field. "What we do for ourselves benefits others and what we do for others benefits us" (Watson, 2008, p. 10). This suggests that when nurses care for the family they also care for the patient, and when nurses care for the patient they also care for the family. The theory of human caring supports relational ontology versus separatist ontology (Watson, 2006). Rather than using a separatist ontology where the patient is viewed as an object with a disease and the family is viewed as a problem to be worked around or ignored, the theory and our study results support using relational ontology where patient and family are viewed as human beings, open to caring relationships and transpersonal caring moments. The theory of human caring recognizes and supports the basic human need for affiliation: belonging, family, social relations, and culture (Watson, 2008). The patient needs his or her family's presence along with needing the nurse to honor their common humanity. Meeting this basic need by providing nursing care for the patient and family enhances awareness of caring and supports wholeness and healing for all. There are limitations to the study, indicating the need for further research. The results suggest that family can be used as proxy in only one institution. Also, different statistical procedures might be used; for example, a paired t test used to measure individual patients' perceptions while concurrently measuring the patients' family members' perceptions of care to determine difference within the same family. This is in contrast to the independent t test that was used for this study, comparing a group of patients and a group of family members.

CONCLUSION

The results of this study offer quantitative support for the unitary nature of the theory of human caring. When care for the patient is provided with loving kindness and equanimity, the universal field of consciousness is transformed and elevated. Love is the highest level of consciousness (Watson, 2005). Love is the greatest source of healing (Watson, 2008). The patient's family is an intimate component of the holographic universal field surrounding the patient and the caring moments that emerge through caring relationships. In the relational paradigm, our findings support that family can be used as proxy to measure caring.

REFERENCES

Benzein, E. G., Hagberg, M., & Saveman, B-I. (2008). "Being appropriately unusual": A challenge for nurses in health-promoting conversations with families. *Nursing Inquiry, 15*, 106–115.

Burkhardt, M. A., & Nathaniel, A. K. (2008). *Ethics & issues in contemporary nursing* (3rd ed.). Clifton Park, NY: Delmar Cengage Learning.

Demir, F. (2008). Presence of patients' families during cardiopulmonary resuscitation: Physicians' and nurses' opinions. *Journal of Advanced Nursing, 63*(4), 409–416.

Eggenberger, S. K., & Nelms, T. P. (2007). Being family: The family experience when an adult member is hospitalized with a critical illness. *Journal of Clinical Nursing, 16*, 1618–1628.

Eicher, J. M., & Johnson, B. H. (2003). Family-centered care and the pediatrician's role. *Pediatrics, 112*(3), 691–696.

Fisher, C., Lindhorst, H., Matthews, T., Munroe, D. J., Paulin, D., & Scott, D. (2008). Nursing staff attitudes and behaviours regarding family presence in the hospital setting. *Journal of Advanced Nursing, 64*(6), 615–624.

Hodges, L. P. (2009, August). Patient-, family-centered care helps decrease LOS. *Hospital Case Management*, 121–122.

Levack, W. M. M., Siegert, R. J., Dean, S. G., & McPherson, K. M. (2009). Goal planning for adults with acquired brain injury: How clinicians talk about involving families. *Brain Injury, 23*(3), 192–202.

Levine, C., & Zuckerman C. (1999). The trouble with families: Toward an ethic of accommodation. *Annals of Internal Medicine, 130*, 148–152.

Levine, C., & Zuckerman, C. (2000). Hands on/hands off: Why health care professionals depend on families but keep them at arm's length. *Journal of Law, Medicine & Ethics, 28*(1), 5–18. Retrieved from http://www.ncbi.nlm.nih.gov/pubmed/11067632

Li, H. (2005). Hospitalized elders and family caregivers: A typology of family worry. *Journal of Clinical Nursing, 14*, 3–8.

Marco, L., Bermejillo, I., Garayalde, N., Sarrate, I., Margall, M. A., & Asiain, M. C. (2006). Intensive care nurses' beliefs and attitudes towards the effect of open visiting on patients, family and nurses. *British Association of Critical Care Nurses, Nursing in Critical Care 2006, 11*(1), 33–41.

Meyers, T. A., Eichhorn, D. J., Guzzetta, C. E., Clark, A. P., Klein, J. D., Taliaferro, E., & Calvin, A. (2004). Family presence during invasive procedures and resuscitation. *Topics in Emergency Medicine, 26*(1), 61–73.

Sjöblom, L., Pejlert, A., & Asplund, K. (2005). Nurses' view of the family in psychiatric care. *Journal of Clinical Nursing, 14*, 562–569.

Van Horn, E. R., & Kautz, D. (2007). Promotion of family integrity in the acute care setting. *Dimensions of Critical Care Nursing, 26*(3), 101–107.

Watson, J. (2005). *Caring science as sacred science*. Philadelphia, PA: F. A. Davis.

Watson, J. (2006, May 9). *Philosophies and theories of caring*. Lecture presented at the International Caring Certification Program at the University of Colorado Health Sciences Center School of Nursing, Boulder, CO.

Watson, J. (2008). *Nursing: The philosophy and science of caring* (Rev. ed.). Boulder, CO: University Press of Colorado.

Yetman, L. (2009). Caring for families: Double binds in neuroscience nursing. *Canadian Journal of Neuroscience Nursing, 31*(1), 22–29.

Preceptor Caring Attributes as Perceived by Graduate Nurses

Robin L. Testerman

*T*his research examined the perceived caring of preceptors as experienced by graduate nurses hired by Winter Haven Hospital between January 2007 and May 2009. Caring as a premise of professional nursing has existed since the days of Florence Nightingale. Williams, Dean, and Williams (2009) state that "both the American Nurses Association and the Royal College of Nursing emphasize caring [is] intrinsic to the modern nursing role" (p. 162). It is believed by the author of this current writing that integration of caring behaviors into professional practice must begin with the training of new nurses into their professional role. It was the desire to understand if caring behaviors were perceived by newly hired nurses within their respective preceptor–preceptee relationship.

This study was conducted at Winter Haven Hospital (WHH), a 525-bed, rural hospital founded in 1926 in Polk County, Florida. Nurse theorist Jean Watson's model of caring has come to represent the philosophy of nursing at WHH; it is the foundation upon which WHH has built nursing practice and has led to a Magnet designation. WHH has attempted to take Watson's caring science and her 10 Carative Factors (CFs) and integrate them into an "ethical-moral-philosophical values guided foundation" (Watson, 2008, p. 29).

Retention and recruitment are essential to the success of any hospital and clinical excellence can be accomplished only by providing care that is competent, professional, and caring. The Florida Center for Nursing (FCN) released a report in January 2009 that forecast the Florida nursing shortage of full-time equivalent RNs to be 52,000 by 2020. FCN also estimated that the cost of replacing a nurse ranges from "50% to 200% of annual salary" (FCN, 2009, p. 2).

Turnover statistics were of primary interest to WHH as the retention rate had declined from a high of 93% in 2006 to a low of 80% in the spring of 2009. A review of the literature by a graduate nurse task force at WHH revealed that an intervention for improving retention was to improve the transition of new graduate nurses into their professional role (Beaty, Young, Slepkov, & Isaac, 2009; Salera-Vieira, 2009). Considering the philosophy of Caritas at WHH, it was deemed appropriate to examine the presence of Caritas within the preceptor–preceptee relationship of new graduates and experienced nurses training the new nurses. The task force hoped that understanding the state of Caritas within the preceptor–preceptee relationship would assist with action planning for successful transition of new graduates to their new professional role and setting.

BACKGROUND

A careful examination of the literature regarding caring demonstrated by nurse preceptors revealed a multitude of studies on caring as it related to the nurse-patient relationship, creating a caring culture, and how we educate nurses in caring. However, no studies were found related to caring behaviors of preceptors and the resulting impact on organizational outcomes.

Considering no literature or instruments were found that related to caring behaviors of preceptors, it was decided that an instrument would need to be developed to explore caring behaviors of preceptors. While several tools were evaluated, a validated tool, the Caring Factor Survey (CFS), was in place and being used to measure the caring of nurses as perceived by patients and families. Developers include John Nelson, president of Healthcare Environment, nurse theorist Dr. Jean Watson, Dr. Karen Drenkard, and Gene Rigotti (Nelson, Watson, & Inova Health, 2009). The original tool had 20 items (two each addressing the 10 Caring Factors [CFs] of Watson) and was eventually reduced to 10 items (DiNapoli, Nelson, Turkel, & Watson, 2010). The 10 CFs measured by the CFS were those of the practice of loving kindness and instilling faith and hope (Watson, 2005).

To measure caring of preceptors, the 10-item CFS was adapted to examine the preceptees' perceptions of how the preceptor behaved during orientation (CFS-CP). For example, the first item on the CFS states, "Overall, the care I have received from the staff at this facility has been provided with loving kindness." This item was modified to "Every day I was with my preceptor(s) I was treated with loving kindness." One of the developers of the original CFS, John Nelson, was contacted to request permission to modify the 10-item CFS and permission was given.

PURPOSE OF THE STUDY

The purpose of this study was to examine the perceived caring of preceptors as experienced by graduate nurses hired by WHH. Training of graduate nurses occurred between January 2007 and May 2009. Thus potential responders were asked to respond as they recalled their training experience during this period.

METHODOLOGY

Institutional review board (IRB) approval was granted from the WHH IRB and the Florida Southern College IRB for this nonexperimental, quantitative study. Data were collected from the participants using self-report. Submission of the electronic survey was considered consent to participate in the study. Respondents were asked to rate their preceptors' level of caring using a 7-point Likert-type scale. The scale ranged from 1, *strongly disagree*, to 7, *strongly agree*. Respondents could select 4 if they had a neutral stance.

SAMPLE

The database of the graduate nurses (GNs) to be surveyed was organized by unit (e.g., orthopedics, emergency department, surgical intensive care, operating room) and resulted in a potential 156 respondents. The electronic survey was launched January 15, 2010, and closed May 4, 2010. Those GNs currently employed by WHH received a hand-delivered letter of introduction and instructions of how to access the anonymous survey site with an encrypted link and an assigned pass code. These letters were delivered by the researcher along with a $1.00 dessert coupon to the hospital cafeteria or a candy bar for those nurses off-site. The addresses for GNs who had resigned or terminated during the survey period were obtained from the State of Florida Board of Nursing website, which posts this as public information.

RESULTS

The result from this study demonstrated a Cronbach's α (alpha) of 0.98, significantly high reliability (Figure 4.4). A "high" value of alpha is often used as evidence that the items are closely related. An examination of a zero-order correlation table also revealed strong inter correlations among the concepts in this survey. Forty-three of the 156 nurses responded, which represents a 28% response rate, and 17 of the hospital units responded. GNs ranked preceptors highest for teaching and learning and the lowest for healing environment (see Figure 4.4).

Upon looking at the variance of scores more closely, it was noted that all 10 factors ranged from 1 to 7, indicating that there was varied experience during orientation as reported by the orientees. All scores were above 4.0, indicating a general "average" sense of caring (Table 4.1).

There was a moderate negative correlation of age and the CFS-CP ($r = -.432$), which demonstrated that the younger nurses tended to report higher caring behaviors. This was statistically significant at .01. This means younger nurses perceived more caring behaviors.

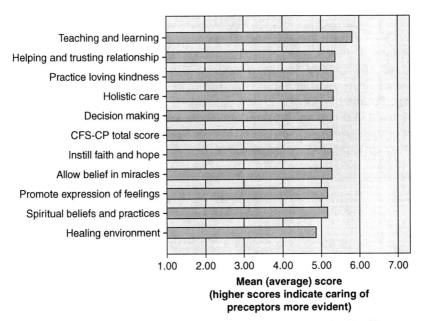

FIGURE 4.4 Rank order of caring behaviors of preceptors as perceived by GNs.

DISCUSSION AND IMPLICATIONS

This study used average (mean) scores, and considering the wide variance of scores, it would be interesting to use Parato mathematics to

TABLE 4.1 Descriptive Statistics from CFS-CP

	DESCRIPTIVE STATISTICS				
	N	MINIMUM	MAXIMUM	MEAN	STD DEVIATION
Teaching and learning	43	1.00	7.00	5.8140	1.67979
Helping and trusting relationship	43	1.00	7.00	5.3721	1.92754
Practice loving kindness	43	1.00	7.00	5.3256	1.65789
Holistic care	43	1.00	7.00	5.3256	1.71438
Decision making	43	1.00	7.00	5.3023	1.79331
Allow belief in miracles	43	1.00	7.00	5.2791	1.57851
Instill faith and hope	43	1.00	7.00	5.2791	1.80377
Promote expression of feelings	43	1.00	7.00	5.1628	1.91399
Spiritual beliefs and practices	43	1.00	7.00	5.1628	1.67517
Healing environment	43	1.00	7.00	4.8605	1.69848
Valid N (listwise)	43				

examine the outliers more carefully. What did those who reported high scores look like? Could the outliers for high scores, all those with 6.5 and higher, be perceiving biases of preceptors? In contrast, those with low scores, all those with 1.0–1.5, may need more training. Further discussion is warranted, but this study launches the possibility of understanding mentoring of caring within the preceptor–preceptee relationship.

It may be useful to use the CFS-CP to measure new graduates and conduct a termination study from hire to time of staff resignation. Termination studies are usually used to study mortality, but they could be applied to the examination of termination of employment. Were GNs who had a caring experience from the very beginning more likely to stay within the organization? It is the use of new mathematics, like Parato mathematics (use of outliers), and innovative procedures, like termination studies to study caring, that will give new insight into the profile and outcome of caring preceptors.

Planning an appreciative inquiry review of the results to continue to improve preceptor preparedness by the education department would assist in honing the clinical and mentoring skills of the preceptor (Challis, 2009). It would behoove the task force to implement a program that surveys all the GNs at regular intervals for a set number of years beyond their first year.

Creating unit incentives as a way to increase survey participation may increase the number of respondents. Having the survey available through a link on the hospital intranet could facilitate participation. Watson (2006) states that "caring and economics, and caring and administrative practices, are often considered in conflict with each other" (p. 87), but studies such as this may assist in demonstrating that "caring and economics are not mutually exclusive." Sharing how we care for our novice nurses is imperative to attracting and keeping our profession alive and thriving.

REFERENCES

Beaty, J., Young, W., Slepkov, M., & Isaac, W. (2009, November 4). The Ontario new graduate nurse initiative: An exploratory process evaluation. *Healthcare Policy, 4,* 22.

Challis, A. M. (2009, July). An appreciative inquiry approach to RN retention. *Nursing Management, 40*(7), 9–13.

DiNapoli, P., Nelson, J., Turkel, M., & Watson, J. (2010). Measuring the Caritas processes: Caring factor survey. *International Journal of Human Caring, 14*(3), 16–21.

Florida Center for Nursing. (2009). *Forecasting supply, demand, and shortage of RNs and LPNs in Florida, 2007–2010.* Retrieved January 13, 2010, from http://www.flcenterfornursing.org/files/RN_LPN_Forecasts.pdf

Nelson, J., Watson, J., & Inova Health. (2009). Caring factor survey. In J. Watson (Ed.), *Assessing and measuring caring in nursing and health sciences* (2nd ed., pp. 253–260). New York, NY: Springer.

Salera-Vieira, J. (2009, July/August). The collegial clinical model of new graduate nurses: A strategy to improve the transition from student nurse to professional nurse. *Journal for Nurses in Staff Development, 25,* 174–181.

Watson, J. (2005). *Caring science as sacred science.* Philadelphia, PA: F. A. Davis.

Watson, J. (2006, July–September). Caring theory as an ethical guide to administrative and clinical practices. *JONA's Healthcare Law, Ethics, and Regulation, 8,* 87–91.

Watson, J. (2008). *Nursing; The philosophy and science of caring.* Boulder, CO: University Press of Colorado.

Williams, G., Dean, P., & Williams, B. (2009). Do nurses really care? Confirming the stereotype with a case control study, *British Journal of Nursing, 18,* 162–165.

Nurses' Perceptions of Being Cared For Within the Hospital Environment: Adapting the Caring Factor Survey to the Bon Secours St. Francis Caring Work Environment Survey

Christi Harley, Tanya Lott, Elizabeth Clerico,
Erin Kosak, Winnie Hennessy, and Yvonne Michel

*B*on Secours St. Francis (BSSF) Hospital adopted the Watson theory of caring in 2007 as its foundational theory of nursing practice. From this inspiration, the BSSF Nursing Research Council (NRC) realized that caring is not a self-renewing resource and began investigating the phenomenon of nurses' perceptions of being cared for within the hospital work environment. Instrument development included modifying the Caring Factor Survey (CFS). The modification was based on measurement of four domains: physical needs, spiritual needs, intellectual stimulation, and authentic relationships. The items of the CFS were modified from measuring patients' perception of being cared for by providers to measuring nurses' perception of being cared for within their work environment. The modified survey was piloted in one unit. Based on the pilot responses and experts' review, the BSSF Caring Work Environment Survey was finalized and administered to nurses hospital-wide to establish baseline data. The survey is now repeated annually and provides feedback toward the continuous development of a caring hospital work environment.

Design: Descriptive, pre- and post-survey. The hospital institutional review board (IRB) granted this study exempt status.

Measurement: BSSF Caring Work Environment Survey.

Definitions: Environment of caring: the work culture of the employee and all entities affecting this culture, not limited to the organization.

Hospital environment: All aspects of the work environment contributing to the organizational mission and values.

Health care team: all individuals who contribute to the organization, not limited to employees.

Data Collection/Survey Development: The CFS (© 2006 Nelson, Watson, & INOVA Healthcare) is a patient survey designed to measure patients' perceptions of caring by their care providers. The original CFS consisted of 20 items, using a 7-point scale, from *strongly disagree*

53

TABLE 4.2 BSSF Caring Work Environment Survey

PHYSICAL NEEDS	SPIRITUAL NEEDS	INTELLECTUAL STIMULATION	AUTHENTIC RELATIONSHIPS
MY HEALTH CARE TEAM AT BON SECOURS ST. FRANCIS . . .			
has created an environment that encourages my physical health.	is respectful of my individual spiritual beliefs and practices.	solves unexpected problems well.	treats me with loving kindness.
allows me the opportunity for breaks.	has created an environment that encourages spiritual health.	is good at problem solving to meet needs and requests.	honors my feelings, no matter what they are, and I can talk openly and honestly about what I am thinking.
has created an environment that recognizes the connection between mind, body, and spirit.	encourages me to practice my own individual, spiritual beliefs as part of my self-caring and health.	is responsive to how I learn and whether I am ready to learn when teaching something new.	makes me feel someone is there if I need them.

(1) to *strongly agree* (7). The NRC modified the original 20 items of the CFS to elicit responses from nurses related to their perception of feeling cared for within the hospital work environment. The first modification was piloted in one hospital unit. The NRC further refined the survey based on responses from the pilot and experts' review. Throughout the process, the NRC sought to maintain the integrity of the original survey. The finalized BSSF Caring Work Environment Survey consisted of 12 items and was reviewed and approved by Dr. Jean Watson and John Nelson. The final survey is displayed in Table 4.2.

With the survey development completed, the BSSF Caring Work Environment Survey was administered to all nursing staff in the fall of 2008 and 2009. The hospital's electronic Learning Management System was used to conduct the survey.

INTERVENTION

Originally interested in evaluating the effect that the new meditation garden would have on the nurses' perception of their work environment as caring, the NRC began to look at the effect of other caring initiatives as well. Caring interventions in 2009 included an annual Blessing of the Hands ceremony during Nurses' Week, the use of a designated nursing resource center, the opening of two new meditation gardens on the hospital campus, and several renovated unit break rooms.

ANALYSIS

For the first administration of the caring survey, factor analysis using principal component analysis produced a single factor, indicating that the four domains were highly correlated. Cronbach's alpha was 0.935, indicating reliable internal consistency for the 12 items. Factor analysis of the second administration of the caring survey supported the first, producing a single factor with a Cronbach's alpha of 0.941.

RESULTS

The 2008 baseline study had a total of 324 surveys completed, reflecting an 81% response rate. The postsurvey in 2009 had a total of 269 surveys completed, reflecting a 70% response rate. The mean survey score in 2009 was 5.6, an increase from the 2008 survey of 5.3. ($p < .0005$). Figure 4.5 provides the 2009 mean results by survey item.

Two items of the survey ("respectful of my spiritual beliefs," and "allows me the opportunity for breaks") had the least changes between the 2008 and 2009 surveys. "Respectful of my spiritual beliefs" was the highest rated survey item in 2008 and, therefore, had little room for improvement. In the case of "allows me the opportunity for breaks," no change occurred in allowing time for breaks.

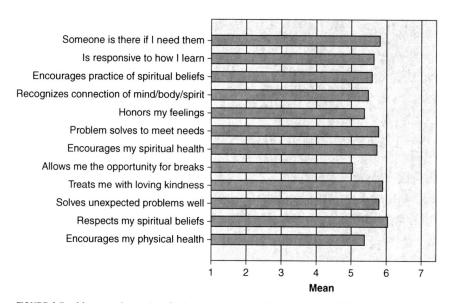

FIGURE 4.5   Mean caring rating for individual survey items for the 2009 survey.

DISCUSSION

This study demonstrates evidence to suggest that the modified survey, the BSSF Caring Work Environment Survey, is reliable, valid, and sensitive to nurses' perceptions of being cared for within a hospital work environment. The survey results provide evidence that BSSF nurses do feel cared for within their work environment.

The NRC plans to administer the survey annually and this year plans to invite another hospital within its health care system to participate. Development of caring interventions and the impact of those interventions on nurses' perceptions of feeling cared for within the work environment will be ongoing as the BSSF Environment of Caring study continues and expands.

Anecdotally, the NRC feels strongly that the experience of conducting this research has had additional and unexpected benefits. The theory of caring, authored by Dr. Jean Watson, was selected because it was consistent with, and provided a framework for, the caring that was already an integral part of the BSSF hospital culture. This led nurses to engage in discussions addressing caring as a resource that is not self-renewing but needs "active planning"—both internally and externally. These ideas led to the implementation of a research structure and process to measure nurses' perceptions of the hospital work environment as caring. The research experience heightened nurses' awareness of caring within their environment, helped to create a language related to caring concepts and principles, and resulted in both individual and group actualization of the caring theory.

Development of the Caring Factor Survey–Caring of Manager (CFS-CM)

Lynda Olender and Sheri Phifer

Over the last two decades, a small but increasing body of knowledge related to caring within an administrative context has been emerging. These empirical studies and manuscripts all support the importance or positive influence of nurse caring within an administrative context, particularly in consideration of the increasing complexity and economic focus of health care agencies (Duffy, 1993; Nyberg, 1989; Ray, 2006; Turkel, 2003, 2007; Turkel & Ray, 2004; Watson, 2006, 2009). Much of this scholarly work has been qualitative in nature, with the aim of exploring the perceptions of nurse manager caring behaviors as perceived by nurse managers (Turkel, 2003; Uhrenfeldt & Hall, 2009), by key supervisory staff (Kramer et al., 2007), and by staff nurses (Kramer et al., 2007). The caring attributes identified within these studies have included the manager/supervisor being present, approachable, and authentic and having the ability to promote group cohesion and teamwork. These attributes all foster the creation of a healing environment and are consistent with attributes within the Caritas framework as informed by Watson's theory of human caring within an administrative context (Watson, 2006, 2009).

A number of studies examined the influence of nurse manager caring and caring attributes quantitatively and have resulted in significant findings related to staff satisfaction, intent to remain with the organization (Duffy, 1993; Hall, 2007; Kleinman, 2004; Longo, 2009), and related negative correlations with outcomes such as occupational stress and somatic complaints (Hall, 2007). These studies used measurement tools that assessed supervisory support (Hall, 2007), leadership behaviors (Kleinman, 2004), and the organizational climate for caring (Longo, 2009). They adapted caring tools with applicability toward manager caring such as the use of the Nyberg Caring Assessment tool (Nyberg, 2009; Wade et al., 2008). Based on this increasing study interest, tools specifically designed to measure the staff nurses' perception of nurse manager caring behaviors have emerged (Duffy, 1993; J. Nelson, personal communication, December 8, 2009). The later tool, the Caring Factor Survey–Caring of Manager (CFS-CM) (J. Nelson, personal communication, December 8, 2009), assesses staff nurses' perception of nurse managers' caring behaviors in accordance with Watson's most recent iteration and enrichment of the theory of human caring as it related to the Caritas Processes. A description of the evolution, development, and testing of this tool follows.

THE CARING FACTOR SURVEY–CARING OF MANAGER (CFS-CM)

The CFS-CM measures staff nurses' perception of the nurse manager's caring behaviors in accordance with the Caritas Processes integral within Watson's theory of human caring (Watson, 2008). The 10 Caritas Processes are an evolution of Watson's original work describing caring attributes as Carative Factors (Watson, 1979) and currently describe these behaviors as Caritas Processes (or ways of being) indicative of a deeper connection of *love*—in this case, between the nurse manager and staff.

Comparatively, the statements within the Caring Factor Survey (CFS) and the CFS-CM are similar. The CFS is worded in the first person and pertains to the respondent's perception of his or her own caring attributes. The CFS-CM is also similarly worded and describes the staff nurses' perceptions of the nurse manager's caring attributes. Like the CFS, each of the 10 items of the CFS-CM is positively worded and corresponds to 1 of 10 Caritas Processes. For example, the Caritas Process of the practice of loving kindness and spiritual regard (as integral to the humanistic-altruistic system between the one who is caring and the one being cared for) is depicted within the statement, "Every day I am here I see my manager treat employees with loving kindness." Choices for the respondent include *strongly disagree, disagree, slightly disagree, neutral, agree, slightly agree,* and *strongly agree.* Scores of each of the 10 items are added, tallying scores from each item (Likert-style dependent scoring) with higher scores indicative of increased caring attributes. Additionally, the tool also includes an open-ended question asking participants to "describe nurse manager attitudes, behaviors, and/or actions. . ." that led the participants to their answers. This open-ended question enables the researcher to have added perspectives to the rationale for the answers provided by the participants and can be categorized and examined for themes using grounded theory methods.

Psychometric Evaluation

Originally, the derivative tool, the CFS, was a 20-item instrument having two items for each of the 10 concepts of caring/Caritas Processes (Nelson, Watson, & Inova Health, 2009). The tool was originally formulated by Nelson and face validity established by Watson (2006). Assessment and review by content experts in the Caritas Processes, including Watson (Drenkart, Rigotti, Nelson, & Watson, personal communication, December 12, 2010), established the tool's content validity. Criterion validity was established by measuring the CFS against a well-validated and similar caring tool, the Caring Assessment Tool (CAT-II) (Duffy, 2002). Pearson correlations between the CAT-II and the CFS were assessed and considered a strong correlation (Glasnapp & Poggio, 1985) at .80 when measured at the same time on the same unit. An evaluation of internal consistency reliability was established via Cronbach's alpha of .96 (Nelson, 2008). Inter item reliability was established with correlations ranging from .80 and above, with the exception of one paired statement related to the promotion of feelings (.74) from patients and support of spiritual belief and the creating of a healing environment (.77 and .75, respectively), and internal consistency for item-to-total correlations for all 20 statements ranging from .80 to .93.

The 20-item CFS was tested in three studies in the United States with a high Cronbach's alpha ranging from 0.97 to 0.98. The latest citation assessed the patients' perception of nurse caring in an acute care setting within a large, metropolitan, acute care facility in accordance to Watson's most recent theory of Caritas (Persky, Nelson, Watson, & Bent, 2008). In this study of 85 patient-nurse pairs, reliability of the CFS was reported as having a Cronbach's alpha of 0.97. Subsequently, to reduce survey burden yet remain true to the tenets of Watson's (2006) theoretical concept of Caritas, the CFS and then the CFS-CM were reduced to 10 items. During factor analysis proceedings, shared variances between paired items on the CFS allowed for a reduction of items to 10 items, one item for each of the Caritas Processes (DiNapoli, Nelson, Turkel, & Watson, 2010). Reliability for this revised tool has been reported in a group of 450 nurses in three facilities via a Cronbach's alpha of 0.89 with individual factor loadings ranging from 0.833 to 0.891. One factor, loving kindness, accounted for 66% of the variance. Psychometric evaluation for the CFS-CM (J. Nelson, personal communication, December 8, 2009) is currently under way.

PSYCHOMETRIC EVALUATION OF THE CFS-CM

Content and face validity were established by a review by the original author of the CFS (Nelson, personal communication, December 12, 2010). The tool was then tested/piloted on a sample of staff nurses in the southeastern portion of the United States ($n = 10$) for content validity (S. Phifer, personal communication, February 11, 2011). Scores for each of the 10 concepts of Caritas ranged from 6.1 to 6.9 on the Likert-type scale (with scores ranging from 1.0 to 7.0). The highest ranked item reported was support for decision making; the lowest ranked concept of Caritas related to spiritual support. Each item had a small-moderate ($r = .20$ to $.40$) to strong ($r = .80$ or greater) correlation with the total CFS-CM score of all items combined as measured by a Cronbach's alpha of 0.81 ($r = .37$ to $.91$).

THE APPLICATION OF THE CFS-CM TO ASSESS THE RELATIONSHIPS BETWEEN MANAGER CARING AND WORKPLACE BULLYING

A large landmark study designed to assess the relationship between the staff nurses' perceptions of nurse manager caring behaviors and their exposure to workplace bullying using the CFS-CM is in process (Olender, 2011). Olender posits that with the perceptions of nurse manager caring behaviors via the application of the 10 Caritas Processes, the recipient/participant of the caring encounter (the staff nurse) will feel caring/Caritas in a way that considers body, mind, and spirit and within the application of compassionate and caring service to others and thus be negatively correlated with the staff nurses' exposure to workplace bullying.

SECONDARY STUDY AIMS

In anticipation of this being a landmark study for the use of this tool, a second open-ended question at the end of the CFS-CM will ask staff nurses to describe a caring moment between the manager and themselves. It is hoped that responses to this question will provide deeper insight into caring connections reciprocally promoted between the manager and staff nurses. Comments will be reviewed and themes identified using grounded theory methods. Additionally, within the background information solicited from participants, the study will also assess religion, the practice of religion, and the staff nurses' opinions as to whether spirituality adds to the perception of caring. These questions will be included within the background information/demographic survey and may provide salient information as to the rationale for pilot study results having the lowest ranking between the concept of Caritas related to spiritual support.

Importantly, the assessment of the relationship of staff nurses' perceptions of nurse manager caring behaviors and workplace bullying in nursing will contribute new knowledge to the increasing body of science related to caring, specifically informed by Watson's theory of human caring (1979, 1985, 1988, 2006). Study results may also lead to shifting work priorities and related mindfulness and intentionality so that managers will have the time and availability to create a caring and healing environment for patients and for staff alike. Lastly, study findings may also support the need for the design and implementation of caring curriculum and caring competencies critical for the nurse manager's role within the clinical practice environment.

REFERENCES

DiNapoli, P. P., Turkel, M., Nelson, J., & Watson, J. (2010). Measuring the Caritas processes: Caring factor survey. *International Journal of Human Caring, 14*(3), 15–20.

Duffy, J. (1993). Caring behaviors of nurse managers: Relationship to staff nurse satisfaction and retention. In D. A. Gaut (Ed.), *A global agenda for caring* (pp. 365–378). New York, NY: National League for Nursing.

Duffy, J. (2002). Caring assessment tools. In J. Watson (Ed.), *Instruments for assessing and measuring caring in nursing and health sciences* (pp. 125–138). New York, NY: Springer.

Duffy, J. (2009). Caring assessment tools and the CAT-admin. In J. Watson (Ed.), *Assessing and measuring caring in nursing and health sciences* (2nd ed., pp. 131–147). New York, NY: Springer.

Glasnap, D. R., & Poggio, J. P. (1985). *Essentials of statistical analysis for the behavioral sciences.* Columbus, OH: Merrill.

Hall, D. S. (2007). The relationship between supervisor support and registered nurse outcomes in nursing care units. *Nursing Administrative Quarterly, 31*(1), 68–80.

Kleinman, C. (2004). The relationship between managerial leadership behaviors and staff nurse retention. *Hospital Topics, 82*(4), 2–9.

Kramer, M., Maguire, P., Brewer, B., Chmielewski, L., Kishner, J., Krugman, M., ... Waldo, M. (2007). Nurse manager support: What is It? Structures and practices that promote it. *Nursing Administrative Quarterly, 31*(4), 325–340.

Longo, J. (2009). The relationships between manager and peer caring to registered nurses' job satisfaction and intent to stay. *International Journal for Human Caring, 13*(2), 26–33.

Nelson, J. (2008). Development of the caring factor survey (CFS), An instrument to measure patient's perception of caring. In J. Watson (Ed.), *Assessing and measuring caring in nursing and health science* (2nd ed.). New York, NY: Springer.

Nelson, J., Watson, J., & Inova Health (2009). Caring factor survey. In J. Watson (Ed.), *Assessing and measuring caring in nursing and health sciences* (2nd ed., pp. 253–258). New York, NY: Springer.

Nyberg, J. (1989). *Caring in nursing administration.* Boulder, CO: University Press of Colorado.

Nyberg, J. (2009). Nyberg caring assessment scale. In J. Watson (Ed.), *Assessing and measuring caring in nursing and health sciences* (2nd ed., pp. 113–116). New York, NY: Springer.

Olender, L. (2011). *The relationship between staff nurses' perceptions of nurse manager caring behaviors and their perception of exposure to workplace bullying in nursing within multitude healthcare settings.* Unpublished dissertation. Seton Hall University.

Persky, G., Nelson, J. W., Watson, J., & Bent, K. (2008). Creating a profile of a nurse effective in caring. *Nursing Administration Quarterly, 32*(1), 15–20.

Ray, M. A. (2006). Marilyn Ann Ray's theory of bureaucratic caring. In M. E. Parker (Ed.), *Nursing theories & nursing practice* (2nd ed., pp. 360–368). Philadelphia, PA: F. A. Davis.

Turkel, M. C. (2003). A journey into caring as experienced by nurse managers. *International Journal for Human Caring, 7*(1), 20–26.

Turkel, M. C. (2007). Dr. Marilyn Ray's theory of bureaucratic caring. *International Journal for Human Caring, 11*(4), 57–72.

Turkel, M. C., & Ray, M. (2004). Creating a caring practice environment through self renewal. *Nursing Administration Quarterly, 28*(4), 249–254.

Uhrenfeldt, L., & Hall, E. O. C. (2009). Caring for nursing staff among proficient first-line nurse leaders. *International Journal for Human Caring, 13*(2), 39–44.

Wade, G., H., Osgood, B., Avino, K., Bucher, G., Bucher, L., Foraker, T., . . . Sirkowski, C. (2008). Influence of organizational characteristics and caring attributes of managers on nurses' job enjoyment. *Journal of Advanced Nursing, 64*(4), 344–353.

Watson, J. (1979). *Nursing: The philosophy and science of caring*. Boston, MA: Little, Brown.

Watson, J. (1985). *Nursing: Human science and human care*. Norwalk, CT: Appleton-Century-Crofts.

Watson, J. (1988). *Nursing: Human science and human care. A theory of nursing*. New York, NY: National League for Nursing. (Original work published 1985.)

Watson, J. (2006). Caring theory as an ethical guide to administrative and clinical practices. *Journal of Nursing Administration, 8*(1), 87–93.

Watson, J. (2008). *The philosophy and science of caring* (Rev. ed.). Boulder, CO: University Press of Colorado.

Watson, J. (Ed.). (2009). *Assessing and measuring caring in nursing and health sciences* (2nd ed.). New York, NY: Springer.

SECTION II

Measurement and Methods for Connecting Nurse to Patient

5

Measuring Caring in Primary Nursing

Georgia Persky, Jayne Felgen,
and John Nelson

*I*t is likely that during a patient's hospital stay the nurse is the caregiver who spends the greatest amount of time with the patient and thus has the greatest opportunity for "caring moments." This opportunity is amplified in the professional practice model, Primary Nursing. This chapter describes the tenets, or elements, of Primary Nursing; its care delivery operating system; vital education processes; and the importance of clarity in the nurse's understanding of self, role, and systems. Illustrations of these elements of Primary Nursing are provided via the description of the implementation of Primary Nursing at New York-Presbyterian Hospital/Columbia University Medical Center (NYP/CU) in New York City and research at that facility that examined Primary Nursing as it relates to caring moments

TENETS OF PRIMARY NURSING

The four tenets of Primary Nursing are: (a) allocation of patient care to one nurse; (b) case method assignment of patient care; (c) interdisciplinary communication; (d) the caregiver as care coordinator. These tenets are supported by a set of principles that assist the staff in integrating Primary Nursing into their practice with the goal of the tenets becoming operational and sustainable. Following is further detail about each of the four tenets.

Clear Allocation to One Nurse of Care for a Particular Patient and Acceptance of Responsibility for Decision Making About That Patient

This nurse accepts the responsibility and declares his or her commitment to partner with the patient, the family, and the health care team to develop and facilitate the execution of a personalized plan of care. Acceptance of this responsibility is evidenced by the nurse

- discovering the patient as a person;
- proactively sharing pertinent clinical and personal information;

■ employing critical and creative thinking to inform the development of a person- or family-specific plan of care consistent with the nursing process;
■ describing his or her role to the patient and family as primary nurse and expressing commitment to partner with the patient and family in developing and executing the patient's plan of care;
■ coordinating care and engaging the patient and family that culminates in a thoughtful and comprehensive transition plan for the patient's return to home or another care provider.

Case Method of Assignment of Patient Care

Case method assignments are patient- and family-centric rather than task based. Professional practice exists when the primary nurse continues to provide care for the primary patient when the nurse returns from absence or that patient has been moved to another room on the unit. By contrast, assignments based solely on geographic pods or zones represent a task-based technical practice. The primary nurse's commitment to the relationship with the patient and family is embraced by the nurse and trumps continuity of assignments in terms of importance.

Creating and Supporting Direct Channels of Communication Between the Patient, Family, Physician, and Health Care Team

"This element was developed to correct the data distortion . . . as a problem inherent in the communication 'pyramid' of task based practices" (Manthey, 1980). It avoids the "middle-man" wherever possible and enhances the quality and quantity of communication by providing team members the most pertinent information by a registered nurse (RN) who is well informed and knows the patient as a person. This element is in place when the primary nurse proactively communicates with the family, physician, other clinical professionals, and colleagues on the unit; communication includes all pertinent information regarding the personalized plan of care that the patient and nurse have developed. Discharge planning conversations directly involve or are directed by the primary nurse.

Caregiver as Care Coordinator

This element raises consciousness about the impact of varied ways of thinking, clinical approaches, levels of expertise, differing educational backgrounds, levels of preparedness, and experience on the patient outcome and on the practical use in the assignment practices of nurses. The decision to integrate the roles of care planner and caregiver forces a different way of thinking about how to assign nurses with different skill levels. "Decisions as to who takes care of which patients should reflect sensitivity to and awareness of each individual nurse's ongoing development" (Manthey, 1980, p. 34; Romano, 2008, pp. 9–10).

Primary nurses can be defined as nurses who have accepted professional responsibility for self, role, and systems at the point of service. These nurses must clearly understand these three interrelated domains to be able to identify effective solutions for overcoming organizational barriers that inhibit providing care consistent with Caritas behaviors (described in Chapters 1 and 2 of this book). The literature is silent on the question of clarity as a function of individual empowerment and professional effectiveness. Research findings from the longitudinal research study described in this chapter provide initial insight into how the implementation of Primary Nursing may foster nurses' clarity about (a) themselves as persons and healers; (b) what it means to be a professional; (c) how to create practice realities that enhance professional intentions. Primary nurses must have a clear understanding of all three domains (self, role, and systems) to achieve an optimal practice environment where caring moments are experienced as the norm.

CLARITY IN PRIMARY NURSING

This includes clarity of self, role, and system (Felgen, 2007; Koloroutis, 2004). Each is a critical element of being an effective primary nurse within a Relationship-Based Care (RBC) model.

Clarity of Self

The professional's level of self-awareness may strongly influence his or her recognition of self as an instrument of caring and healing. The professional may perform certain functions efficiently and in a kind and respectful manner without an overt sharing of self. In contrast are those professionals who are self-aware—whose actions are mindful, compassionate, loving, intentional; and linked to their personal sense of purpose, self-image, and spirituality. They are acutely aware that what they do, and why and how they do it, have a profound effect on self, patients, families, and others.

Clarity of Role

Several factors have a significant influence on the degree of professional autonomy and effectiveness experienced by the nurse: (a) depth of understanding of the multiple dimensions of professional nursing practice; (b) the scope and meaning of the nursing professional role; (c) the practical functions related to that role; (d) similar knowledge regarding the roles of others on the health care team. Nurses must understand the implications and expectations of all three realms of their role: (1) dependent, where the nurse, serving the patient as a full and mutually respected partner within the dependent realm with the physician, enhances patient outcomes (Knause, Draper, Wagner, & Zimmerman, 1986); (2) independent, where beyond medically delegated functions, the nurse must also be aware of and act upon the expectation to bring to the patient care experience unique to nursing, the science, the art, and the ethics of the role through independent function; and (3) interdependent, where the nurse also is uniquely positioned to collaborate with all allied health professionals in the interdependent coordination of care for patients and families. Performing at the highest levels in each of these realms is consistent with being an empowered professional who is clear about his or her role.

Nurses must be clear about the professional boundaries and expectations of their role, their scope of practice, and the specific guidelines within their professional position. They must also be clear about the responsibility that their license allocates to them as well as their level of authority to make decisions on patient care.

Clarity of System

The degree of alignment in the care delivery system in support of patient care and the professional role will determine whether the nurse's actions achieve optimal results. If the patient–nurse assignments are task or convenience driven, the practice is not a professional one. Furthermore, if assignments are task or convenience driven, patients likely will experience more providers during their length of stay and may thus experience effects of fragmentation within a highly complex acute care system. Fragmentation creates difficulty in understanding or applying the patient's context and the meaning of this illness or health event; thus, it becomes more challenging to create caring moments.

A nurse colleague once described the effects of "fragmentation" she observed during her mother's hospitalization:

> During one of my mother's many hospitalizations she received care over five and a half days on a busy telemetry unit where the nurses worked 12-hour shifts. The clinical and technical care was timely and accurate and the providers were courteous. But, this care was provided by ten different nurses.
>
> While each nurse was kind and skillful with accurate IV medication titration and arrhythmia management, the fragmented scheduling and assignment systems conspired to challenge their ability to track my mother's clinical condition changes in order to create a synthesized picture that could inform her future care needs. Most certainly, this compromised the nurses' ability to provide fully present, compassionate, and intentional caring. Not one of these nurses uncovered my mother's chief fear, how would she continue to care for my father at home with early Alzheimer's disease?—a caring moment missed.
>
> Had each of those nurses had a high level of self-awareness as a healer and been also abundantly clear and empowered in their professional role, there may have been even more caring moments. Because the systems of care were fragmented, those moments occurred more by default than by design.

Manthey (1980) wrote about Primary Nursing: "Primary Nursing is a delivery system for nursing care at the unit level that facilitates professional nursing practice despite the bureaucratic nature of hospitals. . . . It is not a staffing system, not an assignment system, but a responsibility relationship. . . . Accepting responsibility is the key to professionhood . . . the key that unlocks power. Legitimate autonomy for nurses is the by-product of accepting responsibility" (p. 1).

PRIMARY NURSING AT (NYP/CU)

In 2005, the Department of Nursing at NYP/CU was in a state of transition on both the organizational and local levels. It was a period of new, corporate, and hospital leadership within the Department of Nursing. There were several vacancies at all levels of the nursing structure including new campus-specific nursing leadership, Directors of Nursing, and Nurse Managers. Other challenges facing the Department of Nursing at NYP/CU included an undefined care-delivery model, centralized nursing processes, and preexisting patient and staff satisfaction initiatives.

Soon after assuming the role of Vice President of Patient Care Services, Georgia Persky introduced a comprehensive patient care-delivery model that sought to address the aforementioned challenges. A defined, professional nursing-practice model was introduced to the staff nurses with the implementation of RBC.

To this end, professional practice—grounded in the knowledge, skills, and education that conform to the ethical standards of the profession and its scope of practice—applies to the behavior, integrity, compassion, and respect awarded nursing. Professional practice, coupled with Caritas principles (see Chapters 1, 2, and 3), is the cornerstone of nursing and the assumed individual and community nursing code for patient care.

Nurse leaders at NYP/CU agree that autonomous practice is critical to professional practice because it gives nurses the opportunity to voice concerns and share in the decisions that they then carry out. This leads to confidence in the nurses' competence, so that they can establish themselves as professionals with the expertise necessary to deliver high-quality nursing care incorporating Caritas behaviors. With autonomy, nurses can exercise the authority necessary to allow control over their practice. This is operationalized through a mature, Shared Governance Model (see Chapter 9), recognition by providers (especially physicians), and an egalitarian organization of nursing practice.

A supportive work environment is critical for primary nurses to have the time to develop and carry out therapeutic relationships and care plans. As a resource-driven practice, Primary Nursing requires critical-thinking skills to prioritize immediate patient needs for now, today, and the entire hospitalization. A concerted effort must be made to optimize care processes (food delivery, housekeeping, materials management, social work, security, physical therapy, respiratory) that support patient care and minimize distractions to caregivers for routine needs. This can be accomplished through a full understanding of the essential need of the patient for a primary nurse and an understanding at every level of the organization that supporting that role is essential to the hospital mission. The unit manager and support staff must understand the Primary Nursing Model, and their roles within it, to enhance the primary nurse's role and the shared goal of patient care.

NYP engaged in an extensive educational program to prepare for the implementation of Primary Nursing. The Primary Nursing educational components of this program, some of which have been described in detail earlier in this chapter, were:

- Primary Nursing practice
- Professional practice:
  - Leadership at the point of care
  - Autonomy
  - Accountability, responsibility, and authority
  - Negotiation, delegation, and conflict resolution
  - Care coordination
  - Work complexity
- Human dynamics:
  - Reigniting the spirit of caring
  - The art of care delivery
  - Narrative nursing discussions (like narrative medicine)
  - Journaling
  - Therapeutic relationships
  - Team building

EDUCATION FOR PRIMARY NURSING

A thorough understanding of professional practice, the primary nurse model, and its related care-delivery system is essential for staff who take on a larger responsibility: designing their professional practice environment. This includes: (a) learning about concepts of responsibility acceptance, levels of authority, and reflective practice as a measure of accountability; (b) how to establish and maintain a therapeutic relationship; (c) the art of care delivery; (d) the unique role of the nurse in coordinating care; and (e) developing skills in delegation, negotiation, conflict resolution, collaboration, and facilitating change.

A series of learning experiences was offered to enhance clarity of self, role, and system:

- Leading an Empowered Organization (LEO) prepared the managers to optimize the shared governance processes on their units.
- A Reigniting-the-Spirit-of-Caring retreat enabled all staff to focus on caring for themselves, their colleagues, and their patients and families through the lens of Watson's (2008) Caritas Processes. The 10 Caritas Processes are, in brief: practice of loving kindness; honoring faith and hope; spiritual knowing and support; building a trusting relationship; being present for and supporting expression of patient's feelings; creatively using self in expression of caring; facilitating the discovery of meaning; creating environments of healing interpersonally, in practice, and in physical space; tending to basic needs as a sacred act of caring; and allowing belief in miracles. These concepts are described more fully in Chapters 1 and 2.
- The Work Complexity Assessment provided staff with the ability to articulate the unique practice in their unit using Nursing Intervention Classification language, and to envision optimal ways to work together.
- Leadership at the Point of Care continued the process of self-discovery, the application of that insight into team behaviors, and the implications for patient practices in their departments. Reflection, journaling, group sharing, narrative discussions, music, motion, and art methodologies were successful in engaging staff. Periodic progress checks—where staff publicly discussed the status of their efforts to organize for practice change and the innovations used to embed those changes into operations—also served to inform and inspire staff throughout the implementation process.

One practice to sustain focus on exceptional patient and family outcomes, while reinforcing the professional role of the primary nurse, is the staff's regular presentation of their reflection on their Primary Nursing experience to colleagues from all disciplines. The primary nurse provides brief, clinical content but focuses on the challenges and resolutions of providing care (what worked and why) before engaging colleagues in a professional dialogue designed to elicit even more effective strategies for future use.

RESEARCH STUDY OF PRIMARY NURSING AT (NYP/CU)

This study was the first to thoroughly investigate the implementation of Primary Nursing and shared governance within a model of RBC and its impact on outcomes of the nurse and patient. At the time of this writing, this study had examined the implementation of Primary Nursing over a 4-year period at NYP/CU within the operational model of Relationship-Based Care premised on theories of caring (see Chapter 9). Both qualitative and quantitative measurement processes were used to validate the operations of Primary Nursing and establish an understanding of its evolution and impact. The following section describes the measurement processes.

EVIDENCE AND EVALUATION

The evolution and impact of the primary nurse within patient care is evaluated at NYP by the collection of discharge questionnaires (post-cards), the Primary Nursing Self-Assessment and Primary Nursing Exemplars and Primary Nursing Audit Tool, Caring Factor Survey (CFS) results, and the Healthcare Environment Survey (HES) results. Outcomes from regularly administered Press Ganey patient satisfaction surveys, nursing quality of care indicators, and responses to discharge follow-up telephone calls are communicated to staff to provide a comprehensive picture of the patient experience. The results of the HES also are presented to each unit for action planning for change at the unit level. Staff's direct engagement with data and these stories of the patient care experience can offer continual inspiration and serve as a charter to the staff to raise and continuously improve the level of care and quality.

Primary Nursing Discharge Questionnaire

The Primary Nursing Discharge Questionnaire is a real-time measure to assess the patients' ability to identify who their primary nurse was, indicate whether or not their identified needs were met, and rate their level of satisfaction with the overall experience during their hospital stay. This real-time feedback is used to assess the impact of nursing staff interventions and to provide continued inspiration for maintaining professional practice (see Figure 5.1).

The Primary Nursing Discharge Questionnaire and a tally form to trend responses within a unit over time were developed at NYP as a unit-based strategy to assess quality improvements in the individual patient perceptions of care and awareness of the name of the individual nurse. Upon discharge, the patient was requested to respond to four questions: (a) Who was your primary nurse? (b) Did you have a caring and supportive relationship with that nurse? (c) How well were your needs and concerns met? (d) How can we do better? Results of these responses were useful to the Patient Care Director in understanding the individual performance of the primary nurse and the patient's perceptions of care. These results have demonstrated that 85% of the patients know their primary nurse and that their needs were met; both scored 4.6 for a scale of 5.0.

---

1. Who was your primary nurse? _____

2. Did you have a supportive and caring relationship with your primary nurse?
   ☐ Yes ☐ No

3. How well were your needs and concerns met?
   ☐ 1 = None of my needs were met
   ☐ 2 = Some of my needs were met
   ☐ 3 = I do not know
   ☐ 4 = Most of my needs were met
   ☐ 5 = All of my needs were met

4. How can we do better? _____
   _____

Unit: _____ MRN#: _____

Date: _____ Completed by: _____

FIGURE 5.1   Discharge questionnaire.

Primary Nursing Self-Assessment

The Primary Nursing Self-Assessment (Romana, 2008) is an adjunct assessment to the RN employee evaluation (see Figure 5.2). This evaluation was created from the four elements of Primary Nursing and prompts the nurse to self-evaluate his or her individual performance on 13 specific behaviors of a primary nurse. If the vision is that every patient will have a primary nurse, then meaning to that role must be continually self-generated and framed for the patient and nurse in a meaningful manner (Manthey, 2002).

Initially, nurses who are new to the primary role are asked to self-evaluate their performance. This self-evaluation is then shared with the Patient Care Manager in an educational discussion of the opportunities and challenges in this role. This assessment and further discussion and evaluation are incorporated into the annual nurse performance evaluation from that point forward.

Primary Nursing Exemplars

To generate ongoing inspiration for Primary Nursing, staff nurses are encouraged to maintain an individual professional journal on experiences (positive and negative), circumstances, and patient stories that are meaningful. A journal is kept on each unit for nurses to contribute these stories and express appreciation to the entire team for situations that were meaningful (see Figure 5.3). The Primary Nursing exemplars form is for stories that are generalizable to the role of all primary nurses and caregivers and that provide inspiration to the unit team and the community of nurses at NYP/CU. These exemplars are shared in departmental meetings, key personnel meetings, bi-annual RBC symposia, and the annual RBC celebratory booklet that formalizes the work and progress of the prior year.

Name: _____   Unit: _____

Date: _____

Relationship Based Care has evolved from the basic tenet of Primary Nursing. This tenet presumes that there is a continuous therapeutic relationship of a nurse with an individual patient over a period or time. It also presumes that as leaders at the point of care, we are to take responsibility, accountability, and authority for professional nursing practice.

This form is used to verify your competency related to primary nursing within the framework of Relationship Based Care. Take time to reflect on the skills you apply to the elements of this system by reviewing the criteria and then providing examples of how you have expressed each element.

1. Allocation and acceptance of individual responsibility for decision making to one individual	
Questions to ask	**Ways I demonstrated this:**
Did I involve the patient and family in developing the plan of care for admission? Did I plan the care of the patient's assigned to me?	Examples of family input into plan of care.
Did the patient, patient's family, the physicians, other nurses and members of the health team know I was the primary nurse for my patients? ■ Documented as care provider ■ White Boards ■ Business Cards ■ Unit Boards	Did I engage with team to discuss the patient care needs?
Did I communicate the care requirements of my assigned patients to other members of the health care team? ■ Handoff/report ■ Primary Nurse POC	Give specific examples of times when specifics were passed.

FIGURE 5.2 Primary Nursing self-assessment 2008.
Source: NYP/CU.

(continued)

2. Assignments of daily care by case method	
Questions to ask	Ways I demonstrated this:
Did I consider the unique needs of the patient when deciding who should meet the needs of the patient?	Look at delegation of work, collaborating with support staff.
Did I consider the strengths and abilities of staff members available to care for the patient when delegating patient care?	Are you considering nurse's skills in assignment of primary patient and in devising daily assignments? If so, how?
Did I resume the Primary Nurse role with my previous patients if readmitted?	Is this being monitored? How is this handled?

3. Direct person-to-person communication	
Questions to ask	Ways I demonstrated this:
Did I provide a complete report, including Primary Nurse Plan of Care, at change of shift to staff assuming care for the patient?	Have the staff describe in detail patient care examples where these questions were addressed.
Did I consistently communicate directly with other members of the health team who either had or needed information regarding the patient's condition?	Consider attaching a copy of the Primary Nurse Plan of Care.
Did I spend 5 minutes with each patient at the beginning of each shift to identify their goal for the day?	Participation in patient care rounding and disposition planning.
Were my responses appropriate and responsive to the patient's communications?	Identify specific goals described by patients and how staff met these goals.
Did I respond to requests from the patient and the patient's family for information regarding the patient's condition from admission to discharge?	Assist staff to identify if they were "present" with their patients. (Swanson's caring processes)
Did I communicate the patient's need for knowledge to other members of the health care team who could meet those needs?	Highlight the importance of communication in all forms, both written and verbal.

The above examples reflect my contributions to the Relationship Based Care Primary Nursing Model.

Signature: _____

NewYork-Presbyterian
The University Hospital of Columbia and Cornell

DIVISION OF NURSING
COLUMBIA UNIVERSITY MEDICAL CAMPUS

Name: _____   **Unit:** _____
Title: _____   **Date:** _____

Relationship-Based Care has evolved from the basic tenet of Primary Nursing. This tenet presumes that there is a continuous therapeutic relationship of a nurse with an individual patient over a period or time. It also presumes that as leaders at the point of care, we are to take responsibility, accountability, and authority for professional nursing practice.

An **exemplar** is a story you tell or write about what you did. Please share your story about how you actualized the role of primary nurse within the context of Relationship-Based Care.

Using the box provided on the next page, describe one or more situations that demonstrate your accountability to the Primary Nursing Care Delivery Model. Your descriptions should include one or more of the components of Primary Nursing listed below.

- The nurse–patient relationship engenders trust, and provides consistency and advocacy.
- Continuity of care is provided.
- There is coordinated and efficient planning for transitions to other sites of care.
- There is an explicit plan of care focused on meeting identified outcomes.
- Effective communication within the health care team occurs.
- The patient and family are involved in the planning, implementation, and evaluation of care.

FIGURE 5.3   Primary Nursing exemplar form.

Primary Nursing Audit Tool

The Primary Nursing Audit Tool was created to further quantify the presence of the primary nurse's relationship with the patient. The purpose of this tool is to capture data regarding the consistent documentation of the primary nurse and the individualized plan of care and to monitor the continuity of assignment of the primary nurse working with the patient when available. Ten charts are randomly selected from each inpatient unit. The nursing documentation is reviewed for identification of the primary nurse within 24 hours of admission and for the presence of an individualized plan of care. The presence of updates to the plan of care by the primary nurse, even when the nurse is not assigned to the patient, and documentation of nurses meeting with patients for five minutes are considered a representation of a caring relationship with the patient. This act has been identified as one of the five caring behaviors that improve patient satisfaction. Other factors in the Primary Nursing audit include accepting assignment of a patient by an identified primary nurse and clearly documenting the responsibility relationship in the chart, in the patient's room, and on the unit census boards. The audit also seeks to identify how many days the primary nurse was assigned to the patient as the primary caretaker based on the length of admission on the survey. Table 5.1 is an example of the Primary Nursing Chart Auditing Tool.

TABLE 5.1   Primary Nursing Unit Audit Tool

UNIT: _____	# of Patients on the Unit: _____											
# of Nurses working today: _____	# of Nurses working with their primary patients: _____											
Nursing assignment:	1	2	3	4	5	6	7	8	9	10		
Patient room number:												
Patient name:												
Admission date:												
Name of primary nurse:												
Date primary nurse identified:												
Primary nurses identified within 24 hours?												
Number of days primary nurse took care of patient since admission:												
# of days since admission:												
Documentation:												
Eclipsys as provider:												
Unit board:												
White board in patient room:												
Is the individualized primary nurse plan of care indicated in Eclipsys?												
Are there updates to the plan of care by the primary nurse?												
Is there a miscellaneous note capturing the nurse spent 5 minutes with their patient to identify goals?												
If the nurse is not working with their patient, is there documentation that he/she met with their patient for plan of care review?												

Caring Factor Survey

The CFS is an instrument used to assess patients' perceptions of the care they received from nurses, as experienced by a caring and loving consciousness toward them as a whole person, including the unity of mind-body-spirit. An example of an item from the CFS is, "When my caregivers teach me something new, they teach me in a way that I can understand." The CFS, like the HES, uses a 1–7 Likert scale with the same methods for scoring the patient's degree of agreement or disagreement (as described in Chapter 4). The CFS was developed to reflect Watson's most recent theory of Caritas, which incorporates and extends her original Carative Factors as the core of professional nursing (Watson, 2005, 2008). For the purposes of this study, the higher the score reported by the patient on the CFS, the more evidence of Caritas was inferred.

Over the first 3 years of implementation of Primary Nursing at NYP, patients were asked about their perception of caring using Watson's theory of Caritas. The 10-item instrument used in this process, the CFS, has been extensively tested psychometrically and described elsewhere (DiNapoli et al., 2010). Results revealed improved scores for all caring factors and in the total CFS score (Figure 5.4).

Results were statistically significant for:

Caritas Process #1: Cultivating Practice of Loving Kindness and Equanimity Toward Self and Other (layman's term: loving kindness)
Caritas Process #2: Being Authentically Present: Enabling, Sustaining, and Honoring Faith and Hope (layman's terms: faith and hope)

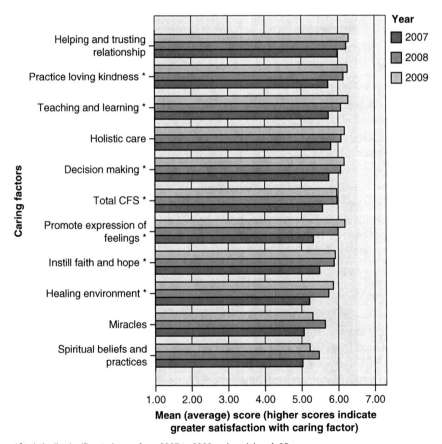

*Statistically significant change from 2007 to 2009, using alpha of .05.

FIGURE 5.4   Caritas (caring) factors, 2007, 2008, and 2009, plus the total CFS score.

Caritas Process #3: Cultivation of One's Own Spiritual Practices and Transpersonal Self, Going Beyond Ego-Self (layman's term: spiritual support)

Caritas Process #4: Developing and Sustaining a Helping-Trusting Caring Relationship (layman's term: helping-trusting relationship)

Caritas Process #5: Being Present to, and Supportive of, the Expression of Positive and Negative Feelings (layman's term: promote feelings, both positive and negative)

Caritas Process #6: Creative Use of Self and All Ways of Knowing as Part of the Caring Process; Engage in the Artistry of Caritas (layman's term: creative problem solving)

Caritas Process #7: Engage in Genuine Teaching-Learning Experience That Attends to Unity of Being and Subjective Meaning—Attempting to Stay Within Other's Frame of Reference (layman's term: effective teaching)

Caritas Process #8: Creating a Healing Environment at All Levels (layman's term: creates healing environment)

Caritas Process #9: Administering Sacred Acts of Caring–Healing by Tending to Basic Needs (layman's term: holistic care)

Caritas Process #10: Opening and Attending to Spiritual/Mysterious and Existential Unknowns of Life-Death (layman's term: allows belief in miracles)

The only two factors that declined slightly from 2008 to 2009 related to spirituality. It may be considered to examine formal religion categories in the next study to determine whether the environment is supporting one religion, denomination, or sect more effectively. The decline in these two factors was sufficient to influence the total CFS score, which, as noted previously, declined slightly from 2008 to 2009.

Healthcare Environment Survey

This instrument is an 81-item environmental assessment based on sociotechnical systems theory. There are 10 demographic questions in addition to the 81 statements that use a 7-point Likert-type scale for response. At NYP the instrument assessed the relationships of staff with physicians, nurses, the entire unit/department coworker team, and the unit manager. The technical aspects that are measured include perception of the model of care (Primary Nursing), staffing/scheduling, workload, autonomy, educational opportunities, executive leadership/vision, and reward structure. The Healthcare Environment Survey (HES) includes measures of organizational commitment (pride and intent to stay in the organization) and job satisfaction. Survey outcomes are presented to the staff on each unit so the staff can reflect, build context-specified research models, and design an action plan within the patient care unit context.

Data from annual administrations of the HES at NYP are subjected to regression analysis to monitor how the work environment is evolving with regard to autonomy, Primary Nursing, and pride in the organization. Workload has also been examined extensively using a time-series study at the unit level. The average response rate by unit has been 90% as staff readily engages with data management processes that assist with shared governance, empowerment, and clarity.

Primary Nursing as a Predictor of Workload and Pride in the Organization

Data revealed that Primary Nursing was the strongest predictor for satisfaction with workload as perceived by nurses. It was hypothesized that Primary Nursing (professional practice model) would increase satisfaction with workload by promoting deepening relationships between patient and nurse. Improved satisfaction with workload was also anticipated if nurses could spend less time each shift orienting to a new patient. It was hypothesized that nurses would not only enjoy their work more by deepening their relationship with the patient, but their perception of workload would improve because they would need less time to orient to each patient.

The analysis of understanding the relationship between workload and other variables began by examining the correlations of 127 independent variables. Unit was the level of analysis. Data from 33 of the 35 patient care units were examined and 15 variables were found to have a statistically significant correlation with perception of workload using an alpha of 0.05. Correlates of workload were entered into a regression equation with the subscale of workload from the HES tool as the dependent variable. Results revealed that 60.4% of nurses' perceptions of workload was predicted by one nurse being accountable for the patient from admission to discharge. This was statistically significant at the 0.05 level. Units whose nurses reported the greatest satisfaction with their workload were those that provided the Primary Nursing experience (accountability from admission to discharge) to the greatest number of patients. Residual diagnostics were conducted and no violations of assumptions were found.

Although these findings supported the hypothesis (i.e., Primary Nursing [professional practice model] would increase satisfaction with workload by promoting deepening relationships between patient and nurse) and predictive validity, the researchers wanted to confirm the findings using other sources of data within NYP. Qualitative data were examined to see what nurses reported they "enjoyed the most" within their job. Approximately 70% of the nurses reported having a connection to the patient and that this was what they enjoyed the most. This finding supports findings from the regression analysis that a deeper connection to the patient by being able to be accountable for care from admission to discharge likely contributes to the improved perception of workload.

A second source of data was examined for additional confirmation that a connection with patients is what nurses enjoy, further explaining the positive impact that Primary Nursing has on perception of workload. Data were examined from surveys of each of the 990 nurses (approximately 90% of nurses) in five "waves" (time periods) at NYP, measurement time-1 (T1), which was year-1, to time-4 (T4), which was year-4. There were five to nine units in each "wave." Primary Nursing was found to be the most consistent predictor of what creates pride in the organization. Primary Nursing explained up to 32% of what makes nurses proud to work in the organization (Table 5.2).

Evolution of Primary Nursing Within Relationship-Based Care

The results described earlier revealed that Primary Nursing relates to improved perception of workload, likely due to the deepened relationship between nurse and patient, which is what nurses enjoy and feel proud of. The researchers wanted to know if continuity of care and scheduling assisted with the nurse–patient connection. To examine this, nurse–patient dyads were examined in the Wave II implementation in 2007. It was hypothesized that nurses who took care of patients more consistently would have higher CFS scores within their respective nurse–patient dyad than those whose patients did not have consistent connections with a primary nurse.

Pearson's correlation was used to examine the relationship between the total CFS score and the number of days the nurse took care of the patient, the number of other nurses who took care of the patient, the number of days the patient was in hospital, and the number of days the patient was on a respective nurse's unit. No statistically significant correlations were found; however, the correlations were in the hypothesized direction for number of days ($r = .077, p = .561, n = 60$) and total hours ($r = .112, p = .393, n = 60$) that the nurse took care of the patient. Thus, as the number of days or hours increased, the report of caring increased. There was a negative correlation, as hypothesized, between the total CFS score and the number of nurses who took care of the patient ($r = -.038, p = .812, n = 42$) and the number of hours that other nurses took care of the patient ($r = -.250, p = .175, n = 31$). This means that caring reported by the patients declined as the number of nurses who took care of the same patient increased.

A replication study was conducted to see if the correlations could be repeated in a larger sample and reach statistical significance. In 2008, 128 nurse–patient dyads were identified and studied, similar to the 2007 study. Results revealed that there was a persistent positive correlation of caring as reported by the patient with the number of days cared for by the same nurse. Interestingly, there was also a positive correlation between the patients' reports of caring and the number of nurses caring for them. This was the second year of implementing Primary Nursing within an RBC model of care. Could it be that as nurses learned how to incorporate case method

TABLE 5.2 Predictors of Pride in the Organization

					EXPLAINED VARIANCE OF PRIDE (AS PERCENTAGE OF TOTAL EXPLAINED PRIDE)						
WAVE	PRIMARY NURSING (%)	EXECUTIVE LEADERSHIP (%)	DISTRIBUTIVE JUSTICE (%)	PROFESSIONAL GROWTH (%)	RELATIONSHIP WITH COWORKERS (%)	AUTONOMY (%)	RELATIONSHIP WITH PHYSICIANS (%)	NUMBER OF HOURS WORKED (%)	STAFFING/SCHEDULING (%)	WORKLOAD (%)	TOTAL VARIANCE (%)
I – T1 (pre)	2.3	9.9	0	21.6	0	0	0	0	0	4.9	38.6
I – T2 (post)	29.0	0	0	10.3	0	0	6.0	0	0	0	56.7
I – T3	26.8	5.1	8.7	0	0	0	0	0	0	1.6	57.9
I – T4	32.4	3.8	1.7	0	0	0	0	0	8.7	0	46.6
II – T1 (pre)	11.4	0	0	0	6.3	0	0	0	0	23.5	41.1
II – T2 (post)	0	45.7	9.8	0	2.3	0	0	0	0	0	57.8
II – T3	1.3	27.9	15.6	3.4	0	0	0	1.4	0	0	49.7
II – T4	3.4	4.9	0	31.8	0	0	0	0	0	0	40.1
III – T1 (pre)	7.0	2.1	0	39.2	0	0	0	0	0	0	48.3
III – T2 (post)	10.0	0	0	33.1	0	0	0	0	0	3.8	46.9
III – T3	6.4	1.3	3.1	40.7	0	0	0	0	0	0	51.5
IV – T1 (pre)	31.8	7.9	0	4.0	0	0	0	0	0	0	45.8
IV – T2 (post)	1.9	28.1	4.9	9.5	0	0	0	0	3.6	0	44.4
V – T1 (pre)	0	2.7	0	25.8	0	5.3	0	0	0	0	33.8

into their concept of Primary Nursing, the nurses became less dependent on having patients assigned to them on their shift but rather were able to coordinate care as both a direct care provider and case manager?

Curiosity about the changed relationship of continuity of care and caring scores initiated a secondary study using another statistical method. A series of regression equations was conducted to examine whether the perception of Primary Nursing as the dependent variable (using the subscale of Primary Nursing in the HES) was predicted as the nurse evolved over time through the benefit of clarity of self, role, and system. It was identified at baseline that Primary Nursing was predicted by nurses' satisfaction with their schedule. One year postinitiation of RBC, the schedule became less predictive for Primary Nursing. In contrast, the nurses' professional knowledge revealed a pattern for increasingly predicting satisfaction with Primary Nursing—from an external source of satisfaction with schedule to an internal source of nursing knowledge. This evolution within the findings from this series of regression equations may explain the change in the direction of the relationship between the number of nurses who care for a patient and the CFS scores. If primary nurses are becoming more dependent on their professional knowledge to execute Primary Nursing, this may suggest that they are more successful continuing with the plan of care and collaboration within the interdisciplinary team as case managers, thus providing enhanced perception of caring as perceived by their patients. Within this case, the RBC program instructs nurses how to use self, role, and system to provide Primary Nursing care. Further inquiry is warranted, but these data from various views and methods appear to be validating one another (Table 5.3).

Summary of Results

- Perception of caring improves over time as Primary Nursing matures within an RBC model of care.
- Nurses who are accountable for the care of a primary patient from admission to discharge are most satisfied with workload.
- Nurses find most enjoyment in their job in connecting to the patient.
- Nurses derive the most pride in their job by taking care of patients.
- Primary Nursing is predicted by scheduling prior to RBC but also predicted by professional knowledge as nurses become more clear in their role after 1 year of learning about themselves, their role, and how to operate within the systems.

DISCUSSION

Caring is a core component of the professional role of the nurse and particularly so for the primary nurse. When nurses are self-aware and embrace the enormous influence they have in the healing experience, they

TABLE 5.3 Predictors for Primary Nursing in Three Waves of RBC, and Amount of Explained Variance (Nurses Only)

WAVE	EXPLAINED VARIANCE OF PRIMARY NURSING (PN)													
	AUTONOMY (%)	EXECUTIVE LEADERSHIP (%)	RELATIONSHIP WITH PHYSICIANS (%)	RELATIONSHIP WITH NURSES (%)	RELATIONSHIP WITH COWORKERS (%)	STAFFING/ SCHEDULING (%)	DISP OPT (%)	PROFESSIONAL GROWTH (%)	PARTICIPATIVE MANAGEMENT (%)	WORKLOAD (%)	UNIT (%)	UNIT YEARS (%)	LEVEL OF EDUCATION (%)	EXPLAINED VARIANCE (%)
I – T1 (pre)	4.7	31.0	0	0	0	0	0	0	0	0	0	0	0	35.8
I – T2 (post)	0	0	7.1	0	0	0	0	22.7	0	0	0	0	0	29.8
I – T3	16.0	3.4	5.0	0	0	0	0	0	0	0	0	0	0	24.4
I – T4	0	2.5	4.8	0	0	0	0	30.3	0	0	0	0	0	37.6
II – T1 (pre)	0	0	0	0	0	8.6	5.2	0	0	0	0	0	0	13.8
II – T2 (post)	0	0	0	0	0	0	0	5.1	0	0	0	0	0	30.2
II – T3	3.6	7.0	0	0	0	1.5	0	22.0	0	0	0	4.9	3.4	42.4
II – T4	23.3	0	0	2.3	0	0	0	2.8	0	0	0	0	0	27.3
III – T1 (pre)	0	0	0	0	0	10.4	0	0	0	0	0	0	0	10.4
III – T2 (post)	0	0	0	0	0	0	2.6	21.4	0	0	0	0	0	24.0
III – T3	5.1	0	0	1.4	0	0	0	24.3	0	1.6	1.7	0	0	34.1
IV – T1 (pre)	0	0	0	6.3	0	0	0	17.8	0	0	0	0	0	24.1
IV – T2 (post)	3.5	7.4	1.5	22.7	1.3	0	0	1.4	0	0	0	0	0	37.8
V – T1 (pre)	0	4.6	0	0	0	2.8	0	0	6.3	0	0	0	0	13.7

are positioned to be more purposeful in carrying out those individual caring moments with patients, families, and colleagues. This multifaceted study reveals that nurses enjoy and feel proud to connect with the patient and are more satisfied with their workload when they are clear about their professional role and the system supports their responsibility for a patient from admission to discharge. This study also reveals that the operations of Primary Nursing are more dependent on knowledge than staffing as nurses acquire knowledge about how to implement Primary Nursing. It is hypothesized that the knowledge is specific to clarity of self, role, and system. Further inquiry is warranted. Finally, the most important finding in this study is that as Primary Nursing matures over time, patients report higher levels of caring. This supports the overall hypothesis of this study that Primary Nursing affords greater opportunities for nurses to enact their professional role most fully and use professional intention to make Caritas moments the norm, not an instance of chance.

REFERENCES

DiNapoli, P., Nelson, J., Turkel, M., & Watson, J. (2010). Measuring the Caritas processes: Caring factor survey. *International Journal for Human Caring, 14*(3), 15–20.

Felgen, J. (2007). *Leading lasting change: I2E2.* Bloomington, IN: Creative Health Care Management.

Koloroutis, M. (Ed.). (2004). *Relationship-Based Care: A model for transforming practice.* Bloomington, IN: Creative Health Care Management.

Manthey, M. (1980). *Primary Nursing.* Boston, MA: Blackwell.

Manthey, M. (2002). *The practice of primary nursing* (2nd ed.). Minneapolis, MN: Creative Health Care Management.

Romana, M. (2008). *Primary Nursing: Resources for a professional nursing practice.* Unpublished manuscript, New York-Presbyterian Hospital.

Watson, J. (2005). *Caring science as sacred science.* Philadelphia, PA: F.A. Davis.

Watson, J. (2008). *Nursing: The philosophy and science of caring* (Rev. ed.). Boulder, CO: University Press of Colorado.

6

Patient and Nurse Perception
of the Individual Caring Relationship

*Patti Leger, Deanne Sramek, Sandra Conklin,
and John Nelson*

The idea of being able to care for and about others is the key motivation for many nurses to enter and stay within the profession of nursing. Caring has been described as the essence of nursing, a core value that has remained constant since Florence Nightingale. Nurses at Wyoming Medical Center (WMC) identified caring as a core value in their professional practice and, subsequently, chose the theory of human caring to provide the structure, language, and foundation to hold and guide our professional practice. A multidisciplinary caring group was formed to create strategies to bring the theory to health care practitioners in ways they could receive it. The strategies developed by this group were designed to encourage reflective practice around the Caritas Processes (Watson, 2008), the foundation of the theory, so that practitioners could enhance awareness of their own unique caring styles in order to transform each patient encounter into a transpersonal caring moment. We believe that caring relationships and caring moments enhance healing for the patient as well as the nurse. During the past five years, the caring committee at WMC has developed many innovative strategies to integrate the caring theory into practice with the hope that each health care practitioner would (1) begin to understand the language of caring; (2) enhance awareness of and implement caring behaviors and attitudes toward self and others; and (3) validate that caring is consistently honored and valued within the organization.

Caring has been evaluated over time at an organizational level using the Caring Efficacy Scale (CES) (Coates, 1997) and the Caring Factor Survey (CFS) (Nelson, Watson, & Inova Healthcare, 2006). These measurements were instituted as a way to, at least partially, measure the effectiveness of the various strategies to bring caring to the forefront within the organization. The CES measures nurses' self-perceptions of caring. This tool was first used in 2005 before any caring interventions were offered and demonstrated a mean score of 5.10 (1–6 Likert scale, $n = 174$). Data were collected again in 2008 using the CES with a mean score of 5.30 ($n = 157$), demonstrating a significant ($p = .012$) improvement. The CFS measures patients' perceptions of nurses' caring behaviors and was used in 2007, demonstrating a mean score of 6.10 (Likert 1–7, $n = 314$). The CFS again was offered in 2009 with a mean score of 5.97 ($n = 337$). These organizational measurements provided useful information regarding caring at a system level and offer direction for future plans. However, they did not measure the caring relationship between the individual nurse and the individual patient directly, something we felt was important to study and share with nurses interested in learning more about their personal caring behaviors and styles.

Nursing scholars and theorists have suggested research guidelines to study both the nurse and the patient within the caring–healing relationship (Quinn, Smith, Ritenbaugh, Swanson, & Watson, 2003). Nurse researchers have used a variety of qualitative and quantitative designs to study caring from the nurses' perspectives (Becker et al., 2008; Dyson, 1996; Lindahl, Norberg, & Söderberg, 2008; McCartan & Hargie, 2004; Patistea, 1999; Sumner, 2008; Wade & Kasper, 2006; Wiman & Wikblad, 2004) and from the patients' perspectives (Baldursdottir & Jonsdottir, 2002; Erci et al., 2003; Finch, 2006; Halldorsdottir, 1991, 2008; Henderson et al., 2007; Oermann, 1999). There have been some studies that have examined caring from both the nurse and patient perspectives in general (Carter et al., 2008; Hegedus, 1999). A few studies have used paired nurse–patient dyads as a method to examine caring in different contexts (Larsson, Peterson, Lampic, von Essen, & Sjödén, 1998; McCance, Slater, & McCormack, 2008; Persky, Nelson, Watson, & Bent, 2008). However, a literature review did not reveal any previous studies where an individual nurse–patient relationship was examined using the patient's and the nurse's perspectives within the context of the theory of human caring.

The overall aim of this study was to examine patterns of caring as perceived by the nurse and the patient. Patterns of caring were examined as reported by both the patient and the nurse in the same relationship as it pertains to the caring behaviors of a specific nurse. This aids in understanding the dimensions within the nurse–patient relationship as it pertains to caring within the theory of human caring.

METHODS
Study Participants

Following approval from the internal review board, six nurse volunteers were recruited for the pilot study via an e-mail invitation to every nurse within the organization. The volunteers were chosen to provide diversity by specialty area. The study design was explained, consent obtained, and a photograph taken of the individual nurse to be shown to patient participants to verify the specific nurse who had cared for the patient.

Following a random shift worked by the nurse, a list of patients the nurse cared for was requested. Patients from this list who met the criteria were asked to identify their perceptions of the individual nurse's caring behaviors. The nurse was notified of patient participation and then, within 24 hours of caring for the patient, identified self-perceptions of caring with the specific patient as well as providing demographic and environmental information. Six patients were recruited for each nurse, making the sample size 36.

Instruments

Patients or family members completed the Caring Factor Survey–Specific Care Provider (CFS-SCP) instrument. Developed by John Nelson and Dr. Jean Watson from the original CFS, this tool measures patient perception of an individual nurse's caring behaviors. The CFS–SCP is a 10-item, 7-point Likert scale quantitative instrument with a 1-item qualitative question added. Content validity has been verified. The nurse volunteers completed the Caring Factor Survey–Care Provider Version (CFS–CPV), which is a 20-item, 7-point Likert scale instrument to measure the nurse's self-perceptions of caring with the specific patient. Johnson describes the CFS–CPV in detail in Chapter 4. Content validity and reliability have been established. Demographic data were also collected.

Definition of Terms

Caritas Process #1: Cultivating Practice of Loving Kindness and Equanimity Toward Self and Others (layman's terms: loving kindness)

Caritas Process #2: Being Authentically Present: Enabling, Sustaining, and Honoring Faith and Hope (layman's terms: faith and hope)

Caritas Process #3: Cultivation of One's Own Spiritual Practices and Transpersonal Self, Going Beyond Ego-Self (layman's terms: spiritual support)

Caritas Process #4: Developing and Sustaining a Helping-Trusting Caring Relationship (layman's terms: helping-trusting relationship)

Caritas Process #5: Being Present to, and Supportive of, the Expression of Positive and Negative Feelings (layman's terms: promote feelings, both positive and negative)

Caritas Process #6: Creative Use of Self and All Ways of Knowing as Part of the Caring Process; Engage in the Artistry of Caritas (layman's terms: creatively problem solving)

Caritas Process #7: Engage in Genuine Teaching-Learning Experience That Attends to Unity of Being and Subjective Meaning—Attempting to Stay Within Other's Frame of Reference (layman's terms: effective teaching)

Caritas Process #8: Creating a Healing Environment at All Levels (layman's terms: creates healing environment)

Caritas Process #9: Administering Sacred Acts of Caring–Healing by Tending to Basic Needs (layman's terms: holistic care)
Caritas Process #10: Opening and Attending to Spiritual/Mysterious and Existential Unknowns of Life-Death (layman's terms: allows belief in miracles)

Statistical Analysis

Correlations were used to examine the individual nurse and individual patient score of caring. Different scores between patients and nurses were also examined to see if and to what extent the patients and nurses differed. Qualitative data were analyzed by relating written comments to the constructs within the caring theory. Finally, demographics that were suspected of relating to caring were examined.

RESULTS

Pearson's correlation of the six nurses and their six paired patients over the course of the study demonstrated no correlation ($r = .038$). Upon deeper examination of the relationship between the patient report and the nurse report of caring for four of the six nurses, it was noted that the correlation was strong at 0.81 for only one of the nurses in the study. In addition, three of the correlations for three different pairs of patient–nurse were found to have a negative correlation, which indicates that the nurses and patients were reporting quite different scores for caring. Furthermore, each individual patient–nurse dyad had varied responses of caring from their respective six patients.

Demographics that correlated with positive difference scores included: hospital years ($r = .31, p = .074$), years as a nurse ($r = .31, p = .075$), working more than scheduled hours ($r = .138, p = .429$), and workload ($r = .261, p = .130$). To clarify, nurses reporting higher scores than patients had more hospital years, more nurse years of experience, worked over scheduled hours, and felt satisfied with workload. Demographics that correlated with negative difference scores included: working later shifts ($r = -.138, p = .476$), and number of days taking care of patient ($r = -.129, p = .459$).

To understand the differences in the patient and the nurse reports of caring, the mean score of the patient was subtracted from the mean score of the nurse, thus creating a difference score. Within the paired scores of this current study, it was identified on average that patients reported higher scores than did nurses. The difference scores of patient and nurse reports of caring is noted in Table 6.1.

The final item on the patient's survey invited a description of the nurse's attitude, behavior, and/or actions that led to answers on the 10 quantitative items. Analysis of these comments provided themes

TABLE 6.1 Correlation and Differences of Patient and Nurse Reports of Caring

	RN1	RN2	RN3	RN4	RN5	RN6	ALL RNs
Correlation CFS-CVP & CFS-SCP	.49	.21	−.36	−.22	−.13	.81	.038
RN response of RN caring (Average score for all nurses)	5.80	6.42	6.21	6.36	5.86	5.69	6.06
Patient response of RN caring (Average score for all patients)	6.31	6.08	6.07	6.40	6.90	6.10	6.31
Difference	−.51	.34	.14	−.04	−1.04	−.41	−.25
RN response: Patient 1	5.95	6.95	5.70	6.40	5.25	5.50	6.07
Patient 1 response: RN	7.0	6.80	6.40	7.00	7.00	5.20	6.52
Difference	−1.05	.15	−.70	−.60	−1.75	.30	−.45
RN response: Patient 2	5.60	6.35	5.95	6.35	6.15	5.75	6.03
Patient 2 response: RN	5.70	7.00	6.30	6.10	7.00	5.80	6.32
Difference	−.10	−.65	−.35	.25	−.85	−.05	−.29
RN response: Patient 3	5.75	5.85	5.90	6.55	5.95	5.55	5.93
Patient 3 response: RN	5.90	5.40	6.50	5.50	7.00	5.00	5.88
Difference	−.15	.45	−.60	1.05	−1.05	.55	.04
RN response: Patient 4	5.65	6.20	6.50	6.45	5.85	5.60	6.04
Patient 4 response: RN	6.70	7.0	6.65	6.40	7.00	6.00	6.64
Difference	−1.05	−.80	−.30	.05	−1.15	−1.0	−.61
RN response: Patient 5	5.90	6.70	6.65	6.00	5.95	5.85	6.18
Patient 5 response: RN	5.90	6.0	6.30	6.40	6.40	7.00	6.34
Difference	0	.70	.35	−.40	−.45	−1.15	−.26
RN response: Patient 6	5.95	6.45	6.55	6.40	6.05	5.90	6.22
Patient 6 response: RN	6.70	4.30	5.82	7.00	7.0	7.00	6.02
Difference	−.75	2.15	2.45	−.60	−.95	−1.10	.20

that were consistent with 8 of 10 Caritas Processes (specific Caritas Processes #s 1, 2, 4, 5, 6, 7, 8, 9). For example, comments related to Caritas Process #1 included: "She's very thorough; she is a wonderful nurse, very caring, very loving." Comments related to Caritas Process #9 included: "She is totally supportive of all my needs, the best nurse I had." Some patients noted that "God never came up in the conversation" or "survey questions concerning spirituality did not arise during care," which may indicate that patients did not receive or notice components of what might be considered spiritual care (Caritas Processes #s 3, 10).

DISCUSSION

The motivation for this study was (1) to provide feedback to an individual nurse about his or her personal caring style and behaviors from the patient's perspective so that the nurse could reflect on the similarities and differences from his or her own perspective and (2) to attempt to test each of the Caritas Processes in the context of a caring relationship/ connection. The results of essentially no correlation between the patient's and the nurse's perceptions of caring were surprising and confusing. The concept of a caring relationship would, logically, seem to imply a connection, a bond, and a correlation between the nurse and the patient. However, the data analysis suggests that there was no relationship, no connection. This conclusion seems inaccurate. Nurses know, at an intuitive level, that there are deep connections and this knowing was supported by the mean results and by the qualitative comments from the study. It seemed that caring occurred on some level; however, it seemed not to have occurred in a predictable, linear, statistically supportable manner. Why was that? And what might these results mean?

The lack of correlation between the patterns of caring perceived by the nurse and the patient is consistent with other studies that have paired the patient and the nurse, although research designs were different (Larsson et al., 1998; McCance et al., 2008). Nurses and patients do not see the nurse–patient relationship in the same way (Halldorsdottir, 2008). Each person, the nurse and the patient, brings a unique perspective and life experiences to the interaction. Nurses and patients view things differently, based on the patient's experience and the nurse's training, so that the correlation of caring, using the same construct, does not correlate. The lack of correlation supports the unitary, transformative paradigm of Caritas consciousness/relationship within the theory of human caring. In such a paradigm, the phenomenon of a caring encounter between a nurse and a patient is viewed as a unitary, self-organizing field embedded in a larger, self-organizing field. "Knowledge is personal and involves pattern recognition. It includes perceptions and what I would call the 'phenomenal field'—the subjective and intersubjective meanings of both participants. Thus, any phenomenon has to be viewed as a whole, not as an additive sum of the parts to make a whole" (Watson, 2008, pp. 78–79). The lack of correlation in our results suggests that we cannot dissect and reconstruct portions of caring from the patient's and the nurse's perspectives; instead each encounter, each moment, must be viewed as a whole. The surprise and confusion was based on an attempt to apply a separatist paradigm to a unitary phenomenon.

Our results suggest that caring and caring relationships cannot be prescribed or reduced to a recipe or script.

> In the nursing literature there is an ongoing search for the core of nursing and claims are being made that it is indeed to be found in the "therapeutic use of self" and in a "therapeutic relationship between nurse and patient." Unfortunately, however, the interpersonal aspects of nursing are often devalued or reduced to a set of behavioral skills. As Askinazi has claimed, however, there is "a mystery to nursing," "a secret energy" that forms in the nurse–patient relationship. "It's powerful and important and it may be the essence of life itself . . . The mystery of the nurse–patient relationship lies in the transforming potential of caring." (Halldorsdottir, 2008, p. 644)

Watson noted "the deeply human and spirit-filled nature of professional nursing and an acknowledgement of the spiritual, mysterious, and sacred dimensions often silently residing in the margins of our work and our life" (2008, p. 81). The lack of correlation suggests that this mystery, the sacredness of caring between a patient and a nurse, remains just that—an elegant, elusive mystery.

Despite the lack of correlation, there are patterns in the results that provide direction for future organizational interventions. Four of six nurses consistently scored themselves lower than their patients scored them. These four nurses had less than five years of experience as a registered nurse, which were similar to previous internal results from the CES when self-perceptions of caring were examined based on years of experience. The results in this pilot study, along with previous results using a different instrument, strongly suggest that nurses with less than five years of experience rate self-perception of caring lower than nurses with more experience. The results from this study indicate that patients cared for by these relatively inexperienced nurses did not share their nurse's self-perceptions; instead they gave high scores, often very high scores, to this group of nurses. This invites the question, what can we do to help less experienced nurses recognize their own caring and caring potential? Would recognition of their caring gifts help them stay in the profession and find internal value in their professional practice? Gathering focus groups with this demographic group of nurses as well as clinical educators, mentors, and clinical nurse specialists will, hopefully, begin to answer this question.

Another useful component to this study involves sharing the individual results with the six nurses who volunteered to participate in the research. Nurses were recruited for this study by asking if they were interested in finding out if their patients perceived them to be as caring as they perceived themselves. A mean caring score of 6.30 from the patient perspective, compared to a mean caring score from the nurse perspective of 6.06, suggests that these particular nurses were often more caring during patient encounters than they thought. The mean caring score of 6.30 is higher than previous organizational caring score means of 6.10 and 5.97, suggesting that the nurses in this study were more caring than the average nurse in the organization. Before the study began, the likelihood that our most caring nurses would be drawn to this type of research was recognized. The data support that the nurses in the study were caring exemplars, which in turn may make the results more meaningful. It alludes to the use of using outliers within Parato mathematics to understand elements of success.

The answer to the research question—Are nurses' self-perceptions of their own caring behaviors similar to their patients' perceptions of caring behaviors?—would seem to be *no*. However, when examining the mean scores and analyzing the qualitative comments, it appears that deep and profound caring moments did occur. Perhaps these nurses were alert and responsive to what was present and emerging for the patient in the given-now-moment they were together. Perhaps these nurses used transpersonal Caritas consciousness to expand caring and, in some instances, this acquired skill of *being present-in-the-now* reduced the demands for caring (Watson, 2008). This suggests that the mystery, sacredness, and wholeness of caring moments that make up caring relationships are difficult or even impossible to measure, articulate, or completely understand.

There are several limitations to this study. The sample size was small and the nurse participants' caring behaviors were skewed toward highly caring. The nurse participants practiced in very different settings, including one from an outpatient emergency fast-track setting designed to limit the quantity of time that the patient and nurse interacted. However, mean scores from this nurse and her patients were higher than previous organizational means, suggesting that caring moments and caring relationships do occur in an environment where time is purposefully limited to 90 minutes or less.

CONCLUSION

The study demonstrates that every nurse–patient relationship is unique. Each patient brings his or her life history, experiences, and varying levels of vulnerability to every encounter with a nurse. Each nurse brings his or her experiences, training, and ways of knowing to every encounter with a patient. The mean scores from the study suggest that caring connections occur frequently; however, the nurse and the patient view such connections differently. Each individual's perceptions within the caring relationship have value in the context of the whole. Although this study supports the idea that nurses and patients do not view caring the same way, it also supports the idea that caring occurs in abundance despite differing perceptions. The study also has implications for further organizational research at WMC. It strongly suggests that we cannot assume that patients' perceptions of caring reflect nurses' self-perceptions of caring or vice versa. Each perspective must be examined independent of the other while valued within a paradigm of the whole. This operational study reaffirms that caring and caring relationships are complex, mysterious, and meaningful to patient and nurse. It also suggests that we need to go beyond the more logical Gaussian mathematics (statistics/averages) when designing caring research and move toward other methods like pattern analysis, Parato mathematics, nonlinear geometry, and qualitative data to gain knowledge within the unitary/holographic paradigm of caring science.

ACKNOWLEDGMENTS

The authors express their deepest appreciation and gratitude to the nurses who volunteered to participate in this research. It showed enormous courage to willingly invite potential positive and negative judgments about the core of who you are and what you do. As authors and leaders in caring science at our facility, we continue to be amazed by your courage, grace, and caring hearts.

REFERENCES

Baldursdottir, G., & Jonsdottir, H. (2002). The importance of nurse caring behaviors as perceived by patients receiving care at an emergency department. *Heart & Lung, 31*(1), 67–75.

Becker, M. K., Blazovich, L., Schug, V., Schulenberg, C., Daiels, J., Neal, D., . . . Smith, M. O. (2008). Nursing student caring behaviors during blood pressure measurement. *Journal of Nursing Education, 47*(3), 98–104.

Carter, L. C., Nelson, J. L., Sievers, B. A., Dukek, S. L., Pipe, T. B., & Holland, D. E. (2008). Exploring a culture of caring. *Nursing Administration Quarterly, 32*(1), 57–63.

Coates, C. (1997). The caring efficacy scale: Nurses' self-reports of caring in practice settings. *Advanced Practice Nursing Quarterly, 3*(1), 53–59.

Dyson, J. (1996). Nurses' conceptualizations of caring attitudes and behaviours. *Journal of Advanced Nursing, 23,* 1263–1269.

Erci, B., Sayan, A., Tortumluoglu, G., Kilic, D., Sahin, O., & Güngörmüs, Z. (2003). The effectiveness of Watson's caring model on the quality of life and blood pressure of patients with hypertension. *Journal of Advanced Nursing, 41*(2), 130–139.

Finch, L. P. (2006). Patients' communication with nurses: Relational communication and preferred nurse behaviors. *International Journal for Human Caring, 10*(4), 14–22.

Halldorsdottir, S. (1991). Five basic modes of being with another. In D. A. Gaut & M. M. Leininger (Eds.), *Caring: The compassionate healer* (pp. 37–49). New York, NY: National League for Nursing Press.

Halldorsdottir, S. (2008). The dynamics of the nurse–patient relationship: Introduction of a synthesized theory from the patient's perspective. *Scandinavian Journal of Caring Sciences, 22,* 643–652.

Hegedus, K. S. (1999). Providers and consumers; Perspective of nurses' caring behaviours. *Journal of Advanced Nursing, 30*(5), 1090–1096.

Henderson, A., Van Eps, M. A., Pearson, K., James, C., Henderson, P., & Osborne, Y. (2007). "Caring for" behaviours that indicate to patients that nurses "care about" them. *Journal of Advanced Nursing, 60*(2), 146–153.

Larsson, G., Peterson, V. W., Lampic, C., von Essen, L., & Sjödèn, P. (1998). Cancer patient and staff ratings of the importance of caring behaviours and their relations to patient anxiety and depression. *Journal of Advanced Nursing, 27*, 855–864.

Lindahl, E., Norberg, A., & Söderberg, A. (2008). The meaning of caring for people with malodorous exuding ulcers. *Journal of Advanced Nursing, 62*(2), 163–171.

McCance, T., Slater, P., & McCormack, B. (2008). Using the caring dimension inventory as an indicator of person-centered nursing. *Journal of Clinical Nursing, 18*, 409–417.

McCartan, P. J., & Hargie, O. D. W. (2004). Assertiveness and caring: Are they compatible? *Journal of Clinical Nursing, 13*, 707–713.

Nelson, J., Watson, J., & Inova Healthcare. (2006). *Dr. Jean Watson's theory of human caring Web*. Retrieved December 10, 2006, from http://hschealth.uchsc .edu/son/faculty/jw_caritaspractice.htm

Oermann, M. H. (1999). Consumers' descriptions of quality health care. *Journal of Nursing Care Quality, 14*(1), 47–55.

Patistea, E. (1999). Nurses' perceptions of caring as documented in theory and research. *Journal of Clinical Nursing, 8*, 487–495.

Persky, G. J., Nelson, J. W., Watson, J., & Bent, K. (2008). Creating a profile of a nurse effective in caring. *Nursing Administration Quarterly, 32*(1), 15–20.

Quinn, J. F., Smith, M., Ritenbaugh, C., Swanson, K., & Watson, M. J. (2003). Research guidelines for assessing the impact of the healing relationship in clinical nursing. *Alternative Therapies, 9*(3), A65–A79.

Sumner, J. (2008). Is caring in nursing an impossible ideal for today's practicing nurse? *Nursing Administration Quarterly, 32*(2), 92–101.

Wade, G. H., & Kasper, N. (2006). Nursing students' perceptions of instructor caring: An instrument based on Watson's theory of transpersonal caring. *Journal of Nursing Education, 45*(5), 162–168.

Watson, J. (2008). *Nursing: The philosophy and science of caring* (Rev. ed.). Boulder, CO: University Press of Colorado.

Wiman, E., & Wikblad, K. (2004). Caring and uncaring encounters in nursing in an emergency department. *Journal of Clinical Nursing, 13*, 422–429.

7

Profile of a Nurse Effective in Caring

Georgia Persky, John Nelson,
Jean Watson, and Kate Bent

*T*he core assumption of the model of Relationship-Based Care (RBC)*
is that those who care for the most vulnerable populations do so
because they want to provide care that is competent and compassionate.[1] This study of the profile of caring nurses was done prior to implementation of the Relationship-Based Care (RBC) delivery model within
a professional practice framework at New York-Presbyterian Hospital/
Columbia University Medical Center.

This secondary analysis of the baseline assessment of the work environment prior to implementation of RBC provides a profile of the nurses
who were reported to convey care and love during care delivery. Both
qualitative and quantitative data were used to identify the demographics
and environmental perceptions of those care givers who received the
highest score of caring as identified by the patients they served. Eighty-
seven nurses who provided the majority of care to selected patients were
paired with those patients to form 85 dyads. Nurses responded to the
Healthcare Environment Survey (HES) while patients responded to the
Caring Factor Survey (CFS) at the same time.† Correlations of the 85 pairs
were examined to identify the relationship of the nurse's report of the
environment to the patient's report of caring. Resultant data may be used
for future research to examine the impact of nurses who are effective in
caring on patient and organizational outcomes.

---

*Relationship Based Care is a program of Creative Health Care Management, Minneapolis,
MN, USA.
†The copyright for the HES is owned by Healthcare Environment. The copyright for
the CFS is co-owned by John Nelson, Jean Watson, and Inova Health System.

BACKGROUND

This baseline profile analysis and report are part of a larger initiative to integrate Relationship-Based Care (RBC) within patient services at New York-Presbyterian Hospital/Columbia University Medical Center. The RBC program is premised on a patient-centered care-delivery model that focuses on relationships among three roles: the patient, nurse colleagues, and the nurse-self as caregiver. The specific intention of the program is to create a culture of caring that is pervasive across all employees and processes of New York-Presbyterian Hospital/Columbia University Medical Center. By early 2009, all 23 inpatient units of the New York-Presbyterian Hospital/Columbia University Medical Center will have implemented RBC.

The structure of RBC incorporates a professional nursing-practice model, promotes collegial relationships among all members of the team, and provides a framework for the organization of patient care and resource utilization. Collegial relationships within RBC are fostered through the development of Unit Practice Councils (UPC) on each participating unit. A critical success factor of the RBC change process for all staff involves an educational retreat, Reigniting the Spirit of Caring, a three-day inspirational/educational experience that enhances awareness of the dimensions of caring essential to RBC, and promotes healthy interpersonal relationships.

It is vital for care givers to understand what patients value in care so they can apply that knowledge in practice to help patients feel cared for. Interviews with over 6,000 hospitalized patients from 62 different facilities revealed that, more than anything, patients desire the "soft" side of health care—a relationship with their care provider(s) during hospitalization.[2]

Nurses and patients agree that caring behaviors of the nurse enhance the desirable nurse–patient relationship.[3] However, studies of patients' and nurses' descriptions of caring relationships indicate that perceptions differ between the two groups.[4-12] Hegedus[7] found that, at every level of patient anxiety, depression, quality of life and perception of health, patients desired behaviors that recognized them as individuals and welcomed family involvement, whereas nurses valued helping patients express and/or vent their feelings. Larsson et al.[9] found that patients and nurses did agree that anticipatory and comforting behaviors were among the most important aspects of caring.

One reason for the difference between patients' and nurses' perceptions of a caring relationship is that the needs for care change during the period of illness; physical care, emotional care and spiritual care needs come and go as the state of the patient changes. A key related finding in several studies, consistent with Watson's Theory of Caring, was the alignment of patients' needs with Maslow's Hierarchy of Needs. Essential physical needs were reported by patients to be most important to them in the caring relationship, followed by the higher order needs of emotion and love.[11,13-15]

It has been proposed that nurses care from a variety of perspectives, based on the theoretical framework each respective nurse was taught within nursing school.[16] Some researchers have proposed that it is possible that the intentionality of the nurse and patient in the relationship may predict agreed upon caring behaviors.[3,17] These proposals and the findings reported below from the current study indicate there could be considerably more to learn about differing perspectives of caring behavior.

PURPOSE

Healing is related to the patient-caregiver humanistic caring relationship and interaction.[18,19] The intent of this study was to create a profile of nurses who are effective in caring within Watson's[18,19] recent framework of *Caritas*: that is, acknowledging caring and love as integral aspects of a dynamic, mutual, humanistic caring interaction. Identifying the essential characteristics within such a dynamic, patient-nursing humanistic context that portrays caring and love has implications for understanding the power of human health and healing, as well as for gaining knowledge of the environment in which this level of *Caritas* nursing can occur.

METHODS

Setting

The setting for this study was New York-Presbyterian Hospital/ Columbia University Medical Center. Both qualitative and quantitative data, collected using the Participative Action Research (PAR) process, were used to create a profile of caring nurses, consistent with Watson's notion of *Caritas* and loving kindness as context for healing relationships. Nurses were selected based on the amount of time they cared for a patient during his or her inpatient stay. Patients were selected based on their admission to six medical-surgical-patient units and one mental health unit that were about to embark on efforts to integrate RBC to improve care. All study procedures were approved by the IRB, and both patients and nurses signed either a paper or electronic consent to participate.

Data Collection

Measurements of unit-based employee job satisfaction and patients' perceptions of caring were used to understand the baseline status of nurses and patients in the care-delivery environment. In conjunction with the PAR process, the Healthcare Environment Survey (HES) was distributed to managers, nurses, nursing attendants, ICU technicians, and unit assistants of each unit studied to understand the unique aspects of the work environment as perceived by these respective staff members. The HES is a valid and reliable 86-item instrument used to obtain staff members' perceptions of the work environment, including relationships with coworkers, unit manager, physicians and nurses, professional patient care, autonomy, staffing and scheduling, executive leadership, learning opportunities, organizational rewards, pride in the organization, intent to stay with the organization, and workload. Nurses used a 1-7 Likert scale to report degree of disagreement or agreement with the statements provided. An example of an item from the HES is, "My nurse manager often gives me recognition for a job well done." The more staff agrees with the statement, the higher the score, while disagreement is noted by lower scores. Respondents can use the number "4" to denote neutrality. Reliabilities of the HES have been shown to perform adequately in reliability testing, with Cronbach's alpha of .96.[20]

The HES also has items about staff demographics, hours worked, and employee disposition. The instrument collects responses to statements about what staff enjoy about their work, what creates the most stress for them within their work, what makes them want to leave the organization, and what makes them want to stay. Responses to each of the four statements were examined for themes.

The second instrument used in the study, the Caring Factor Survey (CFS), is a 20-item instrument used to assess patients' perceptions of the care received from nurses who indicated a caring and loving consciousness toward them as a whole person, including unity of mind-body-spirit. An example of an item from the CFS is, "When my caregivers teach me something new, they teach me in a way that I can understand." The CFS, like the HES, used a 1-7 Likert scale with the same methods for scoring degree of agreement or disagreement. The CFS was developed to reflect Watson's most recent theory of *Caritas*, which incorporates and extends her original Carative Factors as the core of professional nursing.[19] Reliabilities of the CFS have been shown to perform adequately in reliability testing, with Cronbach's alpha .97.[20] For purposes of this study, the higher the score reported by the patient on the CFS, the more evidence of *Caritas* was inferred. That is, the patient viewed the more caring nurses as those who honored their individual wholeness and unity of mind-body-spirit.

Data Analysis

To create a profile of nurses who patients reported to be the most caring, dyads consisting of a patient and his or her nurse were formed, and data from the two instruments were linked for each dyad. Correlation tables were used, using Pearson's *r*, to identify what environmental and demographic data as reported by nurses related to the CFS scores of patients within the 85 dyads. The primary interest was to understand which nurse factors related to the CFS score. Descriptive statistics and comparisons of environmental and demographic data using t-tests and analysis of variance were used to understand nurses who received high scores of caring by the patients they cared for.

Qualitative data from the HES was themed and examined for factors reported most often by nurses who received a high score from the patient they cared for. Due to the sample of 85 patient-nurse pairs, the analysis required an alpha of .15, power of .8 and effect size of .25.

Results were later presented to managers and staff from the participating units. Participative Action Research (PAR) was used to design, collect, examine, and interactively present the findings in relationship to the operations and infrastructure. The outcomes from this research will assist the application of findings into the process of organizational improvements. In addition, managers and practitioners may be able to provide useful interpretation of the data and how it coincides with their daily operations that the researchers who conducted this study were previously unaware of.

RESULTS

The HES and CFS used in this study both provided good reliability, with a Cronbach's alpha of .95 and .97 respectively. The only subscales within the HES that fell below .70 were staffing and scheduling, disposition and intent to stay, which revealed a Cronbach's alpha of .58, .56, and .65 respectively.

The researchers examined demographic, quantitative, and qualitative data about nurses who received high scores on the CFS to create a profile of nurses who were effective in caring. Data from nurses with high CFS scores were compared to data from nurses with low CFS scores.

The cumulative findings were used to create a profile of nurses who were perceived as caring by the patients for whom they provided care. Nurses reported to be caring by their patients were found to
- report the greatest frustration with every work environment variable measured, especially workload;
- have the most hospital and professional experience;
- work their scheduled hours of work, not more than scheduled hours;
- be of any age, not just older or younger nurses;
- be the most affected by stress in the relationship with the patient, especially "difficult patients";

- be those who most enjoyed coworker relationships;
- be those who most often provided continuity of patient care from admission to the respective unit through discharge.

Patients within this study were hospitalized from one to twenty-seven days, with a mean (average) number of hospital days of seven. It should be noted that a mental health unit was included within this study, thus extending the mean. The mode (most commonly reported number) was two days in the hospital. Nurses who were paired with these patients were the primary care provider anywhere from one to sixteen of the days the patient was hospitalized.

DISCUSSION AND IMPLICATIONS

There were several unexpected and interesting results in this study. Primary among these is the negative relationship of every variable in the HES with the CFS. These negative relationships were previously identified by one of the authors of this study in a study of caring and the work environment that was conducted for another organization. However, the findings from that study were thought to possibly be due to chance because of a small sample size (eight units), with the unit as the level of analysis. The current data reveal similar negative correlations of the HES and CFS, but with a much larger sample size, while using paired dyads of nurses and patients. The authors of this study speculate that nurses who received the highest CFS level of caring/love may be frustrated because the health care environment and practices are incongruent with values and goals of caring. Further, frustration among high CFS nurses may also arise from recognizing that authentic caring ("*Caritas* nursing") takes more time and resources than are available.

These findings of a negative correlation between CFS factors and HES factors warrant further inquiry and hypothesis testing. Authors of this study seek to repeat the above study with additional controls to validate that the caring is contained within the humanistic interaction of the patient and nurse. In addition, New York-Presbyterian Hospital/Columbia University Medical Center is seeking to increase continuity of care by implementation of Primary Nursing within a model of Relationship-Based Care and restudy the impact of continuity of care on the perception of caring as reported by the patient.

The authors of this report proposed that understanding the profile of "*Caritas* nurses" (those who receive high scores from their patients on the Caring Factor Survey) is an essential step to understanding and refining work-environment systems and processes of caring and healing. Results were presented to managers and staff to identify the findings within each participating unit that are most meaningful for relationships between nurses and patients on that unit. Success factors and needs, which varied from unit to unit, were used to create action plans and allocate resources based on unit-specific operational strengths and vulnerabilities.

Limitations

There were limitations to this study. This is the first study the authors are aware of that has examined the attributes of nurses who are reported to be effective in caring by the patients they care for. Because this is such a new area of inquiry, midrange theory about caring attributes is also in very early and developmental stages. Because the theoretical structures are not yet fully developed, there are several potentially confounding variables that were not measured, as they do not yet have a "place-holder" within any proposed theoretical structure. Another limitation is that liberal statistical parameters were used, including an alpha of .15, power of .80 and effect size of .25. These liberal parameters were required because of the small sample size of 85 patient-nurse pairs.

CONCLUSION

Creating a profile of so-called "*Caritas* nurses," who are reported by patients to be effective in caring, has implications for further testing of the theory that caring and love are important, if not critical, elements of healing and patient outcomes. Further, understanding the characteristics of a "*Caritas* nurse" may assist educators in their evaluation and development of a curriculum that seeks to prepare future nurses in *Caritas* competencies consistent with patient needs and new professional practice models of caring–healing. In addition, preceptors who understand competencies in caring will be able to coach new nurses according to what has become understood about the profile of effective caring. Lastly, findings from future studies that connect the profile of effective caring to patient outcomes such as healing, pain control, symptom management, and length of stay can be used to show the relationship between caring and cost outcomes. These data can be used in helping hospitals and practitioners alike to restore core values and practices of caring back into health care.

ACKNOWLEDGMENTS

This study was supported by International Caritas Consortium and New York-Presbyterian Hospital.

The authors of this report would like to acknowledge the editorial contribution of Diane Maki, PhD, the operational assistance of Sheila Anane, BA, MPH, and the caring staff nurses who participated in this new area of research.

REFERENCES

1. Felgen J. *Leading Lasting Change: I2E2*. Bloomington, MN: Creative Health Care Management; 2007.
2. Gerteis M, Edgman-Levitan S, Daley J, Delbanco TL. *Through the Patient's Eyes*. San Francisco: Jossey-Bass; 1993.
3. Turkel MC, Ray MA. Research issues. Relational complexity: from grounded theory to instrument development and theoretical testing ... synthesis of the research findings from a 5-year program of qualitative and quantitative studies. *Nurs Sci Q*. 2001;14:281–7.
4. Proch ML. *The development and validation of caring competencies for hospital staff nurses* [Dissertation]. University of South Florida; 1997:122.
5. Bassett C. Nurses' perception of care and caring. *Int J Nurs Pract*. 2002;8:8–15.
6. Kyle TV. The concept of caring: a review of the literature. *J Adv Nurs*. 1995;21:506–514.
7. Hegedus KS. Providers' and consumers' perspective of nurses' caring behaviours. *J Adv Nurs*. 1999;30:1090–1096.
8. Drake E. Discharge teaching needs of parents in the NICU. *Neonatal Netw*. 1995;14:49–53.
9. Larsson G, Widmark V, Lampic C, von Essen L, Sjoden P. Cancer patient and staff ratings of the importance of caring behaviours and their relations to patient anxiety and depression. *J Adv Nurs*. 1998;27:855–864.
10. Widmark-Petersson V, von Essen L, Sjoden P. Perceptions of caring among patients with cancer and their staff: differences and disagreements. *Cancer Nurs*. 2000;23:32–39.
11. von Essen L, Sjoden P. The importance of nurse caring behaviors as perceived by Swedish hospital patients and nursing staff. *Int J Nurs Stud*. 2003;40:487–497.
12. Chang Y, Lin Y, Chang H, Lin C. Cancer patient and staff ratings of caring behaviors: relationship to level of pain intensity. *Cancer Nurs*. 2005;28:331–339.
13. Baldursdottir G, Jonsdottir H. The importance of nurse caring behaviors as perceived by patients receiving care at an emergency department. *J Heart Lung Transplant*. 2002;31:67–75.
14. Mullins IL. Nurse caring behaviors for persons with acquired immunodeficiency syndrome/human immunodeficiency virus. *Appl Nurs Res*. 1996;9:18–23.
15. Holroyd E, Cheung Y, Cheung S, Luk F, Wong W. A Chinese cultural perspective of nursing care behaviours in an acute setting. *J Adv Nurs*. 1998;28:1289–1294.
16. Patistea E. Nurses' perceptions of caring as documented in theory and research. *J Clin Nurs*. 1999;8:487–495.
17. Sherwood GD. Meta-synthesis of qualitative analyses of caring: defining a therapeutic model of nursing. *Adv Pract Nurs Q*. 1997;3:32–42.
18. Watson J. *Caring science as sacred science*. 1st ed. Philadelphia: F.A. Davis; 2005.
19. Watson, J. University of Health Sciences School of Nursing [homepage on the Internet]. Available from: http://www.uchsc.edu/nursing/caring.
20. Nelson JW. *Annual Business Report*. Minneapolis: Healthcare Environment, Inc; 2006.

8

Making the "Quantum Leap": Biochemical Markers of Human Caring Science

Dax Andrew Parcells and John Nelson

*C*aring is the essence, moral ideal, and foundation for nursing practice (Boykin & Schoenhofer, 2001; Leininger & McFarland, 2006; Watson, 2005). As a central construct in the nurse–patient relationship, caring purportedly enhances quality health care delivery and improves patient safety measures in clinical practice (Duffy, 2009; Mitchell, 2008). However, further validation of the role of caring in patient healing hinges on the identification of biochemical markers responsive to caring nursing. Therefore, this chapter explores the proposed link between the human science of caring and the biochemical milieu, investigating the idea that "caring moments heal" (Watson, 2005) as a juxtaposition of caring nursing and quantum mechanics.

CARING IN NURSING

The American Nurses Association (ANA) defines nursing as "the protection, promotion, and optimization of health and abilities, prevention of illness and injury, alleviation of suffering . . ., and advocacy in the care of individuals, families, communities, and populations" (ANA, 2003, p. 6). Noticeably, the definition emphasizes health outcomes for nursing care yet fails to integrate the construct of caring as outlined by major nursing theorists (e.g., Peplau, 1997; Rogers, 1992; Watson, 2005). A more meaningful perspective, advanced by DalPezzo (2009), defines nursing care as "a skilled, safe, high quality, holistic, ethical, collaborative, individualized, interpersonal *caring* process that is planned and designed based on the best evidence available, and results in positive patient outcomes, optimization of health, palliation of symptoms, or a peaceful death" (p. 263). Similarly, Fawcett (2005) and Watson (this volume) recognize nursing as an interactive, relational, and holistic practice grounded in a caring metaparadigm.

The ubiquitous nature of the term "caring" in the nursing literature prompted a concept analysis by Brilowski and Wendler (2005). These researchers concluded that caring consists of five core attributes: relationship, action, attitude, acceptance, and variability. Their conceptualization recognizes caring as grounded in competency (an "action" encompassing tasks, touch, and authentic presence). More importantly, they identified antecedents (e.g., trust and rapport were primary prerequisites to the development of a caring relationship between nurses, patients, and families) and consequences (e.g., nurse satisfaction and patient healing) of caring. The foregoing highlights the importance of caring in nursing and provides insight into the necessary foundation for establishing caring as the essence and moral ideal of nursing practice. Finally, DalPezzo's (2009) conceptualization frames nursing as fully grounded in evidence-based practice (*science*) as well as human caring (the creative *art*/individualized approach supported within cocreatedcaring moments; Locsin, 2005; Watson, 2005)—this marriage of art and science in nursing refreshingly emboldens human caring as a science!

In the broadest sense, caring nursing represents the practice of nursing grounded in caring (Boykin & Schoenhofer, 2001; Watson, 2005). More specifically, caring nursing formalizes the conception of professional nursing practice and validates nursing as a discipline of specialized knowledge in the action of caring for and about the patient and family. However, quantitative measurement of the construct of caring in nursing has challenged researchers until recently (for a compendium of instruments, see Watson, 2009). Now with tools to measure caring from the perspective of nurses, patients, and families, researchers must make the *quantum leap* to further validate caring in nursing by investigating the unbounded potential of caring on human healing—a relationship anticipated to be mediated by biochemical markers. The proposed model, based on quantum theory (i.e., the principle of discrete change units in particulate matter; Scarani, 2006), holds that caring nursing positively shifts the vibrational balance within the biochemical milieu, ergo resulting in profound healing (i.e., a therapeutic change within the individual nurse, patient, and family; Peplau, 1997).

CARING–SATISFACTION LINK IN NURSING

Research indicates that caring enhances patient perceptions of quality health care delivery (Lee, Tu, Chong, & Alter, 2008) and also increases nurse retention (Aiken, Clarke, Sloane, Lake, & Cheney, 2008). Historically, patients were assumed incapable of assessing the quality of care received— fortunately, the tide has changed toward patient-centered care based on reports of patient satisfaction and assessments of safety and healing (Carter et al., 2008; Lynn, McMillen, & Sidani, 2007; Watson, 2009). However, the precise definition of the construct of quality remains elusive, potentially limiting research directed at identifying antecedents and consequences of caring in nursing. Nonetheless, several research teams have formulated measurement protocols for quality of care assessment—for example, Patient's

Assessment of Quality Scale (Lynn et al., 2007) and Caring Factor Survey (Nelson, 2006, 2007; Persky, Nelson, Watson, & Bent, 2008). Each instrument reflects the theoretical orientation of the researcher/group; however, several common factors have been identified as components contributing to care quality: individualization of the plan of care, caring holistically, and creation of healing environments staffed by nurses proficient in Caritas Processes (DiNapoli, Nelson, Turkel, & Watson, 2010; Lynn et al., 2007; Quinn, 2009).

Patient Satisfaction

"[C]are provided by nurses is regarded as the most important factor in patient assessments of their satisfaction with health care. In this respect, the nurse is at the forefront of the hospital" (Johannson, Oléni, & Fridlund, 2002, p. 338). Furthermore, patient satisfaction, reflective of the subjective experience of the patient, forms the basis for overall quality of care ratings (Ervin, 2006), and therefore remains a high priority within health care organizations. Overall, a positive relationship has been observed between patients' perceptions of nurse caring and their overall satisfaction with hospital care (Baldursdottir & Jonsdottir, 2002; Karlsson & Forsberg, 2008). For example, a patient explained the engendering experience of personal touch as a valued exemplar of humanistic 'confirmation': "I really appreciated . . . when somebody came and took my hand just like that. You don't think you can make it without that contact. It gives you that warmth from another human being, the closeness, and it's of *crucial* importance I think" (Karlsson & Forsberg, 2008, p. 45).

Patients identify components such as the hospital environment, nurse–patient communication, and nurse medical-technical competency as significant to their satisfaction (Johannson et al., 2002). Based on a comparison of their actual experience to their expectations, patients arrive at a satisfaction rating. Patients in acute care value clinical nursing competency as foremost among dimensions of caring behaviors compared to emotional/affective domains (Baldursdottir & Jonsdottir, 2002). Moreover, patient-satisfaction ratings relate strongly to sociodemographic and psychosocial characteristics—for example, Lee et al. (2008) found that older patients, those with less self-reported depression, and the most functionally improved patients following a myocardial incident, rated their care most satisfactory. These results underscore the importance of a patient- and results-centered approach to nurse caring (Institute of Medicine, 2001) that emphasizes "what matters most" to the patient as pivotal to the delivery of quality nursing care (Boykin & Schoenhofer, 2001) grounded in relationship-based caring science.

Nurse Satisfaction/Retention

The fast-paced, technology-driven culture of nursing, coupled with staffing shortages, increasing patient acuity, and cost containment have the potential to dramatically impede caring in nursing

(Aiken, Clarke, Sloane, Sochalski, & Silber, 2002). Moreover, resultant from a perceived incongruence between nurses' ideals and the reality of the nursing care environment, job frustration and a sense of being overwhelmed abound, leading to nurse stress and/or increased nurse burnout/turnover (Borysenko, 2011; McVicar, 2003; Ray, Turkel, & Marino, 2002). Researchers found high job satisfaction among nurses at hospitals where nursing leadership was represented on the executive board and the administration was supportive/inclusive of nurses through participatory action paradigms. Other factors contributing to nurse satisfaction were staffing adequacy, schedule flexibility, and encouragement of nursing autonomy (Currie, Harvey, West, McKenna, & Keeney, 2005).

Focus group data revealed that novice nurses must grow into the profession, as they initially embrace a "to-do list" mentality: "This is my list. What I do as a nurse is check off as accomplished all these things on my list" (Carter et al., 2008, p. 57). On the other hand, expert nurses report deep valuing of opportunities to care over mere task completion (Carter et al., 2008). Therefore, in order to fully actualize as a "Caritas nurse" (Persky et al., 2008), novices require mentorship—this sentiment was echoed in the report of nurses and suggested as a means of enhancing caring for patients and nurses through relationships built on teamwork, communication, and staff support (Carter et al., 2008). Such an approach potentially reduces nurse turnover, the direct costs of which exceed US$17,000 per nurse in hiring and training alone (Waldman, Kelly, Arora, & Smith, 2010). Moreover, indirect costs (e.g., decreased care quality or increased adverse events) potentially cripple patient recovery/healing and obscure the image of professional nursing!

The New York State Nurses Association (2005) formalized a position statement related to self-care for the professional nurse based on a sound principle: "There *is* a relationship between nurses' ability to care for self and their ability to provide effective patient care." Such a strong statement validates the importance of self-care in reducing nurse stress and potential burnout (Sherman, 2004) as a measure to buttress patient safety. In order to achieve the mission, nurses must continue living and growing in caring (Boykin & Schoenhofer, 2001) through application of the basic premise that "caring begets caring" (Carter et al., 2008)—by supporting one another in a carative fashion in daily practice, nurses serve themselves and, more importantly, protect the rights of patients to the best quality of care. Research shows that nurses engaging in self-care and working in hospitals with a high regard for caring as an expression of nursing experience greater job satisfaction, have less stress and minimal burnout (Aiken et al., 2008; Foley, 2004), protecting the hospitals' bottom line and fulfilling the nurse's call to serve through caring.

CARING BEGETS SAFETY IN NURSING

The Institute of Medicine estimated that medical errors account for between 44,000 and 98,000 deaths annually in hospitals in the United States—upward of 58% of these deaths were rated "preventable" (Kohn, Corrigan, & Donaldson, 2000). This situation requires a concerted effort on the part of the multidisciplinary health care team to ensure patient safety. The "Swiss Cheese Model" provides a visual describing the occurrence of adverse events as a result of the cumulative "lining up" of several failures within a system (Reason, 2000). The complexities of the nursing care culture at the point of care, constrained by organizational resources and infrastructure, impact the ultimate delivery of safe nursing care (Ebright, Patterson, Chalko, & Render, 2003; Wachter, 2008), requiring greater vigilance to factors such as supply accessibility, interruptions, and communications breakdown.

Adverse events (e.g., medication errors, nosocomial infections, and falls) have been found to be directly related to unmet nursing care needs—statistical regression analyses indicated that 23% to 53% of the variance in adverse events in the United States resulted from unmet nursing care activities (Lucero, Lake, & Aiken, 2010). Alarmingly, the research team found that on average two out of seven *essential* nursing care activities remained undone over each shift (based on self-report by nurses in a multisite study). As an initial bolster to patient safety, the evidence-based practice "movement" was launched (Pipe, 2007) and nurses are encouraged to use the best available evidence in diagnosing and treating each patient. An adequate number of nurses with expert knowledge/clinical judgment (Tanner, 2006), trained to respond urgently, serves to enhance the safety of the patient care environment (Aiken, 2010).

A purely competence-based focus in nursing may enhance safety; however, it severely limits the human potential for healing. Moreover, advances in health and nursing technologies create a presumed dichotomy between caring and technological competency as opposing aspects of nursing care. However, the current chapter proposes that nursing practice grounded in caring science reduces the number and disabling sequelae (as a measure of severity) of adverse events. Nurses are charged with treating the whole person in the specific moment (Boykin & Schoenhofer, 2001; Locsin, 2005; Watson, 2005), thus requiring the application of the full spectrum of Roach's six Cs (competence, confidence, compassion, conscience, commitment, and comportment; Roach, 1987). Locsin (2005) proposed the Technological Competency as Caring in Nursing theory as the vehicle for seamless integration of technology and caring in nursing with a promise for improved patient safety and enhanced patient healing.

Technological Competency as Caring in Nursing values the congruence in shared understanding between nurses and recipients of care with respect to valuation of nursing discipline-specific knowledge and professionalism (Parcells & Locsin, under review). Based on the premise "technological knowing," wherein nurses leverage available technologies and focus on patients as participants in their care rather than as objects of care, technological competency affords deeper knowing of persons through the integration of machine competence with caring competence. In knowing persons as caring, mutual trust and respect develop between the nurse and patient, satisfaction scores improve, and the overall quality of care delivered is enhanced—promoting safety and healing through loving kindness (Watson, 2005).

CARING NURSING AFFECTS HEALING

Nurse caring mutually enhances a patient's physical and emotional healing (Watson, 2005) and promotes nurse growth in personhood (Boykin & Schoenhofer, 2001). Conscience and commitment on the part of the nurse imparts trust within the patient (Roach, 1987), transpersonally enlivening the carative bond between the nurse and the patient. Caring in nursing unleashes a dynamic, life-giving interaction between energies that cumulatively enhances loving kindness, reduces physical and emotional stress, and thus manifests the almost magical process of healing (Halldorsdottir, 2008; Watson, 2005). Within healing environments (Quinn, 2009) specifically designed to afford nurses to practice fully through Caritas Processes, profound metaphysical energy transferences occur—"Nursing skills and knowledge are vital to make a nurse, but *compassion* and *caring* are vital to make a great nurse!" (Hudacek, 2004, p. 99).

Several specific and consistent relationships have been found between self-reported patient satisfaction with care received, quality indicators, and safety parameters directly related to recovery and healing (Isaac, Zaslavsky, Cleary, & Landon, 2010)—for example, higher patient ratings of caring correlated with reduced decubitus ulcers, and several domains of the patient experience related strongly to reduced nosocomial infections and recovery from surgical procedures. These physical-healing and health-promotion examples mirror reported effects of caring on emotional well-being: patients report "a sense of support, a sense of security, decreased sense of anxiety and stress, increased sense of control, and a sense of relief" (Halldorsdottir, 2007, p. 33). Similarly, patients with cancer reported the significance of confirmation ("outer" [e.g., being taken seriously] *and* "inner" [e.g., recognition of human dignity and worth]) as critical in mental, spiritual, and existential healing (Nåden & Sæteren, 2006).

Nurses also gain from the experience of caring for others—a caring nurse develops greater tolerance for uncertainty and gains a sense of empowerment (Oudshoorn, 2005). Through the act of caring, a self-renewing energy process unfolds, resulting in greater zeal for the professional discipline of caring nursing (Perry, 2008). Similarly, caring about fellow nurses and auxiliary staff improves workplace safety, promotes coherence among staff, and contributes reciprocally to patient healing and staff growth. For example, musculoskeletal issues among health care workers are reduced by using a team approach to lifting (i.e., minimal lift environments; Matthews, 2006)—through the practice of team lifts, stronger communication and awareness of bigger issues arise, attention to details increases, and workplace obstacles are slowly eliminated. Collectively, the healing effects resulting from nurse caring manifests organically, serving the greater good of society through simple acts of loving kindness—despite (often) being "bound by paperwork, short on hands, sleep, and energy . . . nurses are rarely short on caring" (Hudacek, 2004, p. 121).

MISSING LINK: BIOCHEMISTRY
OF CARING NURSING

Physical and emotional stress result in profound cellular inflammation and immune suppression, and, ultimately, manifest as a wide array of diseases (Federico, Morgillo, Tuccillo, Ciardiello, & Loguercio, 2007; Kiecolt-Glaser, 2010; Wellen & Hotamisligil, 2005). Patients presenting with illness are particularly susceptible to the stress-disease cycle given an already compromised immune state and the level of vulnerability (e.g., relinquishing of control) associated with hospitalization. Therefore, nurses must work diligently to create a healing space to support patients recovering from illness and promote wellness of the whole person (Boykin & Schoenhofer, 2001; Stichler, 2001). Caring nursing sets a critical foundation for healing environments where patients and nurses make deep humanistic connections affording healing and growth (Halldorsdottir, 2007; Quinn, 2009; Watson & Foster, 2003).

Proposed model. The psychosocial reality of caring encounters and the connection to healing has been established using patient reports: caring is ". . . another form of medication of sorts. It's part of the healing, part of the getting the patient better . . ." (Halldorsdottir, 2007, p. 33). However, further elaboration of the psychoneuroimmunological reality requires association of patient and nurse reports on caring encounters to specific biochemical markers as indicators of healing and "human growth." The proposed model (Figure 8.1), articulates caring as a mantra (i.e., vibrational energy quality) embraced by Caritas nurses in all nursing encounters (Persky et al., 2008; Watson & Foster, 2003)—the dynamic interaction between caring nurses, patients, and families effects discrete changes in measurable units (i.e., quanta) of perceived caring and biochemical markers following caring experiences, resulting in healing.

First, Caritas nurses are proposed to exhibit a state of physical, emotional, and mental coherence/synchronicity consistent with a meditative state of

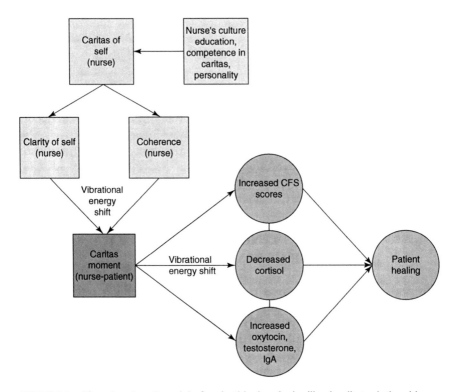

FIGURE 8.1 "Quantum leap" model of caring-biochemical milieu-healing relationship.

Adapted from initial models developed by John Nelson, Lynda Olender, and Kim Richards from meeting in Denver Colorado, December 11, 2010 and from a meeting in Minneapolis, Minnesota, January 26, 2010 with John Nelson and Mary Hauck.

consciousness (McCraty, Atkinson, Tomasino, & Bradley, 2009; Travis & Arenander, 2006) and associated with low stress hormone levels and/or high levels of hormones reflective of caring connectedness (oxytocin in females and testosterone in males; Gray, 2010). Second, these nurses effortlessly imbue caring within nursing situations, creating an environment within which patients and families experience fulfillment of physiological and safety needs, the very foundation of Maslow's needs hierarchy (Powers, 2006). Third, environmental parameters aligned with basic human needs through caring naturally reduce a patient's physical and emotional stress, leading to a deep state of rest, the release of deep physiological stresses, and healing and progression toward self-actualization.

Healing and human growth processes rest on emotional resilience related to anxiety and stress (Eming, Krieg, & Davidson, 2007; Halldorsdottir, 2007); hence, the specific suggestion to examine cortisol as a marker for healing. However, other molecules warrant investigation related to the psychoneuroimmune aspects of healing—for example, oxytocin, testosterone, and immunoglobulin A (IgA). In the final analysis, DNA methylation patterns, as an upstream measure of quantum healing effects, likely change the expression and/or suppression of specific genes implicated for healing (Ornish et al., 2008; Pray, 2004). For example, pioneering research on the frontier of integrative medicine pinpointed an increase in telomerase activity and growth of telomeres (DNA sequences at the ends of chromosomes providing protection from chromosome deterioration related to aging) following lifestyle changes (Ornish et al., 2008). Furthermore, the model recognizes a progression from patient satisfaction to patient safety ultimately coalescing in profound healing—each outcome relating significantly and directly to the perception of caring.

As the basis for human healing, heart-centered connectedness and caring nursing serve as an intrapersonal effector of the physical environment ("outer world") resulting in discrete changes in the biochemical milieu ("inner world"). The dynamics of the outer world filled with caring moments enhance patient satisfaction and nurse job satisfaction, which continues to build a sense of trust and human openness within the nurse–patient relationship as experienced in cocreated nursing situations. This sense of trust manifests yet deeper emotional awareness and reciprocity in the nurse–patient relationship, allowing an energetic shift into the inner world—the personal sanctum that instills hope and drives healing within the biochemical mosaic of hormonal and chromosomal interactions (Lipton, 2005). The overall model builds a strong case for the emergence of psychoneuroimmunology in nursing—through caring, an internal shift occurs that strengthens the psyche, bolsters immunity, and predicates healing (Halldorsdottir, 2007; McCraty et al., 2009).

QUANTUM LEAP: A RESEARCH PROPOSAL

Based on the seminal work of Persky et al. (2008), who argued that the creation of ". . . a profile of so-called 'Caritas nurses' who are reported by patients to be effective in caring has implications for further testing the theory that caring and love are important, if not *critical*, elements of healing . . ." (p. 19), a specific research proposal has been drafted. The overarching premise is to explore the proposed link between the human science of caring in nursing and biochemical markers as mediators of the caring–healing relationship. The theoretical underpinnings of the proposal rest on a melding of caring nursing models validated during the recent history of modern professional nursing (Boykin & Schoenhofer, 2001; Peplau, 1997; Roach, 1987; Rogers, 1992; Watson, 2005). Empirically, the model juxtaposes nursing and quantum theory in explaining the links between perceptions of caring, satisfaction, safety, and healing— each proposed to reflect discrete changes in the human biochemical milieu. The proposal serves to replicate and extend the extant literature in the domains of human caring, quality health care assessments, nurse satisfaction/retention, patient safety, and healing bridged by biochemistry and aspects of quantum physics.

Proposition A. As a precursor to validating the impact of caring moments on patient healing, the profile of a Caritas nurse must be further elaborated. It is important to evaluate the extent to which caring serves as a universal "mantra" in nursing and how nurse caring relates to nurse biochemical indicators reflective of his or her inner world.

1. Nurse self-care is anticipated to vary along a continuum and covary with intrapersonal factors (e.g., level of education, competence in concepts of Caritas, personality variables, and culture). Proposed to reflect an inner state of preparedness to care for and about others (Brown et al., 2005), nurse self-care putatively relates to inner coherence factors. More specifically, nurses high on a scale of self-care (Caring Factor Survey—Caring for Self; Nelson, 2006, 2007) will
   a. express a low perceived stress level (Perceived Stress Scale; Cohen, Kamarck, & Mermelstein, 1983) and high person-centeredness orientation (Person-Centred Climate Questionnaire—Patient Version; Edvardsson, Koch, & Nay, 2009);
   b. exhibit physiological heart-brain coherence (measured by patterns of heart-rate variability and vagal afferent traffic under hyperaroused conditions; McCraty et al., 2009) and low salivary cortisol levels as physiological indicators of emotionality and stress reactivity; and
   c. be perceived by patients as being caring toward others (Caring Factor Survey; Nelson, 2006, 2007) in a fashion congruent with technological knowing from the patient perspective (Technological Competency as Caring in Nursing Instrument; Parcells & Locsin, under review).

Proposition B. Next, the relationship between core attributes of nurse caring (i.e., Caritas Processes/profile of a Caritas nurse) and patient satisfaction, nurse job satisfaction, and safety measures as critical global outcomes warrants detailed investigation.

2. Patient Perceptions of Nurse Caring should relate directly to outer world patient outcome factors, illuminating the external profile of a "Caritas care recipient" (with the recognition of specific covariates, e.g., patient disease state, mental status, and personal values regarding health and wellness)—replicating and extending the findings of several researchers (Baldursdottir & Jonsdottir, 2002; Halldorsdottir, 2008; Johannson et al., 2002; Karlsson & Forsberg, 2008):
   a. Patient satisfaction ratings (Hospital Care Quality Information From the Consumer Perspective Survey; Giordano, Goldstein, Lehrman, & Spencer, 2010) are expected to correlate positively with perceptions of caring nursing (Caring Factor Survey) and

mutually both constructs should indicate a positive sense of security and safety by narrative (qualitative) patient reports.
  b. With regard to patient safety, patient perceptions of caring should correlate with nurse knowledge, skills, and attitudes related to safety competencies (Cronenwett et al., 2007) and predict hospitalization outcomes (i.e., reduced lengths of stay, complications, morbidity, and mortality) and safe discharge (e.g., reduced nosocomial infections) for continued patient recovery and growth.
3. Recursively, patient satisfaction is proposed to increase nurse job satisfaction (Healthcare Environment Survey; Nelson, 2006) via expressions of gratitude shared between the nurse, patient, and family through contextually embedded caring moments in nursing.
4. Furthermore, the expectation is an increased alignment of views and values between patients and nurses surrounding the application of technology in knowing persons as whole and complete in the moment (examining the congruence in expectations and/or experiences relative to Technological Competency as Caring in Nursing; Parcells & Locsin, under review).

Proposition C. Finally, the proposal upholds that caring moments heal (Halldorsdottir, 2007; Watson, 2005; Wing, 1999), warranting examination of the predicted relationship between patient perceptions of Caritas, measured using the Caring Factor Survey, and biochemical markers of the patient's inner world as predictors of patient healing and nurse growth. The literature indicates profound negative effects of stress on human healing (e.g., Eming et al., 2007, found a reduction of wound healing in patients with high levels of stress), supporting the mind-body connection mediated by stress hormones (especially with regard to perceived stress; Parcells, 2010). The remaining research questions provide a thorough test of the proposed quantum leap model (see Figure 8.1), bridging the caring–healing abyss in the nursing literature, afforded by investigation of human physiological correlates of caring nursing delivery.
5. How does the Caritas nurse profile impact patient biochemistry?
    a. Patients who receive care from nurses perceived as caring (Caring Factor Survey) will exhibit
        i. decreased stress hormone levels (i.e., salivary cortisol levels), other hormonal effects (e.g., increased oxytocin and testosterone levels, which further enhance the connectedness between patient and nurse), and immune-enhancing modulation (increased cytokine and immunoglobulin activity), supporting McCraty's psycho-physiological model of synchronicity (McCraty et al., 2009; McCraty, Barrios-Choplin, Rozman, Atkinson, & Watkins, 1998).

      ii. changes in chromosomal expression as a result of caring (e.g., changes in DNA methylation patterns [Pray, 2004] and reversal of acute and chronic conditions resulting from a severing of diathesis—stress relationships and enhancement of psychoneuroimmune resiliency [Ornish et al., 2008]).

    b. Profound patient healing follows based on the physiological shift imparted by the enhanced vibratory quality manifested through the caring relationship:

      i. Patient healing, based on self-reported psychosocial functioning, Global Assessment of Functioning scores (American Psychiatric Association [APA], 2000), and narratives will correlate with perceived nurse caring (Caring Factor Survey), mediated by the foregoing hormonal and chromosomal parameters.

      ii. More profound results are expected in experimental designs in which nurses are specifically trained in Caritas Processes (e.g., in the use of patient family photos and/or display of nurse photos in patient rooms; Legler, this volume) and/or on units where interpersonal coherence is substantiated by self-care practices (e.g., transcendental meditation; Travis & Arenander, 2006).

6. What effect does caring have on nurse physiology? Nurse job satisfaction likely results in further reduction of nurse stress levels and increased states of coherence, precipitating an enhancement of Caritas Processes—nurses who find value in their professional caring role will continue to grow as caring persons (Boykin & Schoenhofer, 2001) and approach self-actualization (Short Index of Self-Actualization; Jones & Crandall, 1986).

CONCLUDING REMARKS

Modern physics recognizes the unified field as the domain in and through which all energy transference processes occur and thus posits a theoretical oneness within the universe (Scarani, 2006). Grounded in dynamic interactionism, the human psychoneuroimmune "complex" (by extension) operates in accordance with universal vibrational energetics at all levels of analysis (Halldorsdottir, 2007; Scarani, 2006). Therefore, the application of quantum mechanics to caring science affords investigation of the natural order in human healing. The current quantum leap model of the caring–healing link (see Figure 8.1) purports a biophysicochemical intermediate at the interfaces of body, mind, and spirit. In the healing transaction, nurses serve as the primary catalyst for the development of trust within the nurse–patient relationship (Brilowski & Wendler, 2005). Subsequently, a shift in the holistic transcendental field sets in motion an unfolding of healing when grounded by Caritas Processes (Watson, 2005).

The link between patient satisfaction and perceptions of caring (Baldursdottir & Jonsdottir, 2002; Karlsson & Forsberg, 2008) provides impetus for continued research on the intra- and interpersonal consequences of caring nursing. The propositions presented in this chapter provide a global examination of the links between caring nursing; quality health care delivery; patient safety; and healing/growth of individuals, families, and communities:

- First, the recognition of caring as central to nursing validates the role of simple acts of loving kindness (i.e., Caritas nursing) in effecting vibrational energy transference (Watson, 2005).
- Second, the research recognizes the recursive effects within the unified field, advancing the concept of interconnectedness in thoughts, deeds, and actions—for example, nurse caring results in patient satisfaction, which enhances nurse job satisfaction and potentially further enhances caring (similar to the "caring begets caring" effect of nurse self-care and culture of caring among nurses; Carter et al., 2008).
- Third, the profound personal and social benefits of Caritas nursing surpass outer world phenomena, eventuating in healing and self-actualization—that is, a heightening of individual and collective consciousness requisite in appreciating the limitless human potential (Halldorsdottir, 2007; Powers, 2006).

Implications for Nursing

DiNapoli et al. (2010) proclaim, "While Watson's (1979) original assertion that caring inspires healing may be difficult to quantify, the use of caritas processes by nurses can be measured." Therefore, the future of human caring science resides at the caring–healing interface, invoking measurement from social and natural sciences to illuminate the relationship. First, a need exists for a deeper appreciation for the uniquely interactive nature of caring in nursing. Second, exploration of the link between quantitative biophysicochemical transactions resulting from caring-nursing delivery and qualitative narratives expressing healing and personal growth serves humanity as a collective. Third, in the current era of health care reform, health care organizations have begun to feel the squeeze applied, for instance, by the Medicare nonreimbursement directive in cases of hospital errors in patient care (Wachter, Foster, & Dudley, 2008)—prompting the need for a paradigmatic shift in the nursing gestalt. Based on the foregoing proposition highlighting the value of caring in nursing, emphasis must remain on the teaching of nursing grounded in caring. This requirement holds for academic curricula at all educational levels and within healing environments (i.e., among nurses in practice) to heighten the care culture in nursing.

Aside from the development of clinical competence/judgment (Tanner, 2006), nursing education (beginning in introductory courses) must nurture a sense of self-confidence (Blum, Borglund, & Parcells, 2010; Parcells & Blum, 2010) directed at unfolding inner potential (i.e., "nurse clarity" and "coherence"—factors essential in the growth of a Caritas nurse living and growing in caring; Boykin & Schoenhofer, 2001; Watson, 2005). Models of "how to" successfully develop Caritas nurses exist (Watson, 2005; Watson & Foster, 2003). Similarly, simulated nursing situations have been designed to teach *safety* in nursing (Henneman & Cunningham, 2005); the utility of teaching caring through modeling and discussion within simulated nursing scenarios has been successfully demonstrated (Blum, Hickman, Parcells, & Locsin, 2010). Ergo, a quantum leap is now required to complete the caring–healing circuit: through the leveraging of nurse self-care and personal/professional development (Schwarzkopf et al., 2007), the actualization of the elusive nature of healing will be manifested and the implications of caring nursing fully realized (Duffy, 2009). Caring has unbounded potential within the unified field to heal, and a transformation of the health care delivery system toward a healing model affords the nurturance of patients, families, and the full complement of the multidisciplinary health care team.

REFERENCES

Aiken, L. (2010). Safety in numbers. *Nursing Standard, 24*(44), 62–63.

Aiken, L. H., Clarke, S. P., Sloane, D. M., Lake, E. T., & Cheney, T. (2008). Effects of hospital care environment on patient mortality and nurse outcomes. *Journal of Nursing Administration, 38*(5), 223–229.

Aiken, L. H., Clarke, S. P., Sloane, D. M., Sochalski, J., & Silber, J. H. (2002). Hospital nurse staffing and patient mortality, nurse burn-out, and job dissatisfaction. *Journal of the American Medical Association, 288*(16), 1987–1993.

American Nurses Association. (2003). *Nursing's social policy statement* (2nd ed.). Silver Spring, MD: Author.

American Psychiatric Association. (2000). *Diagnostic and statistical manual of mental disorder—Text revision* (4th ed.). Washington, DC: Author.

Baldursdottir, G., & Jonsdottir, H. (2002). The importance of nurse caring behaviors as perceived by patients receiving care at an emergency department. *Heart & Lung, 31*(1), 67–75.

Blum, C. A., Borglund, S., & Parcells, D. (2010). High-fidelity nursing simulation: Impact on student self-confidence and clinical competence. *International Journal of Nursing Education Scholarship, 7*(1), Article 18.

Blum, C. A., Hickman, C., Parcells, D. A., & Locsin, R. (2010). Teaching caring nursing to RN-BSN students using simulation technology. *International Journal for Human Caring, 14*(2), 40–49.

Borysenko, J. Z. (2011). *Fried: Why you burn out and how to revive.* Carlsbad, CA: Hay House.

Boykin, A., & Schoenhofer, S. O. (2001). *Nursing as caring: A model for transforming practice.* Boston, MA: Jones & Bartlett.

Brilowski, G. A., & Wendler, M. C. (2005). An evolutionary concept analysis of caring. *Journal of Advanced Nursing, 50*(6), 641–650.

Brown, C., Schwarzkopf, R., Toby-Harris, L., Wertman, C., Voss, D., & Tippett, J. (2005). Caring for self: An action research model. *International Journal for Human Caring, 9*(2), 26.

Carter, L., Nelson, J. L., Sievers, B. A., Dukek, S. L., Pipe, T. B., & Holland, D. E. (2008). Exploring a culture of caring. *Nursing Administration Quarterly, 32*(1), 57–63.

Cohen, S., Kamarck, T., & Mermelstein, R. (1983). A global measure of perceived stress. *Journal of Health & Social Behavior, 24,* 386–396.

Cronenwett, L., Sherwood, G., Barnsteiner, J., Disch, J., Johnson, J., Mitchell, P., et al. (2007). Quality and safety education for nurses. *Nursing Outlook, 55*(3), 122–131.

Currie, V., Harvey, G., West, E., McKenna, H., & Keeney, S. (2005). Relationship between quality of care, staffing levels, skill mix and nurse autonomy: Literature review. *Journal of Advanced Nursing, 51*(1), 73–82.

DalPezzo, N. K. (2009). Nursing care: A concept analysis. *Nursing Forum, 44*(4), 256–264.

DiNapoli, P., Nelson, J., Turkel, M., & Watson, J. (2010). Measuring the Caritas processes: Caring factor survey. *International Journal for Human Caring, 14*(3), 15–20.

Duffy, J. R. (2009). *Quality caring in nursing: Applying theory to clinical practice, education, and leadership.* New York, NY: Springer.

Ebright, P., Patterson, E., Chalko, B., & Render, M. (2003). Understanding the complexity of registered nurse work in acute care settings. *Journal of Nursing Administration, 33*(12), 630–638.

Edvardsson, D., Koch, S., & Nay, R. (2009). Psychometric evaluation of the English language person-centred climate questionnaire—Patient version. *Western Journal of Nursing Research, 31,* 235–244.

Eming, S. A., Krieg, T., & Davidson, J. M. (2007). Inflammation in wound repair: Molecular and cellular mechanisms. *Journal of Investigative Dermatology, 127*(3), 514–525.

Ervin, N. E. (2006). Does patient satisfaction contribute to nursing care quality? *Journal of Nursing Administration, 36*(3), 126–130.

Fawcett, J. (2005). *Contemporary nursing knowledge: Analysis and evaluation of nursing models and theories.* Philadelphia, PA: F. A. Davis.

Federico, A., Morgillo, F., Tuccillo, C., Ciardiello, F., & Loguercio, C. (2007). Chronic inflammation and oxidative stress in human carcinogenesis. *International Journal of Cancer, 121*(11), 2381–2386.

Foley, M. (2004). Caring for those who care: A tribute to nurses and their safety. *Online Journal of Issues in Nursing, 9*(3), 91–103.

Giordano, L., Goldstein, E., Lehrman, W., & Spencer, P. A. (2010). Development, implementation, and public reporting of the HCAHPS survey. *Medical Care Research & Review, 67*(1), 27–37.

Gray, J. (2010). *Venus on fire Mars on ice: Hormonal balance—The key to life, love, and energy.* Coquitlam, Canada: Mind.

Halldorsdottir, S. (2007). A psychoneuroimmunological view of the healing potential of professional caring in the face of human suffering. *International Journal for Human Caring, 11*(2), 32–39.

Halldorsdottir, S. (2008).The dynamics of the nurse–patient relationship: Introduction of a synthesized theory from the patient's perspective. *Scandinavian Journal of Caring Sciences, 22*(4), 643–652.

Henneman, E. A., & Cunningham, H. (2005). Using clinical simulation to teach patient safety in an acute/critical care nursing course. *Nurse Educator, 30*(4), 172–177.

Hudacek, S. (2004). *A daybook for nurses: Making a difference each day.* Indianapolis, IN: Sigma Theta Tau International.

Institute of Medicine. (2001). *Crossing the quality chasm: A new health system for the 21st century.* Washington, DC: National Academy Press.

Isaac, T., Zaslavsky, A. M., Cleary, P. D., & Landon, B. E. (2010). The relationship between patients' perception of care and measures of hospital quality and safety. *Health Services Research, 45*(4), 1024–1040.

Johansson, P., Oléni, M., & Fridlund, B. (2002). Patient satisfaction with nursing care in the context of health care: A literature study. *Scandinavian Journal of Caring Science, 16*(4), 337–344.

Jones, A., & Crandall, R. (1986). Validation of a short index of self-actualization. *Personality & Social Psychology Bulletin, 12*, 63–72.

Karlsson, V., & Forsberg, A. (2008). Health is yearning: Experiences of being conscious during ventilator treatment in a critical care unit. *Intensive & Critical Care Nursing, 24*(1), 41–50.

Kiecolt-Glaser, J. K. (2010). Stress, food, and inflammation: Psychoneuroimmunology and nutrition at the cutting edge. *Psychosomatic Medicine, 72*, 1–5.

Kohn, L. T., Corrigan, J. M., & Donaldson, M. S. (Eds.). (2000). *To err is human: Building a safer health system.* Washington, DC: National Academy Press.

Lee, D. S., Tu, J. V., Chong, A., & Alter, D. A. (2008). Patient satisfaction and its relationship with quality and outcomes of care after acute myocardial infarction. *Circulation, 118*(19), 1938–1945.

Leininger, M., & McFarland, M. R. (2006). *Culture care diversity and universality: A worldwide nursing theory* (2nd ed.). Sudbury, MA: Jones and Bartlett.

Lipton, B. H. (2005). *Biology of belief: Unleashing the power of consciousness, matter and miracles.* Carlsbad, CA: Hay House.

Locsin, R. C. (2005). *Technological competency as caring in nursing.* Indianapolis, IN: Sigma Theta Tau International.

Lucero, R., Lake, E. T., & Aiken, L. H. (2010). Nursing care quality and adverse events in US hospitals. *Journal of Clinical Nursing, 19*(15–16), 2185–2195.

Lynn, M. R., McMillen, B. J., & Sidani, S. (2007). Understanding and measuring patients' assessment of the quality of nursing care. *Nursing Research, 56*(3), 159–166.

Matthews, J. H. (2006, February–March). Safe nursing practice—Protecting ourselves, saving our careers, caring for our patients. *Virginia Nurses Today*, p. 16.

McCraty, R., Atkinson, M., Tomasino, D., & Bradley, R. T. (2009). The coherent heart: Heart-brain interactions, psychophysiological coherence, and the emergence of system-wide order. *Integral Review, 5*(2), 10–115.

McCraty, R., Barrios-Choplin, B., Rozman, D., Atkinson, M., & Watkins, A. (1998). The impact of a new emotional self-management program on stress, emotions, heart rate variability, DHEA and cortisol. *Integrative Physiological & Behavioral Science, 33*(2), 151–170.

McVicar, A. (2003). Workplace stress in nursing: A literature review. *Journal of Advanced Nursing, 44*(6), 633–642.

Mitchell, P. H. (2008). Defining patient safety and quality care. In R. G. Hughes (Ed.), *Patient safety and quality: An evidence-based handbook for nurses* (pp. 1–5). Rockville, MD: Agency for Healthcare Research and Quality.

Nåden, D., & Sæteren, B. (2006). Cancer patients' perception of being or not being confirmed. *Nursing Ethics, 13*(3), 222–235.

Nelson, J. W. (2006). *Inova Health System, results healthcare environment survey.* FallsChurch, VA: Inova Health System.

Nelson, J. W. (2007). Measurement instruments for a caring environment. In M. Koloroutis, J. Felgen, C. Person, & S. Wessel (Eds.), *Relationship-based care: Visions, strategies, tools and exemplars for transforming practice* (pp. 597–605). Minneapolis, MN: Creative Health Care Management.

New York State Nurses Association. (2005, August 30). *Position statement: Self care.* Retrieved from http://www.nysna.org/practice/positions/position22.htm

Ornish, D., Lin, J., Daubenmier, J., Weidner, G., Epel, E., Kemp, C., Blackburn, E. H. (2008). Increased telomerase activity and comprehensive lifestyle changes: A pilot study. *Lancet Oncology, 9*, 1048–1057.

Oudshoorn, A. (2005). Power and empowerment: Critical concepts in the nurse-client relationship. *Contemporary Nurse: A Journal for the Australian Nursing Profession, 20*(1), 57–66.

Parcells, D. A. (2010). Women's mental health nursing: Depression, anxiety and stress during pregnancy. *Journal of Psychiatric & Mental Health Nursing, 7*(9), 813–820.

Parcells, D. A., & Blum, C. A. (2010). Nursing technology vs preferred learning modality. *Academic Exchange Quarterly, 14*(4), 185–190.

Parcells, D. A., & Locsin, R. C. (under review). *Development and psychometric evaluation of the technological competency as caring in nursing instrument: Interfacing technology, caring, and quality nursing.* Manuscript submitted for publication.

Peplau, H. E. (1997). Peplau's theory of interpersonal relations. *Nursing Science Quarterly, 10*(4), 162–167.

Perry, B. (2008). Shine on: Achieving career satisfaction as a registered nurse. *Journal of Continuing Education in Nursing, 39*(1), 17–25.

Persky, G. J., Nelson, J. W., Watson, J., & Bent, K. (2008). Creating a profile of a nurse effective in caring. *Nursing Administration Quarterly, 32*(1), 15–20.

Pipe, T. B. (2007). Optimizing nursing care by integrating theory-driven evidence-based practice. *Journal of Nurse Care Quality, 22*(3), 234–238.

Powers, P. (2006). The concept of need in nursing theory. In H. S. Kim & I. Kollak (Eds.), *Nursing theories: Conceptual & philosophical foundations* (2nd ed., pp. 71–88). New York, NY: Springer.

Pray, L. A. (2004). Epigenetics: Genome, meet your environment. *The Scientist, 18*(13), 14–20.

Quinn, J. F. (2009). Transpersonal human caring and healing. In B. Dossey (Ed.), *Holistic nursing: A handbook for practice* (5th ed., pp. 91–99). Gaithersburg, MD: Aspen.

Ray, M. A., Turkel, M. C., & Marino, F. (2002). The transformative process for nursing in workforce redevelopment. *Nursing Administration Quarterly, 26*(2), 1–14.

Reason, J. (2000). Hazards, defences and losses. In J. Reason (Ed.), *Managing the risks of organizational accidents* (pp. 1–20). Burlington, VT: Ashgate.

Roach, M. S. (1987). *The human act of caring: A blueprint for the health profession.* Ottawa, Canada: Canadian Healthcare Association Press.

Rogers, M. E. (1992). Nursing science and the space age. *Nursing Science Quarterly, 5,* 27–33.

Scarani, V. (2006). *Quantum physics: A first encounter—Interference, entanglement, and reality.* New York, NY: Oxford University Press.

Schwarzkopf, R., Brown, C., Silkin, R., Toby-Harris, L., Torres, M., & Voss, D. (2007). Caring for self: Promoting personal wellness for nursing leaders in the hospital environment. *Nurse Leader, 5*(5), 34–37, 46.

Sherman, D. W. (2004). Nurses' stress & burnout. *American Journal of Nursing, 104*(5), 48–55.

Stichler, J. F. (2001). Creating healing environments in critical care units. *Critical Care Nursing Quarterly, 24*(3), 1–20.

Tanner, C. A. (2006). Thinking like a nurse: A research-based model of clinical judgment in nursing. *Journal of Nursing Education, 45*(6), 204–211.

Travis, F., & Arenander, A. (2006). Cross-sectional and longitudinal study of effects of transcendental meditation practice on interhemispheric frontal asymmetry and frontal coherence. *International Journal of Neuroscience, 116,* 1519–1538.

Wachter, R. M. (2008). *Understanding patient safety.* New York, NY: McGraw-Hill.

Wachter, R. M., Foster, N. E., & Dudley, R. A. (2008). Medicare's decision to withhold payment for hospital errors: The devil is in the details. *Joint Commission Journal on Quality & Patient Safety, 34,* 116–123.

Waldman, J. D., Kelly, F., Arora, S., & Smith, H. L. (2010). The shocking cost of turnover in health care. *Health Care Management Review, 35*(3), 206–211.

Watson, J. (1979). *Nursing: The philosophy and science of caring.* Boston, MA: Little Brown.

Watson, J. (2005). *Caring science as sacred science.* Philadelphia, PA: F. A. Davis

Watson, J. (2009). *Assessing and measuring caring in nursing and health sciences* (2nd ed.). New York, NY: Springer.

Watson, J., & Foster, R. (2003). The Attending Nurse Caring Model®: Integrating theory, evidence and advanced caring–healing therapeutics for transforming professional practice. *Journal of Clinical Nursing, 12*(3), 360–365.

Wellen, K. E., & Hotamisligil, G. S. (2005). Inflammation, stress, and diabetes. *Journal of Clinical Investigation, 115*(5), 1111–1119.

Wing, D. M. (1999). The aesthetics of caring: Where folk healers and nurse theorists converge. *Nursing Science Quarterly, 12*(3), 256–262.

SECTION III

Measurement and Interventions to Facilitate Caritas

9

Measurement of Caring in a Relationship-Based Care Model of Nursing

Georgia Persky, Jayne Felgen,
and John Nelson

*T*his chapter features two studies that implemented and tested patients' perceptions of caring during the implementation of the Relationship-Based Care (RBC) model. The first study reviews the statistically significant improvement over a 5-year time series study as RBC was implemented on 35 patient care units at New York-Presbyterian Hospital/Columbia University Medical Center (NYP/CU). Key findings suggest that the staff-led redesign of day-to-day point of care practice structures, coupled with enhanced role clarity, created an operational context that supported the concepts of caring as a core component of professional practice. The second study illustrates the usefulness of the Caring Factor Survey instrument as a baseline measure before implementing a caring-based care delivery system. It also provides insight into the application of RBC principles and concepts by several clinical professional departments.

> We experience the essence of care in the moment when one human being connects to another. When compassion and care are conveyed through touch, through a kind act, through competent clinical interventions, or through listening and seeking to understand the other's experience, a healing relationship is created. This is the heart of Relationship Based Care. (Koloroutis, 2004)

BACKGROUND

RBC is a professional practice model and a patient-family care delivery system that provides an effective operational blueprint from which committed leaders can achieve organizational transformation resulting in cultures of caring. The model, based on the work of Marie Manthey, presents a philosophy that espouses caring relationships at the heart of healing and the business of health care. Caring objectives are achieved through the intentional focus on the relationships that nurses and other clinical professionals create with patients, their families, their coworkers, and themselves.

This RBC model builds on prior successes with service excellence, process improvement, and Shared Governance initiatives as it focuses on realigning operational infrastructures with individual and organizational caring values. Because RBC is principle based, its concepts have application to all clinical and service support areas where patients and families may experience care. Through a shared decision-making process staff leaders engage their peers in translating these principles to actions in ways consistent with their unique clinical or operational work settings.

The RBC model includes seven dimensions: leadership, teamwork, professional practice, care delivery, resource-driven care, all within a caring and healing environment. Each dimension is linked with specific principles that the staff translates into action, which, in turn, are linked to the strategic vision, operational practices, and individual behaviors. The professional practice dimension is especially appropriate for nurses; increasingly, other clinical professionals are embracing them as well. This expansion of caring expectations and efforts by the entire health care team adds new meaning to teamwork and has the potential to positively impact the patient-family experience while enhancing professional practice.

In the end, a personal commitment on the part of caregivers to therapeutically use themselves in service to others is the most compelling feature of the RBC model. Individuals who make this commitment and engage each other in the systematic redesign of their operational reality collectively make it possible to create extraordinary caring experiences and a sustainable culture of caring.

VISION AND STRATEGY

Before embarking on a major organizational change of this type, it is important for organizational leaders to understand and be grounded in their personal and professional motivations for transformational change and manage their own mindset in an appreciative manner. To succeed, leaders are obliged to consider whether their motivations for implementing meaningful change are personal, career enhancing, or protective, or if they truly want to see and be the change that is necessary. Professional and organizational change takes vision, unwavering commitment, and intentional dedication to improving patient care. The driving force must be focused on patient and staff satisfaction and process improvements rather than on regulatory or reimbursement imperatives that loom large in the immediate future. Courteous behavior on the part of caregivers merely because it is a requirement of their job cannot be sustained over time. The leveraged vision of the organization requires inspiration by leaders and an organization that cherishes and supports patients and their caregivers in every decision—from the bedside to the boardroom.

The guiding principles of RBC are to preserve relationships across all roles and levels, and between all patient and therapeutic and service support departments. It is important to use appreciative inquiry in all discussions. In appreciative inquiry one appreciates what is working as a positive point of understanding before moving on to other opportunities for change. Using influence at all levels of the organization without relevance to position, title, or role enhances the development of the leader in each individual employee.

The RBC model is premised on developing healthy relationships and creating essential infrastructures where high-quality patient care can take place. The evolution of RBC in any organization is dependent on the staff and leadership working collaboratively to identify what is important in the operations of patient care and developing team-oriented plans to make care operational. This process was facilitated by Creative Health Care Management (CHCM), a health care consultation company that uses several educational and leadership programs during the implementation of RBC. These case studies examine the implementation of RBC at two different hospitals. Figure 9.1 illustrates and defines the seven primary dimensions for transformation of a health care delivery system.

INFRASTRUCTURE OF SHARED GOVERNANCE

In an effort to effectively implement Primary Nursing as the professional practice model, the concept of practice autonomy within an infrastructure of Shared Governance fosters the critical element of professional identity and meaning in the service of others. This action provides an opportunity for staff to examine their roles, reflect on their personal practices, and inspire them to seek to achieve a higher level of optimal patient care and caring. Through intensive education about the Shared Governance process and the concept of professional care, the staff creates a shared vision of care delivery on their unit. As part of the implementation of RBC at NYP/CU, unit practice councils evolved to become the localized governance council to represent the needs, sentiment, and vision of the entire unit staff.

Unit Practice Councils (UPC): The creation of UPCs and a two-way communication network enabled 100% of the staff to engage in translating the RBC principles into practice with a priority focus on the elements of Primary Nursing. All staff were expected to participate in translating the RBC principles into practice.

Coordination Council: This multidisciplinary steering team provides oversight and guidance to the staff during the initial and sustaining phases of the 5-year implementation. This council meets monthly with the UPC chairs from each unit and department and representatives of

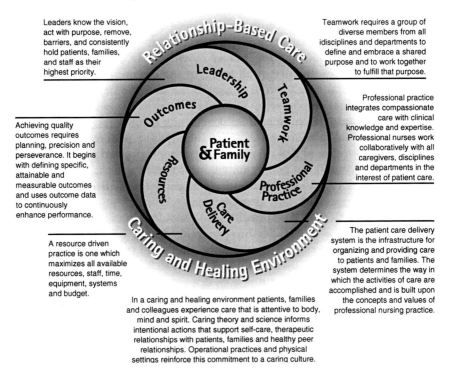

The central focus of Relationship-Based Care is the Patient & Family.
All care practices and priorities are organized around
the needs and priorities of patients and families.
Care is experienced when one human being connects with another.

Leaders know the vision, act with purpose, remove, barriers, and consistently hold patients, families, and staff as their highest priority.

Teamwork requires a group of diverse members from all idisciplines and departments to define and embrace a shared purpose and to work together to fulfill that purpose.

Achieving quality outcomes requires planning, precision and perseverance. It begins with defining specific, attainable and measurable outcomes and uses outcome data to continuously enhance performance.

Professional practice integrates compassionate care with clinical knowledge and expertise. Professional nurses work collaboratively with all caregivers, disciplines and departments in the interest of patient care.

A resource driven practice is one which maximizes all available resources, staff, time, equipment, systems and budget.

The patient care delivery system is the infrastructure for organizing and providing care to patients and families. The system determines the way in which the activities of care are accomplished and is built upon the concepts and values of professional nursing practice.

In a caring and healing environment patients, families and colleagues experience care that is attentive to body, mind and spirit. Caring theory and science informs intentional actions that support self-care, therapeutic relationships with patients, families and healthy peer relationships. Operational practices and physical settings reinforce this commitment to a caring culture.

FIGURE 9.1   Components of a relationship-based delivery system.
Reprinted with permission. © 2011 Creative Health Care Management, Inc.
www.chem.com

the six RBC committees. It is in this forum that innovation and exemplars are shared and ongoing support and education are provided.

   Committee Structure: In addition to the traditional Shared Governance and nursing practice councils, there are six operational councils that directly support an implementation of RBC and collectively represent the majority of members on the coordination council:

- *Caring and Healing Committee* researches, develops, and implements caring and healing practices for patient care generated by the UPCs or the nursing leadership council.

- *Education and Communication Committee* plans the educational needs of all stakeholders, including recruitment, hiring, orientation, and continuing education and ensures they incorporate RBC principles; this group also plans communication strategies that give voice to the goals, vision, and strategies and supports visibility of the RBC principles and implementation.

■ *Physician Relations Committee* engages physicians in the goal to achieve positive patient and family outcomes as well as design and implement strategies to ensure that each attending physician understands the primary nurse role and is provided with pertinent information about patients from the primary nurse.

■ *Integration Committee* collaboratively develops strategies to ensure that RBC principles and UPC innovations are incorporated at all organizational levels and are embedded into the daily fabric of the organization.

■ *Outcomes Committee* outlines the quality measurements needed to assess the status of the RBC implementation, reflecting clinical patient care, safety, and perceptual quality as perceived by patients, families, physicians, and staff and the depth of engagement of specific aspects of caring demonstrations.

■ *Service Support Committee* assesses, designs, and implements strategies to ensure that patients, families, and nurses have the appropriate resources and processes to receive and provide RBC. This committee engages the traditional support departments, for example, dietary, housekeeping, facilities, laundry, respiratory, and admitting.

Department Councils: To broaden the success of RBC, many other therapeutic and support departments have engaged in RBC and Shared Governance to improve the patient experience and staff satisfaction and process improvement within their department and toward positive support of patient care. The success within nursing has stimulated respiratory therapists, nutritionists, physical and occupational therapists, social workers, and pharmacists to apply the RBC professional principles to their practices as well. Attention to empowering the staff to redesign the operational infrastructure that drives practitioners and their practice can, and should, create the conditions for individual providers to show up in ways that are consistent with their intentions and that fully express all professional dimensions of their role. In addition, operational and support departments such as housekeeping, admitting, laundry, and dietary grow to be inspired and fully engaged when they are empowered to elect and develop their own councils and consider their essential role in patient care. These councils engage in intradepartmental quality improvement and support the intentions of Primary Nursing and caring in their contributions to patient care, thus creating one community within a hospital that is aligned to express the principles of RBC and Caritas.

EDUCATIONAL PROGRAMMING

RBC educational opportunities should occur on many organizational levels to ensure that adequate learning precedes action. All nursing and nursing support staff should receive an introduction and in-depth information about the RBC care delivery model and their role in the process to improve care and caring. Regardless of role, educational background, or title, if the care delivery system is to change and reflect professional practice, then everyone responsible for giving care in that environment must have expectations clearly articulated to support role clarity. Everyone deserves to appreciate where their contribution to patient care fits within an RBC model. Education must extend to other nursing practice support staff including nurse educators, clinical nurse specialists, and service line nurse practitioners so they learn how to support the nursing staff implementation. In addition to the Primary Nursing educational programs described in Chapter 5, the programs specific to RBC include an introduction to RBC, the UPC orientation and the RBC Leader Practicum attended by all nurse leaders involved in the RBC implementation.

■ *RBC Introduction*: All nursing and support staff on each unit are invited to participate in a 3-hour introduction about RBC, the goal of cultural transformation, and the concept of Shared Governance.
■ *UPC Orientation*: UPC members receive a 1-day orientation where the RBC implementation guide is reviewed and materials for further education are distributed. The UPCs work together to "Get Smart(er)" and share the learning from the RBC resources available. The orientation includes instruction on how to hold meetings, create an agenda, and take meeting minutes. The development of a communication network is compulsory because this is the venue by which all staff offer and receive feedback about the workings of the UPC and become engaged in planning changes to the care delivery system.
■ *RBC Leader Practicum*: This practical 5-day course provides RBC project leaders with the clarity and competence essential for assembling a collaborative team of change leaders. The program blends a variety of experiential methodologies to develop competencies, integrate learning relative to RBC, and design customized strategies and outcomes for the leaders' individual organizations. The experiential methodologies such as dynamic dialogue, circle and reflection, appreciative inquiry, and action learning ensure that participants are actively involved in the experience and apply their learning through presentations and group discussions.

Case Study 1:
New York-Presbyterian Hospital, New York, NY

Georgia Persky,
Jayne Felgen, and John Nelson

RELATIONSHIP-BASED CARE VISION

New York-Presbyterian Hospital (NYP) is a 2,450-bed academic medical center with five distinct campuses. New York-Presbyterian Hospital/Columbia University Medical Center (NYP/CU) is a 725-bed hospital with all adult, medical, and surgical specialties, including adult cardiac surgery, transplant, neuroscience, and medicine services. NYP/CU implemented the RBC professional practice model in 2006 to create a culture where all interdisciplinary processes support the nurse–patient relationship. This model of care delivery was selected and instituted with the intent to accomplish many objectives: heal and unify professional practice; enhance quality patient care; improve patient satisfaction; engage employees in a Shared Governance model; enhance collaboration and teamwork; focus on the point of care with multidisciplinary oversight; and, finally, to improve caregiver satisfaction and retention.

Implementing RBC at NYP/CU involved 35 patient care units and 10 therapeutic and support departments. The implementation was sequenced in "waves" of cohort groups made up of 8–10 inpatient and procedural units in "waves" every 6 months over the course of 3 years.

The Shared Governance vision at NYP is to be a world-class nursing organization and hospital empowered by a Shared Governance body that sustains a culture of excellence. The Department of Nursing believes that "Shared Governance and clinical decision making are achieved through *partnership, accountability, equity, and ownership* by nurses at the point of care."

INSPIRATION AND INFRASTRUCTURE

Due to the hospital's size and academic complexity, the RBC implementation plan departed from the CHCM suggested implementation of two or three well-supported patient care units or departments per wave or phase. Understanding that momentum and engagement might wane if completion went beyond 3 years, a decision was made to accelerate the normal implementation of this care delivery system with eight patient care units per wave for a total of six waves; a 6-month time line was designed for inspiration, education, and planning for each wave. A director of nursing was responsible for championing all UPC efforts during each wave. A program director and an operations analyst provided oversight to the coordination council and the six different implementation committees and each UPC. The program director and the operations analyst also provided support for the ongoing educational programming.

In an effort to implement Primary Nursing effectively as the professional practice model at NYP/CU, the concept of unit-based Shared Governance was first introduced. Peers elected each council and the chair and/or cochair. This infrastructure engaged point of care staff to participate in how the decisions about patient care delivery were to be considered and put into action. These plans were developed over the first 6 months and presented at a kickoff attended by all councils. These infrastructure changes occurred at NYP/CU through the implementation of RBC and the active engagement of localized Shared Governance councils to represent the needs, sentiment, and vision of the entire unit staff. The ability to improve practice and empowerment of staff to make decisions and learn how to improve their practice serves as an inspirational catalyst to enhance care and caring.

We observed many positive outcomes with the introduction of a defined patient care delivery model and professional practice model. Having a defined practice model was helpful in bringing staff together to identify their shared vision of how caring should occur among nurses. In turn, this inspired the creation of shared meaning and innovation in practice with nurses instrumental in sustaining such inspiration to improve the patient care experience. Here individuals and team members gained a renewed sense of purpose through mutual respect and social and cultural understanding. Again, the result was clear: higher motivation to improve patient care outcomes, patient satisfaction, and professional satisfaction (as evidenced by a shift in unit culture from required courtesy to genuine caring).

Staff is often asked to share their experiences of what intentional caring and professional practice have meant to them and their patients by identifying moments of excellence, storytelling, and letters of recognition sent by the patients about their experience. There has also been a transformational shift in the culture to extend and appreciate the relationships among coworkers on the units and across disciplines. This process has provided an opportunity for shared meaning to be created about the work, the patients served, and the environment in which this occurs. The end result is an environment where expectations are articulated for all staff, collaboration is celebrated, and care delivery that is centered on supporting professional practice is a priority.

In order to sustain the advances in practice and care delivery, nursing leadership continually supports elements of RBC. Nurse leaders at NYP/CU meet regularly with the UPCs individually and the UPC chairs within their division to share new information and exemplars. Nurse leaders discuss issues within their units in balancing and sharing governance so that decision making is not restrictive or laissez-faire. Walking patient-care-unit rounds occur with staff and the nursing leadership team to appreciate the operationalization of Primary Nursing. These same nurse leaders plan monthly meetings with chairs to hear ongoing developments and results through unit outcome dashboards and discuss barriers to care. Each year UPCs and their nurse leaders jointly develop goals and strategies.

Primary patient care delivery has been implemented in every inpatient and outpatient department where patient care occurs, from critical care to ambulatory care. Staff understands that Primary Nursing can occur in minutes in the emergency department, in hours in the operating room or clinic, or weeks in psychiatry and rehabilitation-medicine care units. It is further understood that this care delivery is organized not only around who "owns" the patient primarily, but also which caregiver has the intentional relationships with the patient and how the team organizes care around the patient and this caregiver.

True caring is not about the tasks you perform, but the spirit and love by which you deliver them. For this reason, caring and healing strategies for patients are continually generated and include unit welcome brochures, quiet times each shift so that patients can nap, bereavement baskets and sympathy cards for families of patients at the end of life, patient discharge calls, and hourly patient rounding to provide emotional safety by ensuring that the patient's needs are anticipated. Embracing the notion of the caregiver as a visitor to the patient experience shifts caregivers to understand that the hospital is the patient's home for a period and those who care for patients are the visitors to that experience.

Competence, confidence, and professional pride within a renewed emphasis on *professional practice* have changed the culture within this nursing department. More nurses now seek certification and advanced degrees, assist in developing patient care standards, and readily use the evidence available through the Internet. Many nurses are involved in research studies on their unit and proudly wear new white uniforms with a bright red "RN" embroidered emblem to be the nurse they want to be and help assure their patients that they can trust that they are receiving the best professional nursing care available.

Teamwork is not a skill caregivers learn in training and so it requires education and experiential guidance in sessions like Re-igniting the Spirit of Caring (RSC) for new caregivers or to foster a fresh start within disenfranchised groups. This RSC education has had a dramatic impact on each employee who attended these sessions as a person, colleague, and caregiver. With this opportunity individuals learn that they are not alone, that others care also. As individuals they are reminded that self-care and "friendship with oneself is all-important, because without it one cannot be friends with anyone else in the world" (Lash, 1987). As a team they receive a consistent message on care, care delivery, and professional practice for professionals from widely variable nursing school programs and walks of life. In an effort to socialize teams, many gestures and social events were encouraged to bring teams together as people to foster respect and caring for each other. The UPCs have fostered activities such as birthday acknowledgments; daily huddles to balance the patient care needs and resources; social events on the patient care units and planned events outside the hospitals such as picnics, bowling parties, and trips; improved staff lounges; and caring–healing events such as regularly scheduled masseuse and aromatherapy activities on patient care units for staff teams.

These accomplishments do not occur in a vacuum. For nurse leaders there should be balance when sharing responsibility, authority, and accountability with the nursing care team. Shared Governance is a dance and sometimes leaders stumble into a more rigid stance, and sometimes practice councils overstep their boundaries and lose their appreciative vision. The continuing challenge of needs and resources in patient care such as delivering on budgeted staffing guidelines on every shift and every day requires continuous attention. Today nurses understand that it is a shared responsibility to incorporate creativity and critical-thinking skills to optimize patient care in the moment, hour, or shift. Resources and needs must be triaged and common sense must prevail to ensure that the next most important patient need is met.

EDUCATION

Leading change requires leaders at every level of the organization to share the vision, lead with purpose, remove barriers, and model an intentional focus on patient care. For this reason every nurse leader attended a Leaders Empowering an Organization (LEO) seminar, which is a 3-day leadership retreat led by CHCM. In this session, these leaders learned practical models, skills, and strategies to empower and engage their staffs in the change process and to assist them in managing the shift in governance to a shared system. In addition, each Director of Nursing and Patient Care Manager attended a week-long RBC Practicum to provide an intensive experience on the theories and strategies they would need to know in order to lead an implementation of RBC in their division, department, or unit.

Measuring change is critical to understanding the efficacy of education and the implementation plan. Prior to implementation of RBC, and annually thereafter, each unit participated in a Healthcare Environment Survey (HES) to capture a baseline assessment of staff perceptions about their work environment; relationships among staff, support staff, and other disciplines; and reflections about workload, managerial support, and professional patient care. The results of the survey are shared with staff so that the information can assist with identifying strengths and weaknesses of the unit overall and of staff as individuals, colleagues, and the level of concern regarding patient care.

Assessing the work on each unit is the next step in the process for each UPC. This evaluation was accomplished through their direct engagement in a work complexity assessment. This intensive exercise allows the UPC to examine all of the technical and clinical interventions performed in its respective units with a tool that replaces work tasks with Nursing Intervention Classification (NIC) language. This exercise offers insight into issues related to complexity, intensity, acuity, and delegation of tasks/responsibilities. This is an important step in the implementation of a professional practice model, because it allows nurses to make an accurate assessment about the daily functions of staff on a particular unit, provides a sense of ownership of practice, and generates practical insight about how to reorganize their work to meet the standards of professional practice.

Once the foundation of practice examination was created, education about what constitutes professional practice began at NYP/CU. Book clubs were mobilized by the UPC to study *Relationship-Based Care: A Model for Transforming Health Care* (Koloroutis, 2004) and I_2E_2: *Leading Lasting Change* (Felgen, 2007). Although the staff was introduced to the RBC concept from the initiation of the process, a period of intensive education included the introduction to RBC. UPC orientation and RBC retreats for staff began in 2006 and continue to the present day. The UPCs immersed themselves into numerous multimedia educational resources such as the video "Primary Nursing: What It Is and What It Is Not," narrated by Marie Manthey, RN, and the book, *The Practice of Primary Nursing* by Marie Manthey (2002). These resources reinforced the concepts and tenets of true professional practice. Practical applications of the theory are discussed and reviewed in regular status checks with staff who monitored the progress of each implementation.

EVALUATION

At the center of all innovations in the hospital work environment is the precise measurement that will allow assessment of change over time. Examining the outcomes from such measures fosters a better understanding of variances in the workplace. Understanding the strengths and weaknesses of each work group (as well as the organizational climate/culture) and specific constructs will lead to a unit-based course correction and work stability, and support requirements to create a caring environment where quality patient care can thrive.

With such an integrated implementation, it is impossible to separate the evaluation and outcomes of an RBC implementation from the more specific Primary Nursing outcomes elucidated in Chapter 5. The Primary Nursing measures are directly assessed through the discharge questionnaires, Caring Factor Survey, specific subscales in the HES, and Primary Nursing self-assessment and exemplars. The RBC Evaluation Centers on more broad-based metrics such as the HES Survey Overall Nurse Satisfaction results and specifically the health care environmental support and nurse autonomy subscales. In addition, the Press Ganey Primary Nursing Self-Assessment and Patient Satisfaction Survey results and comments serve to highlight retrospective trends in specific patient-satisfaction areas to assist in understanding positive and negative trends in specific hospital services. Finally, electronic completion of postdischarge telephone calls is monitored (Table 9.1) on each unit to ensure that the attempt rate is high and that the call-completion rate (patient is actually reached) is continually improved. The discharge-call comments of patients assist in understanding patients' perceptions of caring in three ways: (1) they are a more timely (1–3 days postdischarge) way of understanding a patient's perceptions of care while the patient is still known to the caregiver; (2) they are a means to continually inspire staff by the very positive patient response to their call and caring beyond discharge; and (3) they provide a review of patients' health status and frequently important corrections to their understanding of discharge instructions or referrals to their health provider.

At NYP/CU there are many measures to estimate the impact of implementing RBC on caring and patient and staff satisfaction and the

TABLE 9.1   NYP/CU Discharge Call Volume, Fourth Quarter 2010

HISTORICAL DATA	# DISCHARGES	% PATIENTS ATTEMPTED	% PATIENTS COMPLETED
Inpatient overall - October	2,477	93.2%	57.5%
Inpatient overall - November	2,248	91.7%	58.4%
Inpatient overall - December	2,334	85.6%	51.9%
Emergency Dept. - October	4,657	71.8%	48.9%
Emergency Dept. - November	4,481	81.9%	62.3%
Emergency Dept. - December	4,489	84.9%	58.0%
AmbSurg - October	999	83.8%	53.2%
AmbSurg - November	1,112	79.1%	54.8%
AmbSurg - December	976	80.6%	58.0%

implementation of Primary Nursing and care quality outcomes. The staff and patient satisfaction measures have been analyzed independently as well as the relationship of patient perceptions of caring. Some of these measures and the results are described next.

Healthcare Environment Survey (HES)

The HES was selected over the other instruments because it is the most complete work environment instrument compared to other instruments and is sensitive to all work environment disciplines. The electronic format facilitates staff access, completion, and data analysis. At NYP/CU, the HES was used to provide pre- and postimplementation information prior to implementing the new care delivery model, RBC, within 35 inpatient care units and procedural departments. A total of 1,050 nurses were surveyed before and after implementation of RBC using the HES. This survey captures a baseline of staff perceptions about their work environment, including the relationships among staff, support staff, and other disciplines; reflections about workload, managerial support, and professional patient care; and the most essential aspects of the work environment. The results of the survey are shared with staff so that the information generated by the survey can assist with identifying strengths and weaknesses of the staff as a whole. This activity is repeated each year postimplementation to identify any changes in perceptions, identify improvements in staff satisfaction, and highlight any areas requiring further attention such as interdisciplinary relationships. Figure 9.2 reveals the change scores of all respondents from baseline to end of the first year of RBC implementation. Each of the 5 "waves" represents 5–8 units. Change scores were calculated by subtracting the baseline score from the score after year 1. It is noted that all waves had a varied response to RBC with each wave reporting its own successes and remaining needs. It is noted in Figure 9.2 that there are extremely positive as well as negative scores. Parato mathematics were used to understand what the demographics or themes were within these extreme scores to understand actionable change.

Press Ganey Patient Satisfaction

Satisfaction, the ultimate patient outcome, is understood in the literature as influenced by two factors: by an individual patient's perceptions of care and health status and by the volume and demand of other patients on the unit who compete for provider time and attention to care. In addition, health status, morbidity, and mortality are important clinical predictors that can negatively influence patient satisfaction.

The patient satisfaction survey was first developed by Press Ganey Associates in 1987 and was revised in 1997 to a 49-item, self-administered

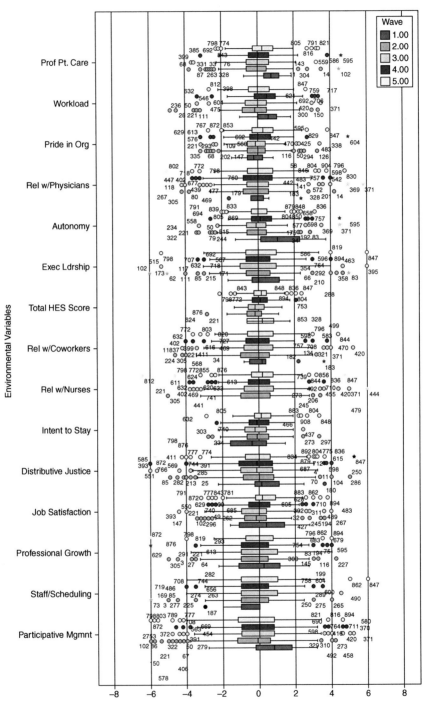

FIGURE 9.2 Pre-post RBC change scores, all HES variables.

survey with a 5-point Likert-type response scale. It was revised in 2007 to correlate with the federally required Healthcare Assessment Patient Satisfaction (HCAPS) survey and was reduced from 49 to 38 items that consisted of 10 internally consistent subscales. Response choices for each question are: "very poor," "poor," "fair," "good," and "very good." The results of this survey are reported as a percentile for each item and an overall average is calculated. Patient satisfaction is measured at NYP using the Press Ganey inpatient survey, which is mailed to all patients who are discharged to their home from NYP. The survey data represent the patients' perceptions of the overall quality of care they received during their hospital stay. This instrument assisted in evaluating not only changes in patient satisfaction but also the impact of RBC.

Over the past 5 years, the Press Ganey overall score (Table 9.2) has improved between two and six points in every area, which is dramatic, considering that most hospitals working to improve patient satisfaction scores advance, on average, one point per year. Clearly RBC has had a major impact on organizational climate; professional culture; and caring among caregivers for themselves, their colleagues, and their patients.

INTEGRATED OUTCOMES DASHBOARD

An outcomes dashboard (Table 9.3) was created by the outcomes committee to create a visual tool for nursing staff to monitor how a professional practice environment impacts the total patient care experience. This graph includes information collected from the discharge questionnaire cards as well as information about patient satisfaction trending and compliance with best practices on the unit. RBC also does impact nursing quality indicators, which are trended separately on nursing dashboards on each unit. This information is included as part of the quarterly report that units are expected to present at the coordination council meetings and also as a tool for communication with other members of the team in the progress of the defined, professional practice evaluation.

UPCs are encouraged to share this information in regular staff meetings to inform their peers of their progress and also as part of their constant reevaluation of the work of the UPC. The dashboard is designed to tell the story of the transformation of unit-based practice and growth of nursing professional practice for each particular unit. In addition, communicating information about clinical outcomes, nursing quality of care, patient satisfaction, and staff satisfaction, which are routinely a part of the Shared Governance appraisal of the work environment, creates shared meaning, commitment, clarity, and inspiration about the work performed.

TABLE 9.2 NYP/CU Press Ganey Results, 2006–2010

QUESTION	MAY 2006 TO APRIL 2007 (N* = 5337)	MAY 2007 TO APRIL 2008 (N* = 4884)	MAY 2008 TO APRIL 2009 (N* = 5067)	BASELINE MAY 2009 TO APRIL 2010 (N* = 5838)	MAY 2010 TO JANUARY 2011 (N* = 4160)
Std overall	80.8	81.4	82.9	83.3	84.2
Std nurses	84.4	85.1	86.1	87.1	87.4
Friendliness/courtesy of the nurses [H]	88.8	89.5	90.1	90.8	91.1
Promptness response to call [H]	81.5	82.0	82.8	84.1	84.9
Nurses' attitude toward requests	85.3	85.9	87.1	88.1	88.2
Attention to special/personal needs [H]	82.7	83.8	85.1	85.9	86.2
Nurses kept you informed [H]	82.0	82.6	83.9	85.1	85.6
Skill of the nurses	87.5	87.9	89.0	89.7	90.1
Staff concern for your privacy	82.5	83.1	84.7	85.1	85.3
How well your pain was controlled [H]	83.6	84.0	85.4	85.5	85.9
Staff addressed emotional needs	78.9	79.7	81.2	82.0	82.8
Response concerns/complaints	77.5	78.4	80.1	80.4	81.5
Staff include decisions re: treatment	80.6	81.0	82.2	83.0	83.7
Staff worked together to care for you	85.5	86.0	87.7	88.2	88.6
Noise level in and around room [H]	70.8	73.0	75.4	75	74.7

KEY (for shading)

Baseline
Gain since Baseline (+0.5 - 1.0)
Gain since Baseline (+1.0 - 2.0)
Gain since Baseline (+2.0 - 3.0)
Gain since Baseline (> 3.0)

Note: N* = Response to overall item; H = Hospital Consumer Assessment of Healthcare Providers and Systems (HCAHPS) measures.

TABLE 9.3 NYP/CU Integrated Unit Dashboard

UNIT: *ENTER UNIT NAME*

PRIMARY NURSING:	2008	2009	Q1 2010	APR '10	MAY '10	JUN '10	Q2 2010	JUL '10	AUG '10	SEP '10	Q3 2010
Primary nurse known by name											
How well patient needs were met											

Press Ganey: Patient Satisfaction

Indicator:	2008	Q4 2009	2009	Q1 2010	Q2 2010	JUL '10	AUG '10	SEP '10	Q3 2010	OCT '10	NOV '10
Overall Patient Satisfaction											
Nurses Overall											
Friendliness/courtesy of the nurses											
Promptness response to call											
Nurses' attitude toward requests											
Attention to special/personal needs											
Nurses kept you informed											
Skill of the nurses											
Staff worked together to care for you											
How well your pain was controlled											
Noise level in and around room											
Staff addressed emotional needs											
2nd MIB Indicator											

(continued)

TABLE 9.3 (*continued*)

Length of Stay (LOS) Performance Analysis:		JAN '10	FEB '10	MAR '10	APR '10	MAY '10	JUN '10	JUL '10	AUG '10	SEP '10
Discharges										
Case Mix Index (CMI)										
Actual LOS (ALOS)										
Expected LOS (ELOS)										
Discharge Phone Calls:	2009	JAN '10	FEB '10	MAR '10	APR '10	MAY '10	JUN '10	JUL '10	AUG '10	SEP '10	OCT '10
Number of calls made											
Number of patients reached											
Clinical Data:	2009	JAN '10	FEB '10	MAR '10	APR '10	MAY '10	JUN '10	JUL '10	AUG '10	SEP '10	OCT '10
Hand hygiene											
Unit-acquired pressure ulcers											

THE ONGOING JOURNEY

"Transformational leadership occurs when one or more persons engage with others in such a way that leaders and followers raise one another to higher levels of motivation and morality" (Burns, 1978). Key to any cultural transformation is the continuing focus on nurturing, sustaining, and cultivating the evolution of change. Caring can only heal in an environment that supports healthy relationships with the patient and among caregivers. RBC has been implemented now on 35 patient care units at NYP and integration continues within each and every patient care unit. At the unit level, new staff and nurse leaders receive consistent orientation and education as their peers did during the implementation. UPC attrition is attended to with an orientation to the concepts by the chair or a member of the council. Attrition is recognized as healthy evolution in the UPC and allows for the development of new champions and new ideas within each unit as well as allows former members to mentor their peers.

The Department of Nursing and Social Services continues to support and develop RBC implementation within centralized patient-centered departments such as respiratory therapy, social services, admitting and registration, food and nutrition, and patient transport. The internal and external environment has evolved from 2006 through the present by engaging unit and department councils to improve patient care and work processes. Within this council structure, the environment is continually reviewed for gaps in care, care processes and standards, and support services. It is through the internal networking of staff on each unit with the councils and the network of council chairs at the monthly coordination councils that improvements are developed and exemplars are shared.

As the nurse evolves in his or her role as the primary nurse and the infrastructure to support patient care improves, so does caring and support for the patient. At NYP, we have restored the core values and practices of caring back into our hospital. Nurse educators and leaders are better prepared to coach caring behaviors. Through a better understanding of the Caritas behaviors, we are better able to continually educate and support nurses on caring competencies "in the moment" with each patient interaction.

> To love what you do. . .to know that it matters. . .How can there be greater joy? (Koloroutis, 2009)

Case Study 2:
Avera Health, South Dakota

Darcy Sherman-Justice, Jill Rye, and Nancy L. Fahrenwald

*A*vera McKennan Hospital and University Health Center is sponsored by the Benedictine and Presentation Sisters and is a member of the Avera Health system. Avera Health comprises nearly 300 locations including hospitals, long-term care facilities, and physician practices located in 95 communities in five Midwestern states. Avera McKennan Hospital and University Health Center has a rich 100-year history of a strong, Christian mission focused on treating each patient in a Christ-like manner. The Avera Health system is guided by the gospel values of compassion, hospitality, and stewardship. The Christian mission has long been a strength that is used to recruit and retain nurses to work at the organization.

In response to the demands for quality patient outcomes and improved patient satisfaction, Avera McKennan embraced two new hospital-wide initiatives in 2004–2005. The first initiative, Process Excellence through LEAN Projects, was an effort to increase efficiency and decrease waste. LEAN principles focus on improving processes by giving the nursing and hospital staff the ability to provide standardized, quality care in the most efficient manner (Kimsey, 2010). The second initiative was Baptist Institute's Service Excellence. Its goal was to implement best practices to improve customer satisfaction (Freifeld, 2009). These two initiatives fit into the organization's strategic plan, which included a focus on improved patient satisfaction and increased efficiency, achieved through five service excellence keys (quality, people, financial stewardship, ministry, and service). The LEAN processes delivered improved efficiencies and cost savings throughout the organization; however, there were varied successes in patient satisfaction. The administrative council for the organization then made the decision to embrace relationship-based care (RBC), and the organization remains committed to improving patient satisfaction by further enhancing the patient and family experience. RBC intertwines customer service and patient- and family-centered care along with caring for team and self (Koloroutis, 2004).

THE RBC JOURNEY

Avera McKennan's RBC journey is chronicled in this section, including a description of the process and the current successes and lessons learned. The RBC journey established its roots in 1993 when the organization formed the first nurse governance councils (NGCs), which are in place today. The NGCs developed the nursing mission and vision based on tenets of Jean Watson's caring theory. Watson's theory focuses on the relationship created when the caregiver interacts with the patient and sees that person as a unique individual. This caring process is described as an interconnection between the one caring and the one being cared for (Koloroutis, 2004, p. 31). Throughout the years the nurse-based councils met at the unit level and sent one representative to a hospitalwide committee. These councils began to practice inconsistently and struggled to solve the emerging patient needs in a rapidly changing health care environment. The increased complexity of patient needs required an interdisciplinary team approach. The all-nurse unit-based council structure could no longer meet these needs.

The organization's nursing leadership maintained a working relationship with Creative Health Care Management (CHCM) and Marie Manthey throughout these years. This was important to the organization as changes in the health care environment continued to evolve. In 2009, a CHCM consultant was invited to the organization to deliver a presentation describing RBC. Over 200 nurses were invited to attend the inspirational and energizing description of RBC. The feedback from the staff who attended the presentation included: "We CANNOT NOT do this, continue to educate the organization as a whole on the model of Relationship Based Care." The message proved to be a catalyst for the organization to continue to improve care and raise the bar on the patient experience. Also, RBC fit naturally into the organization's mission, vision, and values. The approach was adopted as the method by which the organization would strive to achieve its vision for enhanced quality care and an improved patient care experience. The chief nursing officer (CNO) and nursing leaders attended several conferences to gain knowledge on how to implement, RBC in the organization. The decision to implement RBC occurred during a challenging time. Shrinking Medicare and Medicaid reimbursements, coupled with a mission to provide care to all, regardless of ability to pay, left the organization financially challenged. Implementing a new initiative required the vision and support of the CNO and the leadership team. Securing additional funds for a nonbudgeted initiative was a bold request; however, the CNO was passionate about improving the patient experience. Support for implementation of RBC was secured.

Two leaders were selected to receive additional training to facilitate the implementation of RBC. Their enthusiasm and commitment to the effort accelerated the momentum. An RBC results council was organized from throughout the organization and six facilitators were selected to lead 3-day "Reigniting the Spirit of Caring" retreats. When the infrastructure for RBC was in place, the organization was able to take the steps necessary to implement the process. Eight units or departments were selected to be in implementation wave 1. These areas included: acute rehabilitation, neonatal intensive care, adult intensive care, cardiopulmonary, neurology, case management, behavioral health services (BHS) acute adult, and BHS adolescents. These areas formed interdisciplinary unit-based councils. Education was provided on the three core RBC relationships: caring for patients and families, care for self, and care for team. The principles of authority, accountability, and responsibility were described and they began working on how to implement RBC on their unit. Figure 9.3 outlines the RBC implementation timetable.

BEGINNING THE RBC PROCESS AT THE UNIT LEVEL

Staff from wave 1 units attended the "Reigniting the Spirit of Caring" workshops, which focused on caring for self, caring for team, and caring for patients and families. Time was built in to allow participants to reflect on why they chose health care as a profession, how to maintain their passion and energy for the work, and how to care for self. One of the most favorable elements of the retreat involved former patients and family members who shared their personal experiences of caring when they were patients at Avera McKennan. The participants listened to the stories of patients and families and discovered new insights into how caring interactions impacted their hospital experience. The staff that participated in the 3-day workshop evaluated the education regarding RBC as excellent. Comments included: "I am forever changed from this experience"; "I am reenergized"; "It helped me focus on the need to care for myself so I can care for others"; and "Hearing from patients about what their experience was like helped me understand what I could personally do to make it better."

BASELINE ASSESSMENT OF CARING FACTORS

Prior to launch of the RBC initiative on the wave 1 nursing care units, a profile of patients' perceptions of caring nurses was examined using the 10-item Caring Factor Survey (CFS) developed by Nelson (2009). The instrument was derived from a 20-item CFS also developed by Nelson (2006). The scale includes one item to measure each of the caring factors from Watson's theory. Items explore patients' perceptions of the care received from nurses who indicated a conscious approach to caring for them as a whole person, including the unity of body-mind-spirit. The scale reflects Watson's most recent theory of Caritas, which includes and

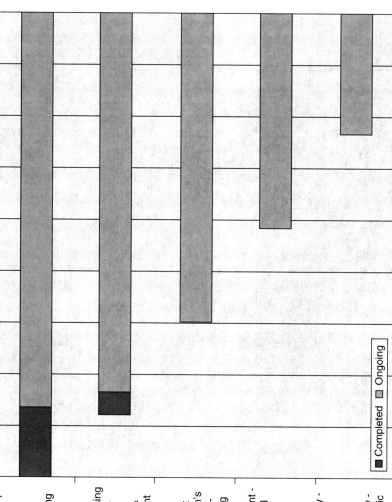

FIGURE 9.3 Relationship-based care implementation.

extends the original Carative Factors as the core of professional nursing (Watson, n.d.). The instrument employs a 1–7 Likert response scale with options that ranged from *strongly agree* (= 7) to *strongly disagree* (= 1). There is a neutral response option (= 4). The 10-item CFS has a strong estimate of internal consistency (Cronbach's α = 0.93) in a population of acute care patients (Nelson, 2009).

This study used a descriptive cross-sectional design. After institutional review board approval, all patients or family member proxies who were discharged from the wave 1 patient care were invited to participate in the study on the day of discharge. A letter that explained the study was given to the patient and family by the clinical nurse educator or alternate caregiver on the unit. Informed consent was implied by completing the survey.

BASELINE ASSESSMENT FINDINGS

There were 126 baseline surveys completed. The overall mean score was 5.67 (±1.92). Mean responses (±SD) to the 10 items within the scale are provided in Table 9.4. The baseline findings indicate a high level of caring in the wave 1 units. A follow-up survey is administered on the units 6 months after the launch of the RBC initiative.

RBC IMPLEMENTATION STRATEGIES

Implementation of RBC across the different wave 1 units varied according to the ideas and strategies proposed by the staff and the unit councils. The following subsections provide an overview of implementation strategies.

REHABILITATION NURSING UNIT

The rehabilitation unit was included in the first wave to implement RBC. The rehabilitation unit serves patients after serious illness or injury. Patients admitted to the unit may have experienced traumatic brain injury, stroke, spinal cord injury, amputation, or multiple trauma. They are cared for in an interdisciplinary team environment. The team members include physical therapy, occupational therapy, speech therapy, community integration, social services, physiatrist, and rehabilitation nursing. The goals for each patient are established in the first three days after admission; these goals are posted in patients' rooms and are changed weekly as patients achieve their goals and set new ones. The therapists and nurses meet daily to discuss patient status, progress, and any medical changes that may affect progress toward their established goals. The unit encourages families to participate in care, and all activities are tailored to help patients achieve their goals.

TABLE 9.4 Caring Factor Survey Item Responses (N = 126)

SURVEY ITEM	MEAN ± STD DEVIATION
1. Every day I am here, I see that the care is provided with loving kindness.	5.67 (±1.92)
2. As a team, my caregivers are good at creative problem solving to meet my individual needs and requests.	5.89 (±1.83)
3. The care providers honored my own faith, helped instill hope, and respected my belief system as part of my care.	5.54 (1.99)
4. When my caregivers teach me something new, they teach me in a way that I can understand.	5.75 (1.97)
5. My caregivers encouraged me to practice my own individual, spiritual beliefs as part of my self-caring and healing.	5.26 (1.97)
6. My caregivers have responded to me as a whole person, helping to take care of all my needs and concerns.	5.90 (±1.85)
7. My caregivers have established a helping and trusting relationship with me during my time here.	5.82 (±1.90)
8. My health care team has created a healing environment that recognizes the connection between my body, mind, and spirit.	5.67 (±1.83)
9. I feel like I can talk openly and honestly about what I am thinking because those who are caring for me embrace my feelings, no matter what my feelings are.	5.71 (1.86)
10. My caregivers are accepting and supportive of my beliefs regarding a higher power, which allows for the possibility of me and my family to heal.	5.24 (±1.99)

Staff members attended the 3-day "Reigniting the Spirit of Caring" education as well as a retreat day that focused on the specifics of RBC and described the formation of a new unit-based practice council. A nurse and occupational therapist agreed to cochair this new council and lead the new council members through the work of implementing the specifics of RBC.

The practice council did a great job of establishing communication networks and getting feedback from their colleagues about implementing RBC. Therapy and nursing teams began to form and primary nurses were assigned to both therapy and nursing teams. New admissions to the rehabilitation unit were placed on teams according to their therapy and nursing needs. While a patient's discharge was being planned, those teams prepared for new patient admissions. Patients' rooms were transformed into supply rooms or therapy offices so the teams would be closer to their patients' rooms. The goal for each team was to establish a relationship with the patient and family consistently throughout their stay. Some of the challenges the council worked through early in the process were how to best keep the teams in balance as several patients were discharged from the same teams. The biggest challenge with consistency was the 12-hour nursing schedule. The rotating 12 day/night schedule made it difficult to know what team they may have worked with earlier in the week. To help solve that issue, the nurse manager altered work schedules around the team framework. Each nurse was assigned a team, which helped when the primary nurses and resource nurses made the assignments for the next shift. The nurses would be assigned to their team and help maintain patient and family relationships.

The unit continues to work on consistency by assigning patients to teams with fewer patients or with planned discharges. The practice council continues to meet monthly to discuss feedback from the staff and make any needed changes in the process. They are more intentional about caring for each other and caring for themselves by ensuring that each staff member has had a break during the day, or checking with coworkers to see if they need assistance. The "Commitment to CoWorkers" document written by Marie Manthey is posted at the nurses' station (Koloroutis, 2004). It provides a daily reminder that our individual conduct and actions impact the unit environment. The rehabilitation unit is committed to continue the goal to provide excellent care to patients and families who require acute rehabilitation.

The rehabilitation unit created three teams, each with a primary nurse/patient care coordinator, associate nurse, physical therapist, occupational therapist, speech therapist, and social worker. The nurses' station is decentralized to place teams in closer proximity to patients. Before scheduling a patient to a team, therapy and nursing staff discuss which team can best meet an individual patient's needs. The rehabilitation physicians are changing their clinic patient times to schedule time to make rounds with their teams at the bedside. This change allows time for the patient and family to discuss any questions or concerns about their care, goals, and discharge plan.

NURSE CASE MANAGEMENT

Case management restructured its department into three areas. The first area is the admission specialist who makes sure that patients are in the correct admission status and reviews all patients in observation status. The second area is the physician-based case managers who are assigned to physician groups and follow patients throughout their stay in all patient care areas. This model has already been in place for about 10 years and has been very successful and satisfying for physicians because they have one "go-to" person who knows the patients well. The physician-based case managers make rounds with physicians and coordinate the patients' plans of care among the multiple physicians. They meet one-on-one with the patient and family to develop a relationship with them and to identify any needs and concerns regarding their hospital stay and discharge plan. They also run interdisciplinary rounds and insurance reviews and provide financial information to patients and families.

Case management has also developed a new, third area: the clinical documentation specialist who reviews charts to ensure that physicians are documenting a clear picture of the clinical course for each patient.

The case management RBC team continues to meet monthly to make changes in its practice from staff and physician feedback. The goals for this group include evaluating the physician groups to ensure that there is appropriate coverage and enhancing the interdisciplinary round documentation. The team meets with other nursing units to discuss how to further enhance the patient experience and ensure that needs are met.

BEHAVIORAL HEALTH SERVICES (BHS), ADULT UNIT

The RBC plan for the BHS adult unit was to assign nurses and social workers to work as a team with psychiatrists. It kept its concept of nurse/technician teams in which one nurse and one technician are typically assigned a group of patients. A primary nurse is assigned within 12 hours of admission and the same nurse is responsible for completing treatment goals and a "My Story" form with each patient within 24 hours. White boards were added to patient rooms to identify the primary nurse and nurse/technician team for that shift, and documentation times were changed from set times to one time per shift. The unit's hope is to develop better continuity of care and improved relationships with families. An additional goal is to ensure that the staff care for themselves and each other by taking a break when needed throughout the day. The physicians appreciate knowing which nurse to contact for patient and family concerns. The teams monitor their success via patient and staff satisfaction survey results.

CONCLUSION

Avera McKennan remains committed to the continued implementation of RBC. The positive responses from the wave 1 staff, along with their commitment to creating a stronger caring environment, have served as an inspiration to continue the journey. The process will continue to be evaluated to ensure that we realize the goals of RBC. Follow-up evaluation of patient perceptions of caring will take place 6 months after launch of the RBC initiative in the wave 1 units.

REFERENCES

Felgen, J. (2007). I_2E_2: *Leading lasting change.* Bloomington, IN: Creative Health Care Management.

Freifeld, L. (2009). Highway to health. *Training, 46*(4), 52–54.

Kimsey, D. B. (2010). Lean methodology in health care. *AORN Journal, 92*(1), 53–60. doi: 10.1016/j.aron.201.01.0105

Koloroutis, M. (2004). *Relationship-based care a model for transforming practice.* Minneapolis, MN: Creative Healthcare Management.

Lash, J. (1987, Spring). Eleanor Roosevelt: Joseph Lash's "Eternal Mother." *Biography, 10,* 107.

Manthey, M. (1990). *Primary Nursing: What it is and is not [VHS tape].* Minneapolis MN: Creative Health Care Management.

Manthey, M. (2002). *The practice of Primary Nursing* (2nd ed.). Minneapolis, MN: Creative Health Care Management.

Nelson, J. W. (2006). *Annual business report.* Minneapolis, MN: Healthcare Environment.

Nelson, J. W. (2009). *Relationship based care symposium.* Paper presented at the annual meeting of Sigma Theta Tau, International, Indianapolis, IN. Retrieved from http://www.stti.iupui.edu/PP07/chcmpresentations/Nelson,%20John.pdf

Watson, J. University of Health Sciences School of Nursing. Retrieved January 3, 2011, from http://www.ucdenver.edu/academics/colleges/nursing/caring/caringinaction/Pages/ThePracticeofCaritas.aspx

10

Integrating Human Caring Science Into a Professional Nursing Practice Model

Karen Neil Drenkard

*C*urrent supply and demand projections for registered nurses (RNs) in the United States paint a picture with many gaps. Efforts have been directed to increasing the supply of nurses through increasing enrollments and increasing the number of new graduate nurses. Challenges, such as faculty shortages, exacerbate the problem, hampering the hard work that has been directed at increasing the number of students so that the subsequent supply of nurses is increased. The other half of the equation is improving the retention rate of nurses, especially in hospitals across the country. The nurse leader is required to pay attention to the work environment and improve the ability of nurses to provide care. This has become more of an imperative for this generation's nursing leaders to impact and improve nursing retention.

Nursing care in hospitals requires a framework of a professional nursing practice model, which is necessary as a foundation for care delivery. The professional nursing practice model needs to include a philosophy of nursing care and be based on a theory of practice that resonates with all of the nurses in the practice site. The nurses executive, working in partnership with the clinicians at the bedside, have a privileged opportunity to give substantive meaning to the philosophy of nursing and mission statement regarding the caring nature of nursing. "A well developed nursing conceptual framework that explicitly grounds nursing service and communicates the uniqueness of nursing as well as its connection to the other sectors of the health care system is the foundation for successful integration of theory into practice."[1] This chapter shares the results of a multiyear Health Resources and Services Administration (HRSA)-funded grant aimed at reducing work intensity for hospital nurses and creating a human caring environment in the acute care workplace.

BACKGROUND

Inova Health System is a nonprofit, integrated health care system in northern Virginia that consists of five hospitals, two long-term care facilities, emergency care centers, and ambulatory services (including mental health and rehabilitation services) that serve a population of almost two million people. Each hospital and the continuum of care services have a chief nurse, and a system chief nurse serves as the corporate representative of nursing at the highest executive level. The system chief nurse has responsibility for strategy and oversight of nursing practice, education, and research across the system.

As part of the nursing strategic planning process, Inova Health System chose to base its nursing practice on a nursing theory, and planned to develop a professional nursing practice model that captured the essence of an American Nurses Credentialing Center (ANCC) Magnet Recognition Program hospital system. The nursing executive team went through a process of reviewing and examining the many nursing theories during a strategic planning process, and used shared governance strategies to engage staff in the decision-making process. Goals and measurement of the theory-based practice model included the improvement of nursing retention.

Through multiple focus groups and open forums, the decision was made to implement a human caring model of care. The philosophy of care was based on caring science, as conceptualized by Jean Watson.[2-4] Watson's[3] work included the identification of 10 caring factors, and has resulted in formal attention to "nursing theory as the disciplinary foundation for nursing science, education and practice." Watson[3] describes the process where any "nurse–patient encounter can be considered a caring occasion or caring moment, if it is conscious, intentional orientation based on humanistic values of kindness, empathy, concern and love." The nurse is described as the guide to the creation of a healing environment and the main therapeutic element in creating this environment for the patient.[5,6] In this caring science environment, "nursing contributes to the preservation of humanity and seeks to sustain caring in instances where it is threatened."[3]

The nursing leadership at Inova engaged the staff in creating a vision for the application of a human caring model. The staff nurses began the work of making the vision a reality. They quickly realized that to create a caring and healing environment, the care units needed to streamline "hassle factors"[7] and gain time back at the bedside to care more directly for patients. What began as a linear process of implementing a philosophy and model of care became a complex interactive process of work that took place over a 4-year time period.

The need to streamline work processes and provide nurses with more time to create a healing environment was a turning point for the work that was ahead. How could the nursing units implement a human caring model if the nurses were "too busy" to engage in the transformation? What strategies and opportunities did this present to the nursing leadership team?

OPPORTUNITIES IDENTIFIED

To create a healing environment, it was clear that the first step was to streamline some of the work processes, reduce work intensity, and eliminate some hassle factors for the nurses. Inova Health System applied for a HRSA grant as part of the Division of Nursing and Bureau of Health Profession, Health Resources and Services Administration, Department of Health and Human Services. Inova received a 4-year, $685,000 award to improve work processes so that a human caring model could be implemented across four hospitals. The project was called "Making Time for Caring." The chief nurse of the system was participating in a Robert Wood Johnson Executive Nurse Fellowship, and used funding that was allocated as part of the fellowship. The chief nurse executive applied these project funds for the dissemination of data and training materials to the nursing leadership community.

LITERATURE REVIEW

A review of the literature provides both methods and processes for engaging in decreasing work intensity to allow nurses more time actually to care for patients. One of the fundamental questions for nursing leadership is: If nurses are able to streamline their work processes, how can one use that time positively to impact nursing practice? This research project hypothesized that if work intensity was reduced, that would free up more time for the nurse to be present at the patient's side, allowing for more time for caring activities. Research is beginning to emerge that suggests that a core factor of a nurse's identity is the ability to respond to patient caring needs.[8] Constant interruptions and chaos in the care setting is a barrier to caring.

To assist nurses who are looking to redesign patient care delivery, the American Organization of Nurse Executives has identified key components of any research activities to examine work processes. They suggest evaluation components that include the determination and collection of baseline data to analyze productivity and then using that data to measure progress toward improvement of productivity.[9] Tools for work sampling are available to assist in this process.[10] Other multisite projects such as Robert Wood Johnson Foundation's Transforming Care at the Bedside, support the assumption that taking the time to figure out what is wrong with care processes and then doing something about it is key to reducing work intensity and designing new processes of care.[11] Responses to streamlining the work of the nurse include innovative approaches to eliminating hunting and gathering activities, and simplifying documentation.[12] Beaudoin and Edgar[7] identified a methodology for assisting in the identification and elimination of hassle factors in an inpatient care unit, and began the link between these hassles and the human cost of inefficiency.

As a result of the literature review, and in response to staff feedback, it became clear that a two-phased approach is required to be successful in implementing a nursing professional practice model based on human caring theory. Phase I involved improving staff nurse satisfaction by decreasing work intensity. Phase II implemented a human caring environment with a goal of reducing nurse turnover and increasing satisfaction of both patients and nurses. By separating the effort into two distinct phases, nurses could see that their request for a streamlined work environment was being met before the implementation of a human caring model. This two-phased approach proved to be an effective strategy in gaining the support of the staff nurses who desired to have more time to interact with their patients, but perceived that they did not have the time to do so.

PURPOSE

The objective of the HRSA Nursing Retention Grant was to improve nurse satisfaction and retention by decreasing work intensity, streamlining cumbersome nursing processes, and creating a human caring environment in the workplace. The study engaged and involved staff nurses in the process.

STUDY DESIGN

This study was a quasiexperimental, between-subjects, naturalistic, longitudinal study on four pilot medical units and four surgical comparison units at Inova Health System. Inova Health System Institutional Review Board (IRB) approval was obtained. The unit of study was the patient care unit, rather than the individuals within the unit, and participants in the groups being compared were different people over time. The units were not randomly selected.

METHODS

The four medical units were chosen across four hospitals. Selection variables that were considered include leadership stability, current nursing vacancy and turnover rates, hours per patient day, and patient complexity.

Four surgical units across the four hospitals were chosen as comparison units, and these units had no interventions during the study period. Preliminary data collection took place before any intervention, and included assessment of nursing turnover rates, patient and staff satisfaction scores, and RN satisfaction indicators from the National Database for Nursing Quality Indicators (NDNQI) data set. There were two phases of the study. Phase I was a process improvement phase where work intensity was decreased on the pilot units, resulting in more time available for staff nurses to provide direct patient care. Phase II was the implementation of caring processes on the pilot units, with premeasurement and postmeasurement of nurse satisfaction, nurse turnover, and patient satisfaction. No interventions except routine data collection occurred on the comparison units during the study time period. Table 10.1 describes the protocol and timeline of the study.

TABLE 10.1 Integrating Human Caring Science Into a Professional Nursing Practice Model: Inova Health System Study Grid

DESCRIPTION OF PROTOCOL	YEAR 1	YEAR 2	YEAR 3	YEAR 4	YEAR 5
Interventional Group					
Preintervention phase					
Selection of study groups (pilot and control) based on variables	█				
Phase I: Decrease work intensity					
1. Work teams identify hassle factors	█				
2. Work teams decide on four processes to address	█				
Phase I: Process improvement interventions					
1. Work teams collect baseline data on each of four processes (time wanding)	█				
2. Work teams develop interventions to address four processes	█				
3. Work teams pilot interventions to address four processes	█				
4. Core process changes implemented throughout Inova inpatient units		█	█		
Phase II: Creation of human caring environment					
1. Nurse caring behaviors identified for pilot testing			█		
2. Integration of 10 Caritas Factors into practice model			█		

(continued)

TABLE 10.1 *(continued)*

DESCRIPTION OF PROTOCOL	YEAR 1	YEAR 2	YEAR 3	YEAR 4	YEAR 5
3. Caring ambassadors selected on four interventional units			▓		
4. Ambassadors participate in 2-day caring science immersion education course: caring coaches designated			▓		
5. All staff members on interventional units participate in caring science educational sessions			▓		
6. Implementation of Caritas Factors into nursing practice			▓		
7. Implementation of Caritas Factors into all inpatient units			▓	▓	
8. Implementation of Caritas Factors on all outpatient and ambulatory care units					▓
Postintervention phase					
Quantitative data collection	▓				
Caring Assessment Tool Version II		▓			
Caring Factor Survey		▓			
Healthcare Environment Survey		▓			
NDNQI Nurse Satisfaction Survey	▓	▓	▓	▓	
Inova internal turnover and vacancy rates	▓	▓	▓	▓	
Qualitative data collection			▓		
Focus groups			▓		
Comparison Group					
Preintervention phase					
Selection of study groups based on variables	▓				
Phase I: Routine Inova data collection					
No targeted interventions; routine organizational processes	▓	▓	▓	▓	▓
Postintervention phase					
Routine Inova data collection and organizational processes	▓	▓	▓	▓	▓

Phase I: Decrease Work Intensity

Once the pilot units were chosen, groups of staff were brought together in work teams. These teams identified hassle factors that impacted the nurses' ability to complete work and resulted in interruptions and daily workflow inefficiencies. Each of the four units had to agree on the top four areas to address. Although there was some overlap in identified hassles, the group voted to come up with four improvement areas: (1) medication administration process, (2) admission-discharge-transfer process, (3) documentation process, and (4) communication process. Process and performance improvement methodologies were used to save nursing time.

Interventions for Phase I

For each of the four processes, cross-hospital teams worked to collect baseline data on the time each process took before any interventions. In addition, workflow diagrams were created. Once baseline data collection was completed, the teams worked together using quality improvement methodologies to develop interventions that would improve each work process. For each of the processes, the interventions and results are identified in Table 10.2. The process changes were implemented on each of the pilot units. Once the final data were collected and results showed improvement, all of the interventions were subsequently included in the strategic plan for the rest of the units across all of the hospital inpatient units. For example, the automated telephone messaging system for report was implemented across 75 inpatient units during year 3 of the study. The technology changes to documentation were also implemented across all of the hospitals and a plan for each unit to go wireless was put in place. Likewise, use of the pharmacy scanning system was initiated in all relevant patient-care areas.

Results From Phase I

Data were collected from each of the pilot units and time was saved in each process area except in documentation, where total compliance scores increased (see Table 10.2). On completion of the process improvement pilots, the nursing satisfaction survey was redistributed to the staff on the four medical units. The nurses' perception of having sufficient time to attend to the emotional and psychosocial needs of the patients improved 16.2%, and a 13.1% improvement was noted in having sufficient time for direct patient care as a result of changes in the admission process.

There was improvement in nurse satisfaction of the role of the admission nurse, which is one element of improving work intensity. The nurses' perception of benefit of the admission role as a result of the pilot was a score of 5.67 overall benefit on a scale of 1 to 6. As a result of all of the process improvement work that was done, core process changes were made to the pilot units and then spread throughout Inova Health System inpatient units during the course of years 2 and 3. Once the pilot units had completed the process improvement changes, Phase II of the studies began.

TABLE 10.2 Improved Work Processes

HASSLE FACTOR AND PROCESS	IDENTIFIED INTERVENTIONS TO SAVE TIME	RESULTS IN TIME SAVINGS
Medication administration process Hassle: "Time for pharmacy to get orders was too long, resulting in delays."	Piloted use of a medication order scanning process to speed time that physician order arrived in pharmacy.	Med Order Scanners streamlined the process from 30–60 minutes per order sheet.
Admission/discharge/transfer process Hassle: "Time to admit patient was too long."	Piloted use of an admission nurse, sole job to admit, discharge and transfer patients on medical unit. Also assisted in "hunting and gathering" activities related to patient admission, including beginning nursing care interventions. Greeted and oriented patient, obtained equipment, documented vital signs and patient history, performed and documented initial patient assessment.	Using an admissions nurse reduced the average time to admit a patient from 75.93 minutes to 56.13 minutes; resulting in 18.2-minute decrease in time for admission.
Documentation process Hassle: "Paper documentation was too redundant."	Automated online documentation system for multiple forms on medical unit, use of "computers on wheels" to facilitate point of service documentation.	Improved compliance with documentation from 85% to 98%.
Communication process Hassle: "Time spent on report was too long; hunting and gathering for report supplies was a waste of time."	Piloted VoiceCare system, a telephone voicemail system for report, allowing for pre-recorded patient history to be repeated each shift.	VoiceCare expedited shift change communication by 3.6 minutes per patient per report, or more than 10 minutes per patient.

Phase II: Creation of a Human Caring Environment

Phase II included the development and implementation of a human caring work environment based on the work of theorist Dr. Jean Watson.[13] In Watson's theory, the patient is an equal partner with health care providers to optimize wellness physically, emotionally, and spiritually. The objective in this phase was to improve staff nurse satisfaction and turnover rates by providing the nurse time to practice the art of nursing in a caring and healing environment within an acute care setting. A review of the literature led to the discovery of caring behaviors that were considered for the pilot.[14–19] Watson worked with Inova Health System to design the translation of the Human Caring processes into key interventions for the study. The interventions were also based on the literature that described the importance of nurse caring behaviors in acute care settings[20–23] and throughout the continuum of care.[24] Finfgeld-Connett[18] shares that a work environment conducive to caring is necessary for caring to occur, and the environmental factors include improvements in coworker support, teamwork, supportive management, learning experiences, and adequate time to care for patients. Behaviors that were well documented in the literature[18] that constitute caring include attentive listening, making eye contact, touching, offering verbal reassurance, being physically and mindfully present, centering on the patient, being emotionally open and available, and taking cultural differences into consideration. Activities include listening, providing information, encouraging expressions of concern, and helping cope with difficult situations. All of these were considered as the interventions were designed to create a healing and caring environment in the study.

In addition, effort was dedicated to determining appropriate measurement tools based on the literature review.[2,25,26] The translation of Watson's Caritas processes into shared language that was developed by Westlake Hospital nursing staff in Melrose, Illinois, was used to help the Inova staff understand that caring is a process.[18] Permission was granted to use the Westlake description of Watson's caring processes throughout the Inova Health System pilot.

The 10 caring (Caritas) factors described in a simplified interpretation developed by Westlake Hospital, Melrose, Illinois, are based on Watson's theory and are included in Box 10.1.

Work teams on Inova's pilot units worked together to determine key factors of human caring, and interventions were developed and then

---

Box 10.1 Translation of Watson's caritas processes: caring factors

1. Practice loving kindness
2. Instill faith and hope
3. Nurture individual spiritual beliefs and practices
4. Developing helping-trusting relationships
5. Promote and accept the expression of positive and negative feelings
6. Use creative scientific problem solving methods for decision-making
7. Perform teaching and learning that addresses the individual needs and learning styles
8. Create a healing environment for the physical and spiritual self that respects human dignity
9. Assist with physical, emotional, and spiritual human needs
10. Allow room for miracles to take place

Courtesy of Westlake Hospital, Melrose, Illinois.

implemented on the pilot units. The interventions included several key efforts at educating and coaching the nursing staff in the implementation of caring activities. Ambassadors on each of the four pilot units were chosen to be the champions of the care changes. These ambassadors participated in a 2-day immersion course led by Watson and Dr. Janet Quinn, where the human caring theory was fully explained and the ambassadors were trained in centering techniques, intentionality exercises, and being more fully present with patients. Training included intentionality or "being in the moment" with patients, caring connection or taking time to care and connect with each patient, and reflection and celebration or honoring the power that lies in service to others based on the 10 caring factors.

The ambassadors were also cultivated into "caring coaches" and were encouraged to develop monitoring capability on their care units. For example, they learned to collect data and give feedback to staff as they served as a role model for caring behaviors in daily work. After the ambassadors were trained, a curriculum was developed for all of the staff on the pilot units. This curriculum content included intentionality and centering techniques (being "in the moment" with patients); breathing techniques that helped to decrease stress and improve concentration for both staff and patients; caring connections (taking time each day to care and connect with each patient); reflection and celebration of positive events through the ritual of hand washing in the care area; participating and leading caring circles to recenter thoughts around the patient; creation of a caring lounge on each patient-care unit for nurses to retreat to find quiet space for recentering and reflection; and monitoring, observing, and evaluating peer activities.

Some examples of practice changes that were implemented and evaluated include the following:

Nurses spent up to 5 minutes each shift with each patient focusing on authentically being present with the patient and interacting with them in this connected space. This time allowed the patient to be a partner in care and helped the nurse understand the patient's perception of need for caring. The nurse spent time in a way that conveyed concern and respect, being present with the patient, face to face, at the eye level of the patient. The nurse used touch as appropriate and was able to relate to the patient on a very human level.

Nurses used the time spent for hand washing and transformed it into a ritual of thanks for having the ability and privilege to care for each patient. For many the hand-washing time became a time to reflect on closure and completion of the human caring experience between patient encounters.

Nurses used motivational signs that were hung over each sink and magnets placed outside the door of each room to help them focus on being intentional in their work before each patient interaction. Each

nurse stopped before entering the room to pause, read the message of hope and healing, and become centered on the patient encounter. Nurses placed posters on each unit with the 10 caring factors in a large display for patients, families, and staff members to be able to visualize the commitment to caring behaviors.
On some units, the nursing staff decided to decrease the lighting level, which impacted the noise level on the pilot units.
All of the pilot units created a centering lounge. Staff used this lounge as a place to center and learn about human caring. Some units called it their nursing "sanctuary" where staff could practice their breathing techniques. Peer coaches identified staff that were stressed and encouraged them to take a break in the centering lounge as a way to recenter around the patients.

At Inova Health System, the goal continues to be the creation of an intentional environment within the hospital setting that addresses the needs of the nurse, the patient, and colleagues. Training interventions began at the end of year 2 and continued through year 5.

Results From Phase II

Measurement tools. Baseline data were collected from several sources, including the review of tools that have been especially developed to measure the impact of human caring activities on nurses and patients.[25-27] For this research study, several measurement surveys were used. To understand better the patient's perception of caring based on Watson's theory of caring, Inova used the Caring Assessment Tool (CAT) Version II developed by Duffy and coworkers[27] at Catholic University. The CAT II tool has established content validity and reliability when used in an acute care setting. The Caring Factor Survey measured the impact of the 10 caring processes on patient's perception of the caring nurse. The Caring Factor Survey was developed by John Nelson[15] and has been used only to test the psychometric properties of the tool (Cronbach's alpha 0.97). Both the CAT II and the Caring Factor Survey measurement tools are based on the Caritas Processes, which are concepts of caring based on the theory and work of Watson.

To evaluate nurse satisfaction, the Healthcare Environment Survey (HES) developed by Nelson was used.[15] The HES is a valid and reliable (Cronbach's alpha 0.96) 86-item instrument used to obtain staff members' perceptions of the work environment, including relationships with coworkers, unit manager, physicians, and nurses; professional patient care; autonomy; staffing and scheduling; executive leadership; learning opportunities; organizational rewards; pride in the organization; intent to stay; and workload.

Other data collection included review of Inova's employee opinion survey and the NDNQI RN satisfaction survey that was being collected at each hospital. In addition, turnover data were collected and evaluated during year 4 of the study.

Patient perception of caring. Results of the CAT II measured a patient's perception of caring, preintervention and postintervention. In the pilot group, there were 134 patients in the predata collection and 155 patients postcaring interventions. Data were also collected on the comparison units that consisted of 141 patients in the pregroup and 127 in the postintervention group. When compared with the preintervention group, patients on both pilot and comparison units reported more satisfaction with care at postintervention. Score differences, however, were not statistically significant for either group (using an alpha of .05). On the pilot units, scores increased 0.12 points on a scale of 1 to 7.

Patient satisfaction. Inova Health System uses Professional Research Consultants (PRC) to measure inpatient hospital satisfaction data. During this study, the investigators used the data from PRC to evaluate patient satisfaction. PRC data are valid and reliable across hundreds of hospitals in the United States. The tool measures scores of percent "excellent." Data comparison on the pilot units from 2005 (preintervention) to 2006 (postintervention) during the time of the caring protocols showed improvement in overall patient satisfaction (Figure 10.1). The percent ranked excellent improved on the pilot units from 9.9% precaring interventions to 79.2% postcaring and from 57.6% precaring to 98.7% postcaring interventions. Improvements were seen in each of the pilot units.

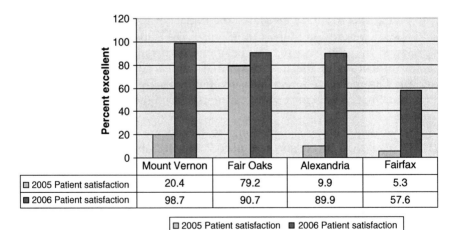

	Mount Vernon	Fair Oaks	Alexandria	Fairfax
☐ 2005 Patient satisfaction	20.4	79.2	9.9	5.3
■ 2006 Patient satisfaction	98.7	90.7	89.9	57.6

☐ 2005 Patient satisfaction   ■ 2006 Patient satisfaction

FIGURE 10.1   Comparison of patient satisfaction 2005 (patient satisfaction) compared with 2006 (patient satisfaction) on human caring pilot units; measures percent ranked "excellent" on Professional Research Consultants data collection tool.

Nurse satisfaction. In November 2004, the HES was distributed to 621 nurses at Inova Health System for the baseline assessment. The "caring protocol" had not been implemented on any unit, but several staff had attended introductory classes at the time of the baseline measurement. One hundred and sixty-five nurses from the pilot units returned the survey (a 52% response rate) and 113 nurses from the comparison units returned the survey (a 37% response rate). Combined, 278 nurses returned the survey (a 45% response rate). Results of the 277 usable surveys were analyzed using various statistical methods. These were considered the predata set.

In February 2006, the HES survey was repeated. A total of 578 staff participated in the sample with 291 staff responding (50% response rate). There were 131 staff who responded to the HES at both premeasurement and postmeasurement (approximately 23% of the staff). Responses of those who participated in both measurements were used within the final paired t-test, comparing the changes of the postintervention scores with the baseline scores. Respondents to the HES were asked to rank their level of satisfaction using a Likert-type scale (ranging from one to seven, strongly dissatisfied to strongly satisfied, respectively) on workforce environmental variables.

The results revealed no significant differences in demographics over time, indicating stability on the unit. The interaction effects of the pilot comparison group that were statistically significant at the 0.05 level (Table 10.3) were the HES total score, relationship with coworkers subscale score, and workload perception subscale score.

Other improvements that were noted, but were not statistically significant, included relationships with physicians, pride in the organization, promotional opportunities being present, and improved relationships with other nurses.

Nurse satisfaction: National Database for Nursing Quality Indicators data (NDNQI). The NDNQI offers an RN satisfaction survey that is conducted annually for those hospitals opting to participate. The question

TABLE 10.3   Positive Improvement in Healthcare Environment Survey Subscores Postintervention of the Caring Protocol

VARIABLE	CHANGE SCORE COMBINED PILOT UNITS	CHANGE SCORE COMBINED COMPARISON UNITS
Healthcare Environment Survey total score	0.09[a]	0.05
Workload	0.21[a]	−0.17
Relationship with coworkers	0.21[a]	−0.16
Promotional opportunities	0.10	0.02
Pride in the organization	0.07	0.02

[a] Statistically significant at 0.05 level.

that the study compared was the Nurse-Nurse Interaction score on NDNQI: "Do nurses help each other, feel at home on the unit, is there teamwork, are nurses friendly to each other?" Comparing the scores of 2005 before intervention and 2006 postintervention on the four medical pilot units, three out of four units improved to a level considered "high satisfaction" by the survey guidelines (Table 10.4).

Turnover and vacancy rates of registered nurses on pilot units. These indicators were by far the most difficult to analyze, because there are many reasons that RNs choose to leave or resign from a care unit. Nonetheless, a comparison of the pilot units during the time period of the study and ongoing has revealed a lower rate of turnover and vacancy, and a decrease of vacancy and turnover rates over time. The primary driver for RN turnover could not be determined, although the relationship with patients remained the nurses' number one source of job satisfaction. Table 10.5 shows a sample of one unit's tracking of retention during the 6-month pilot time period of human caring practice interventions. Although improvement

TABLE 10.4 National Database for Nursing Quality Indicators Nurse–Nurse Interaction Score

UNIT	2005 SCORE	2006 SCORE
Inova Fairfax Hospital Tower 8 Medicine	71.25	72.39
Inova Alexandria Hospital Unit 23 Medicine	63.54	72.72
Inova Fair Oaks Hospital 4 New Medicine	61.91	60.86
Inova Mount Vernon Hospital 3B Medicine	49.27	57.65

Notes: "Do nurses help each other, feel at home on the unit, is there teamwork, are nurses friendly to each other?" Pilot units' comparison between 2005 and 2006.
Scale: <40, low satisfaction; 40–60, moderate satisfaction; >60, high satisfaction.

TABLE 10.5 Example of Retention Results

UNITS	JAN	FEB	MAR	APR	MAY	JUNE	JULY
Control	100	100	77.8	83.3	86.7	77.8	81
Pilot	100	100	100	83.3	86.7	88.9	100

Note: Inova Mount Vernon Hospital Comparison versus pilot units percent registered nurse retention rates, January–July 2006. Includes voluntary and involuntary terminations during time period studied.

was noted compared with the comparison units, there was inconsistency and no statistically significant trends when this was studied across all of the pilot units and comparison units for the health system.

Qualitative data. During the study time period, opportunities to engage staff and hear feedback in focus groups about what was working and what did not work helped to guide the process of education and coaching on the units. Focus groups were held, and surveys were administered that allowed nurses to share their stories about what it was like to practice nursing in an environment where caring processes were encouraged and expected. The following statements capture the essence of the feedback with themes of nurses feeling able to care for themselves, to care for each other as coworkers, and to increase their intentional care for patients.

- "By starting with the present from within me, and coming with a good heart, I am able to deliver the best care I ever thought possible."
- "I am able to take more time to clear my mind and take time to focus on each issue."
- "I am in the process of ordering my private world. I now have the learning tools to cope with situations in a positive way; now I am learning to be in the present."
- "Because we are all doing this together, I know that my patients are going to get great care from my coworkers too."
- "I have felt a renewal of spirituality, love, and caring energy that allows me to care for my patients."
- "This work enhances the caring spirit, which I try to administer with every patient."
- "I gave one of our patients a brief massage the day before yesterday. She truly loved it. It gave her some respite from her physical and mental suffering. Were it not for caritas, I would not have even considered this."
- "I have been a nurse for about 2 years now, and I had been feeling frustrated because I was not able to spend enough time interacting with my patients. I was actually thinking of leaving nursing because I was so discouraged. By being able to have the time to implement the human caring interventions, my perspective has changed and I have the support from my coworkers and nursing leadership to spend time with my patients. It has made all the difference for me, and I cannot imagine being anything but a nurse."

LIMITATIONS OF THE STUDY

Limitations of the study include no random assignment of control and intervention units, which may have led to a systematic bias. Not all of the variables could be manipulated and the caring interventions could not be controlled as the only variables, making it difficult to attribute cause and effect inferences. The lengthy time frame of the study meant that other changes occurred on the care units over the 4-year time period, such as changes in leadership and opening and closing of new units. In addition, there may have been a double Hawthorne effect[28] because some of the surgical units became aware of the changes occurring on the pilot medical units because those units were receiving a lot of attention over time. As a result, causal links and cause and effect inferences need to be made with care.

MOVING BEYOND THE STUDY

Creation of Inova's Human Caring professional practice model has continued beyond the four pilot units. During 2007, education sessions were created and four to six staff nurses from each of the 75 inpatient units attended special sessions to be educated in the practice changes for creating a healing and caring environment. Over 1,000 RNs were trained. Each unit received $1,000 to create a healing lounge area and staff members were very creative in transforming small spaces into special areas for centering. A toolkit was distributed to each of the remaining 70 inpatient units. The toolkit consisted of posters with the display of the 10 Caritas Processes for the unit; magnets for enhancing intentionality to be placed on the door jambs; brochures (education and information); Caritas cards (used for reminder of the caring processes); pins to recognize staff who had attended education sessions; inspirational quotes with suction cups (to be placed in hand washing areas); and the CD "human caring meditations" for use in centering during a shift.

During 2008, the Inova Human Caring model was implemented in the ambulatory and outpatient centers. Educational sessions were held during first and second quarter, with over 200 staff attending from multidisciplinary backgrounds. In addition, the caring processes and interventions are now included in the Inova infrastructure. These include the development of a philosophy of care based on Human Caring Theory, inclusion of the caring processes into orientation for new staff members, integration of caring processes into the job profile and job descriptions of RN 1 to 4 categories and the annual competencies and annual evaluation, the development of a nursing model of care based on caring processes, development of a recognition program called the Caritas Awards, quarterly workshops included in the learning network and education programming, a special internal website devoted to human caring activities, and most recently the introduction of a Human Caring Research Internship Program. This work has also led to the development of an evolving Inova Model of Care based on caring processes, which is in the final stages of completion. These foundational elements are critical to

ensuring that the human caring work continues and that the caring processes are encouraged in an integrated manner across all hospitals and
care settings within Inova.

SUMMARY

The unique contribution of this study is that it involved two distinct
phases of work to improve nursing care at the bedside. Although the ultimate goal was to implement a human caring philosophy, the staff nurses
in the practice environment shared their perspectives about inefficient
work processes and hassle factors in care. Only by improving those processes first could the integrative nursing work of caring and healing be
implemented. Quality improvement and work process redesign should
be a core project activity in every patient care area, with ongoing efforts
at improving efficiency and freeing up the nurse to be more present with
patients.

It is incumbent on nursing-practice leaders, from bedside nurse to
chief nurse, to make space for quality improvement projects that improve care efficiency, so that the nurse can redirect time toward caring
encounters with patients. Caring interventions should be well described,
taught, and coached. The caring interventions described in this study
are not separate activities, but rather integrated activities to be woven
throughout the day, or the visit, or the encounter. Watson describes this
caring as a transpersonal relationship between the nurse and the patient.
This is a special kind of human care relationship, a union with a high
regard for the whole person and their being in the world.[16] Whitmer and
coworkers[17] describe the need for caring as especially evident in the critical care environment, where nurses face the dilemma of a lack of time to
complete nursing tasks and provide comfort.

Although studies are emerging that describe how nurses are spend-
ing their time with nonvalue-added tasks and activities such as hunting
and gathering for supplies,[29] very few have suggested what the nurse
should do with the time saved when processes are improved. Streamlining work processes can gain time back at the bedside, giving nurses
the opportunity to establish a more meaningful, caring connection with
patients. This enhanced ability to provide nursing care in a healing
and caring environment has led to greater work fulfillment, a sense of
belonging, commitment to the care unit, and improved morale. Findings from this study show that nurses are very willing to enhance their
therapeutic relationships with patients and feel more satisfied when they
make that connection.

It is incumbent on nursing-practice leaders, from bedside nurse to
chief nurse, to make space for quality improvement projects that improve care efficiency, so that the nurse can redirect time toward caring
encounters with patients. Caring interventions should be well described,
taught, and coached. The caring interventions described in this study
are not separate activities, but rather integrated activities to be woven
throughout the day, or the visit, or the encounter. Watson describes this
caring as a transpersonal relationship between the nurse and the patient.
This is a special kind of human care relationship, a union with a high
regard for the whole person and their being in the world.[16] Whitmer and
coworkers[17] describe the need for caring as especially evident in the critical care environment, where nurses face the dilemma of a lack of time to
complete nursing tasks and provide comfort.

This study suggests that making time for caring is a necessary step
to maximize the nursing practice contribution. If time is saved, then the
redirection of that time to care processes that allow the nurse to serve

as an agent of healing at the bedside is realized. Being able to create a caring environment is a privileged opportunity for nursing leadership.[1] Understanding nursing as a caring science and the ability to create a caring culture, where the processes of care are grounded in connection with the patients, is the role of every nurse. The ability of nurses to serve as role models so that caring processes and interventions are valued over simple task completion ensures that the next generation of nurses has job fulfillment and that patients are cared for in a holistic manner.

ACKNOWLEDGMENTS

The author acknowledges the contributions of Gene Rigotti, RN, MSN, and Jean Watson, PhD, RN, ANC, BC, FAAN, to the content of the chapter.

REFERENCES

1. Boykin A, Schoenhofer S. The role of nursing leadership in creating caring environments in health care delivery systems. Nurs Adm Q 2001;25(3):1–7.
2. Watson J. Nursing: the philosophy and science of caring. Colorado (CO): University Press of Colorado; 1985.
3. Watson J. Watson's theory of human caring and subjective living experiences: carative factors/caritas processes as a disciplinary guide to the professional nursing practice. Texto and Contexto Enfermagem, Florianopolis. Brazil: University of Santa Catarina; p. 129–35.
4. Watson J, Smith MC. Caring science and the science of unitary human beings: a trans-theoretical discourse for nursing knowledge development. J Adv Nurs 2002;37(5):452–61.
5. McCormack B, McCance TV. Development of a framework for person-centered nursing: nursing theory and concept development or analysis. J Adv Nurs 2006;56(5):472–9.
6. Sumner J. Caring in nursing: a different interpretation. J Adv Nurs 2001; 35(6):926–32.
7. Beaudoin LE, Edgar L. Hassles: their importance to nurses' quality of work life. Nurs Econ 2003;21(3): 106–13.
8. Fagerstrom L. The dialectic tension between being and not being a good nurse. Nurs Ethics 2006; 13(6):622–31.
9. Patient care delivery and work design, pdf manual, May 2003. Available at: www.aone.org/aone/docs/hwe_excellence_initiatives.pdf. Accessed June 29, 2008.
10. Urden LD, Rooder JL. Work sampling: a decision-making tool for determining resources and work redesign. J Nurs Adm 1997;27(9):34–41.
11. Viney M, Batcheller J, Hourston S, et al. Transforming care at the bedside: designing new care systems in an age of complexity. J Nurs Care 2006; 21(2):143–50.
12. Fuller J. Regarding work intensity, less is more. Nurs Manage 2007;28(5):12.
13. Watson J. Caring theory as an ethical guide to administrative and clinical practices. JONAS Healthc Law Ethics Regul 2006;8(3):87–93.

14. Carter LC, Nelson JL, Sievers BA, et al. Exploring a culture of caring. Nurs Adm Q 2008;32(1):57–63.
15. Persky GL, Nelson J, Watson J, et al. Creating a profile of a nurse effective in caring. Nurs Adm Q 2008;32(1):15–20.
16. Rexroth R, Davidhizar R. Caring: utilizing the Watson theory to transcend culture. Health Care Manag (Frederick) 2003;22(4):295–304.
17. Whitmer M, Hurst S, Stakder K, et al. Caring in the curing environment: the implementation of a grieving cart in the ICU. Journal of Hospice and Palliative Nursing 2007;9(6):329–33.
18. Finfgeld-Connett D. Meta-synthesis of caring in nursing. J Clin Nurs 2008;17: 196–204.
19. Hemsley MS, Glass N, Watson J. Taking the eagles' view: using Watson's conceptual model to investigate the extraordinary and transformative experiences of nurse healers. Holist Nurs Pract 2006; 20(2):85–94.
20. Baldursdottir G, Jonsdottir H. The importance of nurse caring behaviors as perceived by patient receiving care in an emergency department. Heart Lung 2002;31(1):67–75.
21. Wang CH. Knowing and approaching hope as human experience: implications for the medical-surgical nurse. Medsurg Nurs 2000;9(4):189–93.
22. Chung LY, Wong FK, Chan MF. Relationship of nurses' spirituality to their understanding and practice of spiritual care. J Adv Nurs 2007;58(2): 158–70.
23. Rosenberg S. Utilizing the language of Jean Watson's caring theory within a computerized clinical documentation system. Comput Inform Nurs 2006; 24(1):53–6.
24. Owens RA. The caring behaviors of the home health nurse and influence on medication adherence. Home Healthcare Nurse 2006;24(8):517–26.
25. Cossette S, Cote JK, Pepin J, et al. A dimensional structure of nursing patient Interaction from a caring perspective: refinement of the Caring Nurse–Patient Interaction Scale (CNPI-short scale). J Adv Nurs 2006;55(2):198–214.
26. Beck CT. Quantitative measurement of caring. J Adv Nurs 1999;30(1):24–32.
27. Duffy J, Hoskins L, Seifert RF. Dimensions of caring: psychometric evaluation of the caring assessment tool. ANS Adv Nurs Sci 2007;30(3):235–45.
28. Polit DF, Beck CT, Hungler BP. Essentials of nursing research, methods, appraisal, and utilization. 5th edition. Baltimore (MD): Lippincott; 2001.
29. Hendrich A, Chow MP, Skierczynski BA, et al. A 36 hospital time and motion study: how do medical surgical nurses spend their time? The Permanente Journal 2008;3(12):25–33.

11

Impact of Intentional Caring Behaviors on Nurses' Perceptions of Caring in the Workplace, Nurses' Intent to Stay, and Patients' Perceptions of Being Cared For

Anna Herbst

Nurse satisfaction, nurse turnover, and burnout remain cyclical concerns among nursing staff outcomes. Researchers from Inova Health System (IHS) hypothesized that they could impact all three outcomes by creating more healing work environments (Drenkard, 2008). A grant from Health Resource and Service Agency (HRSA) was used to implement an environmental intervention of Jean Watson's theory of Caritas (2008). Nurses were asked to do the following: center before each patient encounter, enjoy a 5-minute meaningful encounter with each patient, use hand-washing time postencounter to intentionally acknowledge gratitude and closure, and participate in weekly gatherings called Caritas circles. These sharing circles took place in specially decorated, nurse-healing lounges on the unit, called Caritas lounges. Based on successes in these pilot medical units, the work tools, four caring–healing interventions, and Caritas lounges were implemented on 74 inpatient and 41 outpatient nursing units across the five-hospital health system between 2007 and 2008 (Drenkard, 2008).

In June 2008 the labor and delivery (L&D) unit at Inova Alexandria Hospital (IAH), a 318-bed community hospital within the system, still had not implemented the human-caring portion of the program. Nurses cited lack of time as the cause of delay. Nurse researchers at the hospital seized this opportunity to replicate pieces of the original research and examine some nurse- and patient-subgroup responses to caring–healing interventions.

BACKGROUND

The draw of individuals to the nursing profession has traditionally been less about scientific aptitude and more about altruism. The desire to heal, make a difference, and promote good can describe attributes of a nurse. Persky, Nelson, Watson, and Bent (2008) identified humanistic constructs of caring and love as part of a powerful healing relationship between nurses and patients. Conversely, history has demonstrated repetitive trends of nurse disillusionment, burnout, and, ultimately, exodus from healing at the bedside.

A concern in contemporary acute care is that as patients become sicker and have increased comorbidities, a greater risk for safety events exists within a shorter length of stay. Nursing *care* has adjusted by adding numerous checklists, screening tools, prevention tactics, documentation requirements, technological devices, and delegation of the more rudimentary tasks of physical care. As the nurse is pulled farther away from the bedside, some of the natural, even habitual, ways to altruistically connect with patients are lost. Out of necessity, in a busy environment, nurses may become so focused on accomplishing their work or tasks that mindful attention is not given to the caring relationship. It is theorized that without conscious attention to the development of the caring relationship, satisfaction and optimal healing for nurses and patients are at risk.

All areas of nursing experience staffing shortages, and specialty areas, including L&D, experience critical shortages (Stechmiller, 2002). Retention of nurses has consistently been related to job satisfaction (McNeese-Smith, 1999). Hayhurst, Saylor, and Stuenkel (2005) found peer cohesion and work pressure to be among the reasons nurses report leaving their jobs. Conversely, Strachota, Normandin, O'Brien, Clary, and Krukow (2003) found that environments enhancing a sense of belonging among staff strengthened nurses' commitment to facilities.

THEORETICAL FRAMEWORK

Jean Watson's theory of human caring describes caring as the core of nursing and the nurse–patient relationship as the conduit of caring. Caring is transpersonal and has the potential to grow and change both giver and receiver (Watson, 2008). Intentionality defines the mindful way a nurse connects with a patient and promotes holistic healing in all realms including mind, body, and spirit. *Caritas*, the Latin word for "love," describes the transcendental, universal energy or love that all human beings share. Caritas is how people care or connect on a holistic level. Watson's 10 Caritas Processes demonstrate how the caring connection manifests itself within nursing functions and beyond. IHS adopted Westlake Hospital's (Melrose, IL) simplified versions of the 10 processes:

1. Practice loving kindness.
2. Instill faith and hope.
3. Nurture individual spiritual beliefs and practices.
4. Develop helping-trusting relationships.
5. Promote and accept the expression of positive and negative feelings.
6. Use creative, scientific problem-solving methods for decision making.
7. Perform teaching and learning that address individual needs and learning styles.
8. Create a healing environment for the physical and spiritual self that respects human dignity.
9. Assist with physical, emotional, and spiritual human needs.
10. Allow room for miracles to take place.

SIGNIFICANCE

Inova nursing's philosophy/model of caring is centered on these 10 Caritas Processes and addresses caring outcomes equally in the realms of self, colleague, and patient. Though caring is a core value in nursing, quantitative studies that address caring relationships in acute care nursing environments are rare. There is a need for further research that connects measures of caring with evidence-based practice and patient outcomes (Watson, 2002). Because caring techniques are so ingrained in nursing practice, they are often invisible and impossible to measure (Coates, 2002). Swanson (1999) asserts that nurses who perceived experiences as caring may experience improved clinical skills, reasoning, caring competence, empathy, and professional satisfaction.

Nurses approach their caring in a variety of ways (Vitello-Cicciu, 2001). However manifested, caring happens within interactions. All patient outcomes have the potential for improvement when a healing, caring environment exists. It is theorized that creating a more caring environment can improve retention, stabilize staffing, and enhance patient healing.

PURPOSE

The L&D unit under study at Inova Alexandria Hospital had experienced five interim patient care directors from 2005 to 2008. Nursing turnover and, consequently, vacancy rates were high. The nursing climate was busy and anxious. A "we-they" mentality existed between staff and leaders. Nurse researchers wanted to assist the L&D unit in returning focus to the more satisfying caring aspects of their work. The purpose of this study was to investigate the impact of nurses performing four intentional caring behaviors on nurses' perceptions of their caring, nurses' intent to stay in the current position, and patients' perceptions of being cared for.

The intentional caring behaviors were designed to target all modes of care with the Inova nursing philosophy/model of caring: self, colleague, patient.

RESEARCH QUESTIONS

1. Does performing intentional human-caring behaviors have an impact on nurses' perceptions of their caring in the workplace?
2. Are nurses who intentionally perform human-caring behaviors less likely to leave their jobs?
3. Does performing intentional human-caring behaviors have an impact on patients' perceptions of being cared for?

DESIGN AND METHODS

A quasiexperimental, nonrandomized, between-subjects design with pre- and postintervention surveys of nurses and patients was used. Institutional review board approval was obtained, as was permission to use the following three surveys.

Nurse Surveys

■ Caring Factor Survey–Care Provider Version (CFS-CPV) (Hinshaw, 1987): The 20 items, rated on a 7-point Likert scale based on Jean Watson's 10 Caritas Processes, measure a nurses' perception of self and health care team caring for patients. Higher scores indicate greater perception of caring.
■ Anticipated Turnover (AT) Scale: This 12-item survey, based on a 7-point Likert scale, measures a nurse's self-reported intent to leave his or her current job. Higher scores indicate greater intent to leave.
■ Demographic Information Collection Tool: This tool includes 18 points of personal and professional demographics that were hypothesized by the investigators to influence caring. The hypothesis was influenced by the investigators' collective experience in obstetrics (OB).

Patient Surveys

■ Caring Factor Survey (CFS): The CFS measures the patient's perception of being cared for by staff nurses. It included 20 items rated on a 7-point Likert scale based on Jean Watson's 10 Caritas Processes. Higher scores indicate greater perception of being cared for.

■ Fourteen demographic items were presented to patients. Demographic items were selected by OB staff using professional experience to select those demographics believed to have potential to influence results, thus essential to examine within this study. **Preintervention Phase, August 4 to September 12, 2008:** During a 6-week period in 2008, the two nurse surveys were distributed to all L&D unit staff in order to be inclusive; only registered nurse (RN) staff results were analyzed. Staff was instructed about the study and informed that their participation would be considered their consent to investigators. Subinvestigators gained informed consent of patients and surveyed L&D patients one day after delivery on the postpartum unit. Using a script, subinvestigators informed patients that their responses should refer to their stay in the L&D unit only and would be shared with L&D staff in aggregate form but not for several months. Only patients older than 18 and literate in English were included. All results were confidential. **Intervention Phase, September 15, 2008 to January 10, 2009:** L&D staff and leadership buy-in for participation in the study was gained by describing the caring interventions as one way for nurses to regain caring control of their own practice despite transitional leadership and staffing shortages. Eighty percent of RNs agreed to complete the 30–40-minute human-caring training sessions offered by the principal investigator to introduce Watson's theory and the four intentional caring behaviors. Multiple sessions were given on the unit during the course of normal work. Nurses received a human-caring pin to wear on their name badge once they completed the training. A poster of Watson's 10 Caritas Processes (see Figure 11.1) was prominently displayed at the nurses' station. Investigators monitored 5–10 randomly selected staff nurses each week for 15 weeks to check for nurse performance of the caring processes while on duty and offered further education and support on the unit.

The four intentional caring behaviors that nurses were asked to perform during the normal course of patient care were:

■ **Centering before a patient encounter:** Cued by reading a magnet with a positive saying on the patient door (see Figure 11.2), the nurse takes a deep breath and, with intention, mentally focuses on the particular patient and enters the room.

■ **Five-minute meaningful patient encounter:** The nurse mindfully spends 5 minutes "being with" a patient. This is separate time to build the relationship; nurses are encouraged to make eye-level, eye-to-eye contact.

■ **Hand-washing ritual:** Cued by signs with positive sayings placed at hand-washing stations (see Figure 11.3), the nurse uses the hand-washing time to mentally acknowledge the "care" just given and bring closure before moving on to the next encounter.

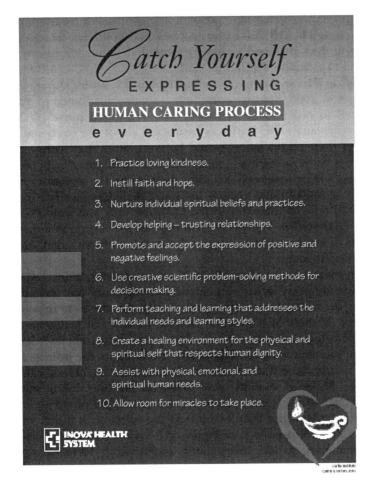

FIGURE 11.1   Ten Caritas Processes poster.

■ **Weekly Caritas Circle:** This is a 15–20-minute, informal staff gathering to center with focused breathing and to share caring moments; it takes place in the centering lounge. Facilitation of weekly Caritas circles was offered on the day shift by the principal investigator; night-shift staff nurses created their own circle time.

Postintervention phase, January 12 to February 21, 2009: This phase consisted of a postintervention survey. Presurvey methods and criteria for both nurse and patient populations were repeated in the 6 weeks immediately following the intervention phase in 2009.

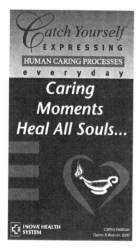

FIGURE 11.2 Sample magnet for patient door frame.

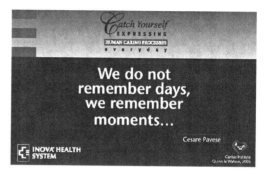

FIGURE 11.3 Sample sign at hand-washing station.

RESULTS

There were 42 nursing staff members preintervention; this increased to 62 nurses postintervention as vacancies were filled. Of the patients, 100 were invited to respond in the preintervention sample and 103 to postintervention. See Table 11.1 for response rates for all participants and surveys.

Reliability for Nurse and Patient Groups

Reliability for the CFS-CPV, CFS, and AT total scores (all subscales per measure combined) was satisfactory in both pre- and postsurveys. The desired Cronbach's alpha was at least 0.70. When examining the subscales for the CFS-CPV, it was noted that the only subscale to perform satisfactorily in both pre- and postintervention was "Allow Miracles," with a Cronbach's alpha of 0.83 and 0.78, respectively (see Table 11.2).

TABLE 11.1 Response Rate by Year, All Instruments

MEASURE	SAMPLE PRE / POST	RESPONSES PRE / POST	RESPONSE RATES PRE / POST
CFS-CPV (nurses)	42 / 62	42 / 30	100.0% / 48.4%
CFS (patients)	100 / 103	86 / 98	86.0% / 95.1%
Anticipated turnover	42 / 62	39 / 30	92.9% / 48.4%

TABLE 11.2   Reliability of Surveys

	CRONBACH'S ALPHA, PRE/POST		
SCALES AND SUBSCALES	CFS-CPV	CFS	AT
Total score (CFS-CPV and CFS)	0.94 / 0.92	0.97 / 0.98	–
Loving kindness	0.65 / 0.88	0.92 / 0.96	–
Problem solving	0.76 / 0.59	0.85 / 0.89	–
Faith and hope	0.86 / 0.62	0.77 / 0.92	–
Teach and understand	0.87 / 0.60	0.92 / 0.86	–
Support spiritual belief	0.32 / 0.50	0.79 / 0.84	–
Healing environment	0.90 / 0.53	0.77 / 0.84	–
Helping and trusting	0.59 / 0.20	0.78 / 0.93	–
Holistic care	0.55 / 0.69	0.86 / 0.95	–
Promote expression	0.93 / 0.63	0.72 / 0.81	–
Allow miracles	0.83 / 0.78	0.81 / 0.89	–
Anticipated turnover, total score	–	–	0.89 / 0.78

Nurse Demographic Data

Several demographics were examined in the nursing staff who responded to the survey. These demographics were selected because the primary investigators and subinvestigators theorized that they may have influence in the responses of the nursing staff. The demographics and descriptions of each are noted in Table 11.3, "Nurse Respondent Demographics."

For the nursing staff group that responded to the pre-CFS-CPV, the average age was 39.2 with a range of 18–59. In the postintervention sample the average age was 40.6 with a range of 23–60. Pre/postrace makeup in samples was predominantly White (56% or 22 nurses/60% or 18 nurses), followed by Black, non-Hispanic (26% or 11 nurses/20% or 6 nurses). Most of the nurses reported being from the Christian/Protestant faith in both pre- and postsamples with 67% ($n = 28$) and 77% ($n = 23$), respectively. Most of the nurses in both samples reported being at the RN 2 level (out of 4) in the clinical ladder promotion program with 52% ($n = 22$) preintervention and 60% ($n = 18$) postintervention. Overall, the demographic impression is similar in both groups.

Descriptive Statistics, Caring Factor Survey–Care Provider Version (CFS-CPV)

When comparing pre- and postscores, the total CSF-CPV score and several of the 10 Caritas Process scores improved ($p < .05$), including support patient's spiritual beliefs, holistic care, allowing miracles, promote expression of feelings, faith and hope, and healing environment. When

TABLE 11.3 Nurse Respondent Demographics

DEMOGRAPHIC	PREINTERVENTION	POSTINTERVENTION
Age	Mean: 39.2 Range: 18–59 Median: 39.0 SD: 11.1	Mean: 40.6 Range: 23–61 Median: 41.0 SD: 10.1
Race	White: 52% ($n = 22$) Black: 26% ($n = 11$) Asian/South Pacific: 5% ($n = 2$) Other: 7% ($n = 3$)	White: 60% ($n = 18$) Black: 20% ($n = 6$) Asian/South Pacific: 7% ($n = 2$) Other: 7% ($n = 2$)
Religion	Christian/Prot: 67% ($n = 28$) Catholic: 10% ($n = 4$) Other: 7% ($n = 3$) Muslim: 7% ($n = 3$) Jewish: 2% ($n = 1$)	Christian/Prot: 77% ($n = 23$) Other: 17% ($n = 5$) Muslim: 3% ($n = 1$)
Full-time or part-time	Full-time: 81% ($n = 34$) Part-time 12% ($n = 5$)	Full-time: 87% ($n = 26$) Part-time 13% ($n = 4$)
Hours worked per week in L&D	Mean: 35.6 Range: 8–50 Median: 36 SD: 7.9	Mean: 36.1 Range: 16–72 Median: 36.0 SD: 9.4
Hours worked per week	Mean: 37.6 Range: 4–72 Median: 40 SD: 11.1	Mean: 37.9 Range: 4–72 Median: 36.0 SD: 11.0
Clinical ladder	Level 1: 12% ($n = 5$) Level 2: 52% ($n = 22$) Level 3: 12% ($n = 5$) Level 4: 5% ($n = 2$)	Level 1: 7% ($n = 2$) Level 2: 60% ($n = 18$) Level 3: 10% ($n = 3$) Level 4: 13% ($n = 4$)
Years in L&D	Mean: 6.9 Range: <1–30 Median: 1.5 SD: 8.7	Mean: 7.6 Range: <1–30 Median: 2.0 SD: 8.9
Units worked before L&D	Mean: 3.0 Range: 0–11 Median: 2 SD: 3.0	Mean: 2.5 Range: 0–10 Median: 2 SD: 2.4
Certified	Yes: 41% ($n = 17$) No: 57% ($n = 24$)	Yes: 40% ($n = 12$) No: 57% ($n = 17$)
Years as RN	Mean: 12.1 Range: <1–40 Median: 6.0 SD: 11.9	Mean: 13.3 Range: <1–35 Median: 6.0 SD: 12.4
Years as RN in L&D	Mean: 9.9 Range: <1–34 Median: 4.0 SD: 10.2	Mean: 11.2 Range: <1–35 Median: 4.0 SD: 11.6

examining the responses, it is noted in both samples that the scores were all above 4.0, indicating more nurse confidence, than lack of it, in nurses' ability to demonstrate caring behaviors with their patients (Figure 11.4).

A two-way ANOVA was used to examine if there was a main effect and/or an interaction effect among the demographics. A **main effect** was used because it compared the difference in both samples, not just

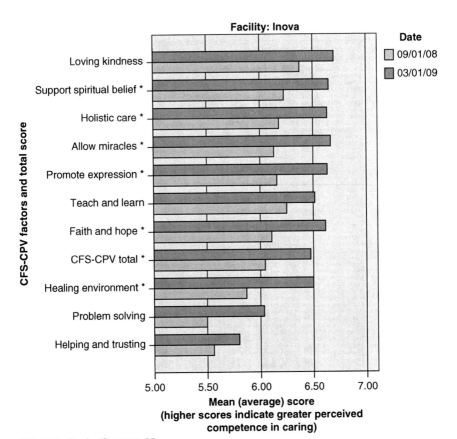

* Statistically significant at .05.

FIGURE 11.4   Mean scores, variables measured by CFS-CPV, 2008 and 2009.

one at a time. The **interaction effect** can be identified if demographic groupings had differing responses to caring within the environment over time (pre- to postintervention). No main effects (using an alpha of 0.05) were found for any demographic subgroups. The only demographic found to have an interaction effect was the number of units worked before L&D. Nurses who never worked on another unit had an increased perception of caring competence over time. In contrast, nurses who worked on other units prior to L&D did not demonstrate statistically significant improvement (Figure 11.5).

Statistics for Anticipated Turnover (AT) Scale

No statistically significant change was noted in AT total scores over time pre- and postintervention (Table 11.4).

The same nurse demographic groupings were used to examine if there were main effects or interaction effects found for any of the variables listed.

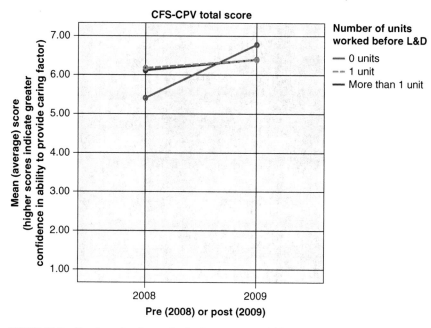

FIGURE 11.5   Number of units worked prior to current L&D unit.

There were no interaction effects ($p < .05$) found for any demographic grouping. Two variables were found to have a main effect (differed in both pre- and postsamples) that was statistically significant at the .05 level: the number of years as an RN. Nurses with less than 3-years experience were more likely to leave, whereas the nurses with more than 4-years RN experience were more likely to stay (Figure 11.6). Additionally, nurses who work 36–40 hours per week in L&D reported being more likely to leave than nurses who reported working less than 36 hour in L&D (Figure 11.7). Nurses were asked in the demographic information pre- and postintervention about their performance of human-caring behaviors (Table 11.5).

Two-way ANOVA between intentional-caring behaviors and human-caring training with pre- and post-CFS-CPV total scores was performed. Only centering demonstrated an interaction effect with the total CFS-CPV score over time.

There were no interaction effects among the four caring behaviors, being familiar with the caring program, or attending human-caring training

TABLE 11.4   Statistics Anticipated Turnover for Total Score (All Subscales Combined)

VARIABLE	MEAN PRE/POST	MEDIAN PRE/POST	MODE PRE/POST	SD PRE/POST	MIN - MAX PRE/POST
Anticipated turnover	4.3 / 4.4	4.4 / 4.3	4.7 / 3.4	1.4 / 1.1	1.5-6.8 / 2.4-6.5

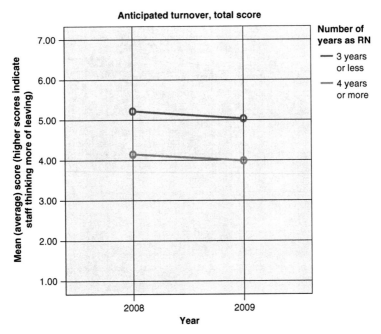

FIGURE 11.6 Main effect of years as RN for anticipated turnover.

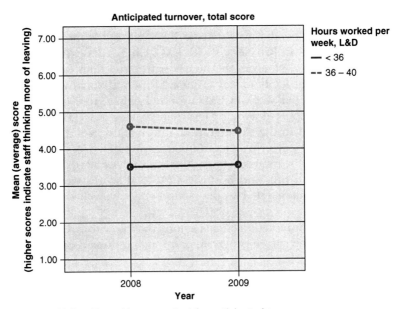

FIGURE 11.7 Main effect of hours worked for anticipated turnover.

TABLE 11.5 Participation in Human Caring Intervention

DEMOGRAPHIC	PREINTERVENTION	POSTINTERVENTION
Do you know what HC program is?	No: 50% ($n = 21$) Yes: 45% ($n = 19$)	No: 5% ($n = 3$) Yes: 37% ($n = 23$)
Have you participated in HC training?	No: 81% ($n = 34$) Yes: 17% ($n = 7$)	No: 35% ($n = 12$) Yes: 47% ($n = 16$)
Do you center?	No: 19% ($n = 8$) Yes: 64% ($n = 27$)	No: 26% ($n = 9$) Yes: 56% ($n = 19$)
Five minutes?	No: 5% ($n = 2$) Yes: 71% ($n = 30$)	No: 5% ($n = 2$) Yes: 62% ($n = 23$)
Hand-washing ritual?	No: 14% ($n = 6$) Yes: 81% ($n = 31$)	No: 11% ($n = 4$) Yes: 61% ($n = 22$)
Caritas circle?	No: 57% ($n = 24$) Yes: 12% ($n = 5$)	No: 65% ($n = 22$) Yes: 18% ($n = 6$)

pre- and postintervention, or with any of the demographics on the AT. The last statistical analysis was a correlation analysis of the CFS-CPV and AT using the Pearson r. No correlation between these two variables was found either preintervention ($r = .146$, p .146) or postintervention ($r = .061$, p .061) (Figure 11.8).

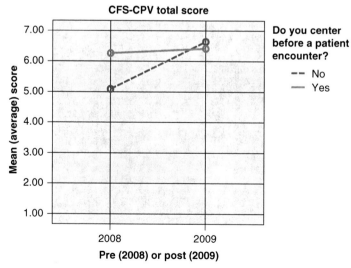

FIGURE 11.8 Interaction effect of centering before a patient encounter on the total CFS-CPV score over time.

Patient Demographics

Several demographics were examined in the patients who responded to the survey because investigators theorized that they may have influence in the responses of the patients. Note that the average age of patients was constant over both years, approximately 31 years. There was a similar makeup in race (White, 53%, 47.5% and Black, non-Hispanic 26%, 35%), religion (Christian Protestant/Catholic, 47%, 49%), multiple experiences with IAH (77%, 80%), support person present (88%, 93%), babies born alive (86%, 89%), satisfactory pain control (85%) for both years. Complete demographics and descriptions of each are noted in Table 11.6.

Caring Factor Survey for Patients

As with nurses' perceptions of their caring competence, patients also reported feeling cared for well above the median (4.0) in both pre- and postsurveys. However, no statistically significant changes in caring process subscales or CFS total score were found when examining the sample groups as a whole.

TABLE 11.6   Demographics of Patients Who Responded to the CFS Instrument

DEMOGRAPHIC	PRE		POST	
Age	Mean: 30.8	Range: 18–44	Mean: 31.1	Range: 18–45
	Median: 30.0	SD: 6.1	Median: 11.0	SD: 6.5
Race	White: 53% ($n = 53$)		White: 47% ($n = 48$)	
	Black, non-Hispanic: 26% ($n = 26$)		Black, non-Hispanic: 35% ($n = 34$)	
	Asian/So. Asian/Pacific Islander: 12% ($n = 12$)		Asian/So. Asian/Pacific Islander: 7% ($n = 7$)	
	Hispanic/Latino: 2% ($n = 2$)		Hispanic/Latino: 9% ($n = 9$)	
	Other: 6% ($n = 6$)		Other: 2% ($n = 2$)	
Religion	Christian/Protestant: 35% ($n = 35$)		Christian/Protestant: 34% ($n = 35$)	
	Catholic: 12% ($n = 12$)		Catholic: 15% ($n = 15$)	
	Other: 40% ($n = 40$)		Other: 42% ($n = 43$)	
	Muslim: 3% ($n = 3$)		Muslim: 3% ($n = 3$)	
	Jewish: 3% ($n = 3$)		Jewish: 2% ($n = 2$)	
	Buddhist: 1% ($n = 1$)		Buddhist: 3% ($n = 3$)	
	Hindu: 1% ($n = 1$)			
	Atheist: 2% ($n = 2$)			
Childbirth (CB) education	Yes: 48% ($n = 48$)		Yes: 42% ($n = 43$)	
	No: 38% ($n = 38$)		No 49% ($n = 50$)	
First labor	No: 48% ($n = 48$)		No: 58% ($n = 60$)	
	Yes: 44% ($n = 44$)		Yes: 28% ($n = 29$)	
First IAH experience	No: 77% ($n = 77$)		No: 80% ($n = 81$)	
	Yes: 17% ($n = 17$)		Yes: 19% ($n = 20$)	

(continued)

TABLE 11.6 *(continued)*

DEMOGRAPHIC	PRE		POST	
Number of IAH experiences	Mean: 7.7 Median: 5	Range: 1-37 SD: 7.2	Mean: 6.4 Median: 5	Range: 1-25 SD: 5.3
Number of admits this pregnancy	Mean: 4.4 Median: 3	Range: 1-18 SD: 3.5	Mean: 4.4 Median: 3	Range: 1-19 SD: 3.9
Chose IAH?	Yes: 89% ($n = 89$), No: 3% ($n = 3$)		Yes: 92% ($n = 93$), No: 5% ($n = 5$)	
Expected provider	Yes: 87% ($n = 87$), No: 4% ($n = 4$)		Yes: 85% ($n = 88$), No: 9% ($n = 9$)	
Support person	Yes: 88% ($n = 88$), No: 3% ($n = 3$)		Yes: 93% ($n = 93$), No: 0% ($n = 0$)	
Who is support?	Family: 5% ($n = 5$) Friend: 2% ($n = 2$) Family and friend: 1% ($n = 1$) Significant other: 53% ($n = 53$) Significant other and doula: 2% ($n = 2$) Significant other and family: 19% ($n = 19$) Significant other, family, friend: 3% ($n = 3$) Significant other and friend: 2% ($n = 2$) Other: 1% ($n = 1$)		Family: 6% ($n = 6$) Friend: 1% ($n = 1$) Family and friend: 2% ($n = 2$) Significant other: 63% ($n = 65$) Significant other and family: 12% ($n = 12$) Significant other, family, other: 4% ($n = 4$) Significant other, friend, and other: 1% ($n = 1$)	
Number of hours in labor	Mean: 6.9 Median: 5.3	Range: 0-45 SD: 7.3	Mean: 7.8 Median: 5.0	Range: 0-48 SD: 9.7
Delivery mode	SC: 20% ($n = 20$) UC: 27% ($n = 27$) V: 45% ($n = 45$)		SC: 24% ($n = 25$) UC: 20% ($n = 21$) V: 50% ($n = 51$)	
Baby status	A: 89% ($n = 89$) N: 4% ($n = 4$)		A: 86% ($n = 89$) A: twins: 1% ($n = 1$) N: 6% ($n = 6$)	
Pain control	Yes: 85% ($n = 85$) No: 6% ($n = 6$)		Yes: 85% ($n = 87$) No: 5% ($n = 5$)	

Note: SC = scheduled cesarean; UC = unscheduled cesarean; V = vaginal; A = admit term nursery: N = NICU admit.

Differences Between Demographic Groupings, Caring Factor Survey

A two-way ANOVA procedure was used to identify main effects or interaction effects among demographic subgroups using an alpha level 0.05. Effects were found based on age, religion, race, and perceived pain control.

Age: There was no interaction effect. Main effect of age group of 18 to 25 years was found for patient's perception of support of spiritual beliefs (Figure 11.9).

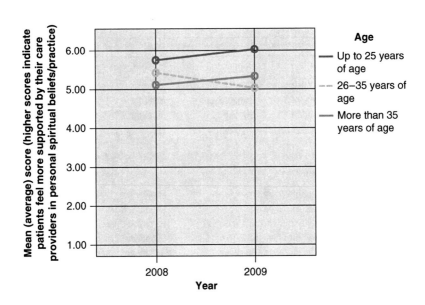

FIGURE 11.9   Support of spiritual beliefs, comparing age groupings by year.

Race: There was no interaction effect. Main effect of race was found for patient's perception of loving kindness, teaching in a way the patient can learn, and building a trusting/helping relationship with the patient. Note that Black patients report lower caring, whereas Asians report higher caring. These patterns are noted in Figures 11.10–11.12.

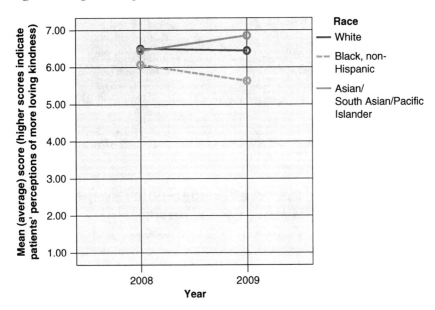

FIGURE 11.10   Loving kindness, comparing race groupings by year.

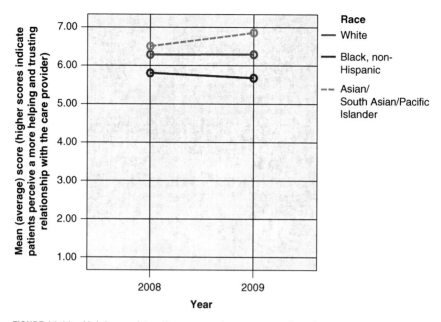

FIGURE 11.11 Helping and trusting, comparing race groupings by year.

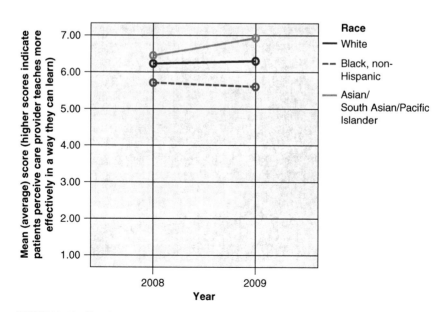

FIGURE 11.12 Teach and learn, comparing race groupings by year.

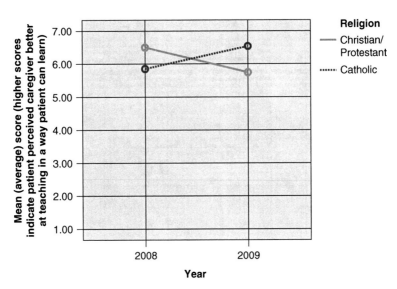

FIGURE 11.13 Teach and learn, comparing religion groupings by year.

Religion: There was a persistent pattern for every caring factor and the total CFS score where Catholic improved pre- to postintervention, whereas the score of Christian/Protestant declined. However, only one variable was statistically significant, teach and learn, which asks patients if the care provider is teaching in a way they can learn. There were no main effects when comparing religion pre- and postintervention (Figure 11.13).

Pain Control: There was a persistent pattern for every caring factor and the total CFS score where the patients who perceived poor pain control had a lower caring score than those who perceived adequate pain control. It should be noted that the sample for those with poor pain control had only six patients preintervention and five patients postintervention. However, the differences between these groups as it relates to caring were striking and worth reporting here despite the small sample size. Main effects were found for loving kindness, teach and learn, healing environment, helping and trusting, holistic care, miracles, and the total CFS score. These finding are noted in Figure 11.14.

DISCUSSION

Nurse Caring on the Unit

L&D nurse participation in the human caring program implementation contributed to nurses' ability to exercise control of their caring practice. As a result, they felt cared for by themselves and each other. Urgencies inherent in care of patients in labor and delivery did not allow

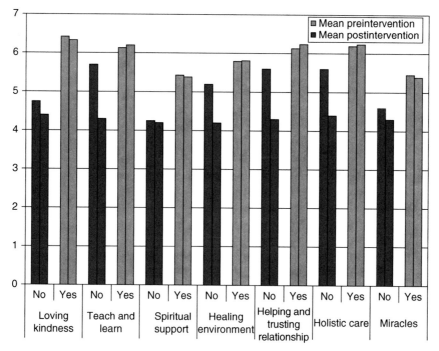

FIGURE 11.14   Perceived pain control.

opportunities on day shift for Caritas circle sharing away from the nurses' station. Unit climate from the nurses' perspective became more caring as evidenced by a significantly improved CFS-CPV total score. Although both pre- and postloving kindness scores approached *strongly agree*, the subscales for healing environment and allowing for miracles showed the widest range of improvement in total score and range of responses. This may suggest that nurses never questioned their personal ability to be loving and kind but found it more effective and satisfying in a healing and hopeful environment.

Even though fewer nurses admitted to practicing centering before a patient encounter postintervention, it is possible that the unit culture was so positively altered that most nurses were consciously working within a more holistic, caring paradigm. Most encouraging was that even the most experienced nurses who perceived themselves as caring competent prior to intervention still achieved higher CFS-CPV total scores postintervention. This suggests that growth and fulfillment within a caring paradigm is not limited.

It should be noted that less-than-optimal unit conditions preintervention may have predisposed staff to readily accept any therapeutic intervention. Postintervention the unit was still without a permanent, patient-care, director, but the number of unit staff had increased by 20 employees (including full-time, part-time, and contract nurses). This also contributes to a more positive work environment.

Novice Nurses

The finding that novice nurses (those who worked in zero units prior to L&D) showed the most improvement in total CFS-CPV scores is interesting. Patricia Benner (2001) has described novices as task oriented, rule bound, and less globally or experientially aware. Without clinical experience to anticipate need and enhance decision making, inexperienced nurses need a list of "things to do" in order to organize and avoid being overwhelmed. By inserting intentional-caring behaviors on the novice's "mental list," conscious focus and practice within a caring paradigm may have taken less time to develop.

Further, whereas novice nurses showed the most caring improvement in total CFS-CPV scores, nurses with the least experience (<3 years) were also the most likely to leave according to the AT scores. These results suggest that increasing caring consciousness simultaneously increases awareness of environmental barriers to caring and healing including noise (e.g., multiple call lights, alarms, phones ringing), limited staffing resources, and inability to meet competing patient needs. This may initially lead novices to frustration and desire to leave. Novice nurses should be fully supported by their colleagues during this vulnerable time.

Anticipated Turnover Model

Performance of intentional-caring behaviors did not significantly change total AT scores. This suggests that additional factors impact a nurse's decision to leave the current job. Part of this model may include unit leadership variables and staffing resources as well as degree of healing environment. In this study, nurses who worked full time were more likely to leave than nurses working part time. In context, this result may suggest that nurses who work more hours in a less-than-optimal work environment have greater exposure to negativity and perhaps less work-life balance, all of which lead to a greater desire to leave. Further research is needed to identify these variables.

Patients

Although nurses report increased caring competence after incorporating the four intentional caring behaviors into their practice, equitable impact should also be demonstrated in the patients' perceptions. However, although pre- and post-CFS total scores for patients were generally high (>4.0), a significant difference in total score was not found. Several demographic subsets did differ significantly from mean total scores.

Cultural Caring

Contrasting demographic group scores may explain the absence of significant change (either positive or negative) in total patient scores but it also identifies a larger issue between cultural context and caring. Asians ($n_{pre}12$, $n_{post}7$), Catholics ($n_{pre}12$, $n_{post}15$), those experiencing their first admission to the IAH ($n_{pre}17$, $n_{post}20$), and those who are ages 18–25 ($n_{pre}15$, $n_{post}^{unknown}$) experienced increased caring. Black, non-Hispanic patients ($n_{pre}26$, $n_{post}24$) experienced less caring both pre- and postintervention particularly related to loving kindness, helping and trusting relationships, and teaching in a way patients can learn. Whereas Catholic patients perceived increased caring, Christian patients did not. Examining the demographic makeup of pre- and postintervention, it is possible that Asian patients in the sample are Catholic, and the Black, non-Hispanic patients are Christian. Regardless, these results suggest that cultural inclinations and barriers exist and can enhance or impede the caring relationship. Further study is needed to determine caregiver and care receiver variables in a cultural caring model. Additionally, follow-up focus groups on this L&D unit may enhance understanding of caring barriers related to age, religion, and race of both patients and nurses.

Perceived Pain Control

Finally, despite the small sample size, patients who reported poor pain control ($n_{pre}6$, $n_{post}5$) consistently reported not feeling cared for across every Caritas Process subgroup and in total CFS score. Poor pain control interferes with optimal healing, as does lack of a caring–healing relationship. Variables to consider investigating in future research include: decreased touching, decreased social interactions, impact of anxiety, time/attention from the caregiver, and lack of patient confidence in caregiver. Further study with a larger sample size is needed to more closely examine the correlation between increased pain and decreased perception of caring and to determine how the caring connection between nurse and patient in pain is lost.

Study Limitation

The decrease in postintervention response rate may introduce bias into the sample depending on which staff nurses responded (those who participated in human-caring implementation or those who did not).

CONCLUSION

Mindful attention by the nurse to building the human caring–healing relationship with the patient does increase nurses' perceptions of their caring competence and contribute to a positive, healing work environment. Caring competence alone does not predict a nurse's intent to stay in the current job. Novice nurses need the most support when consciously developing their caring practice. Patients respond differently to nurse caring based on cultural factors and perceived pain control; more research is needed to develop a cultural caring model.

ACKNOWLEDGMENT

The author acknowledges the contribution of John Nelson, PhDc, MS, RN, to the content of this chapter.

REFERENCES

Benner, P. (2001). *From novice to expert: Excellence and power in clinical nursing practice* (Commemorative ed.). Upper Saddle River, NJ: Prentice-Hall.

Coates, C. (2002). The evolution of measuring caring: Moving toward construct validity. In J. Watson (Ed.), *Assessing and measuring caring in nursing and health science* (pp. 215–241). New York, NY: Springer.

DiNapoli, P., Nelson, J., Turkel, M., & Watson, J. (2010). Measuring the Caritas processes: Caring factor survey. *International Journal of Human Caring, 14*(3).

Drenkard, K. (2008). Integrating human caring science into a professional nursing practice model. *Critical Care Nurse Clinics of North America, 20,* 403–414.

Hayhurst, A., Saylor, C., & Stuenkel, D. (2005). Work environmental factors and retention of nurses. *Journal of Nursing Care Quality, 20*(3), 283–288.

Hinshaw, A. S., Smeltzer, C. H., & Atwood, J. R. (1987) Innovative retention strategies for nursing staff. *Journal of Nursing Administration, 17*(6):8–16.

McNeese-Smith, D. (1999). A content analysis of staff nurse descriptions of job satisfaction and dissatisfaction. *Journal of Advanced Nursing Administration, 29*(6), 1332–1341.

Nelson, J. W. (2007). Measurement instruments for a caring environment. In M. Koloroutis, J. Felgen, C. Person, & S. Wessel (Eds.), *Relationship-based care: Visions, strategies, tools and exemplars for transforming practice* (pp. 597–605). Minneapolis, MN: Creative Health Care Management.

Persky, G., Nelson, J., Watson, J., & Bent, K. (2008). Creating a profile of a nurse effective in caring. *Nursing Administration Quarterly, 32*(1), 15–20.

Stechmiller, J. (2002). The nursing shortage in acute and critical care settings. *AACN Clinical Issues* (13), 577–584.

Strachota, E., Normandin, P., O'Brien, N., Clary, M., & Krukow, B. (2003). Reasons registered nurses leave or change employment status. *Journal of Nursing Administration, 33*(2), 111–117.

Swanson, K. (1999). What is known about caring in nursing science. In A. Hinshaw, S. Fleetham, & J. Shaver (Eds.), *Handbook of clinical nursing research* (pp. 31–60). Thousand Oaks, CA: Sage.

Vitello-Cicciu, J. (2001). *Leadership practices and emotional intelligence of nurse leaders.* Santa Barbara, CA: The Fielding Institute.

Watson, J. (2002). *Assessing and measuring caring in nursing and health science.* New York, NY: Springer.

Watson, J. (2008). *Nursing: The philosophy and science of caring* (Rev. ed.). Denver, CO: University of Colorado Press.

12

Caring at the Core: Maximizing the Likelihood That a Caring Moment Will Occur

Mary Ann Hozak and Maria Brennan

*A*ltruistic caring is the primary focus of nursing. Such caring promotes positive outcomes for patients and nurses alike. The model of care delivery, relationship-based care (RBC) (Koloroutis, 2004), is the model that is based on Watson's (2005) theory of Caritas and was thus used to pursue implementation of altruistic care at the study site, St. Joseph's Healthcare System (SJHS) in Paterson, New Jersey. Involvement of the entire organization was required to satisfy the tenets of this altruistic practice model and care delivery system. Inclusive within this involvement was commitment to developing a structure for caring moments and a process of reflective practice with measured outcomes that would define an organizational culture of caring. Concepts of RBC have been described in detail in Chapters 5 and 9. Baseline measures using four instruments referred to as Caring at the Core helped establish an understanding of what unique successes and needs were existing at the hospital, department, and unit levels. Baseline data also assisted with understanding that there were relationships that existed at SJHS among employee self-care, patient perception of caring, and the work environment. This chapter reviews the RBC launch at SJHS and the initial insights into how caring and infrastructure relate to one another.

BACKGROUND

St. Joseph's Regional Medical Center, a 651-bed teaching hospital, was founded in 1868 by the Sisters of Charity of St. Elizabeth, whose mission is to care for the poor and underserved in the culturally diverse urban community of Paterson, New Jersey. Today it is part of SJHS, which includes St. Joseph's Children's Hospital on the Paterson campus; St. Joseph's Wayne Hospital, a division of St. Joseph's Regional Medical Center, a 229-bed community hospital in Wayne; St. Vincent's Nursing Home in

Cedar Grove; and Visiting Health Services of New Jersey. It has been the honor of the Paterson campus to have been granted Magnet status by the Magnet Recognition Program® since 1999, one of the first 15 Magnet hospitals in the country, and then to receive the 2010 Magnet prize for nursing innovation for the Women's Heart Center.

Guiding and supporting the implementation of the RBC process included staff commitment to high professional standards, strong nursing leadership, a perceptive board of trustees, and supportive executive leadership. There were also reference tools we used to maintain positive energetic progress from the launch into the trajectory of transition to RBC. One of the essential resources was the book I_2E_2: *Leading Lasting Change* by Felgen (2007) that helped us understand *inspiration, infrastructure, education, and evidence*. It should be noted that the I_2 stands for inspiration and infrastructure while the E_2 stands for the education and evidence.

Inspiration

Inspiration starts with the mission of the Sisters of Charity at SJHS and from Dr. Jean Watson's theory of caring (Watson, 2008). The 10 Caritas (caring) Processes serve as the foundation for the structure. Caring is in the heart of each health care worker in the organization, with this practice model and care delivery system. Watson's work (2008) has inspired SJHS to pursue the art of caring with articulated structures and processes that center on care for self and others. Pursuit of the art of caring was perceived to allow all employees to care for patients and families with joy and fulfillment.

Infrastructure

The RBC implementation guide of Creative Health Care Management (CHCM) and the Professional Nursing Practice Council were both used as the hub for the transformation and involved use of a grassroots approach to develop the structure and processes within SJHS. A designated master's-prepared, registered nurse (RN) titled RBC Manager coordinates the project and serves as liaison, coach, and mentor for each department and nursing unit as they start the journey. Each of these groups elects an advisory council consisting of 20% of the staff to develop, implement, and evaluate the practice model and care delivery system specifically designed for the department. A results council was also formed consisting of vice presidents, physicians, directors, managers, and the staff advisory council chairs.

Responsibility, accountability, authority, as well as the guiding principles are defined and agreed upon through consensus by this interdisciplinary team. Having senior leadership involved allows for staff to see the commitment of the organization as well as have immediate decisions made for issues and action plans that the advisory councils bring to the table. Transforming care at the bedside (TCAB) is a problem-solving process used by the councils to brainstorm on issues, then develop and evaluate action plans to solve the identified issues or barriers to care.

Education

Understanding the principles and theory of caring was paramount for everyone, from executive leadership and physicians to staff. Educational sessions thus encouraged a thorough assessment of the mission, vision, and values of the organization on three levels: that of the organization as a whole, each department's role, and a self-assessment for each employee. Once assessed the sessions were individualized for the departments to work on processes to achieve the caring goals set. This most important phase of I_2E_2 (Felgen, 2008) is ongoing. It establishes a strong foundation and commitment to ensure a successful change to a caring culture.

Evidence

Each action plan developed by the departments includes a measurement process. Patient satisfaction or the particular indicators within the satisfaction survey, National Database for Nurse Sensitive Indicators (NDNQI), or department-specific performance improvement tools, are used to uniquely measure outcomes for the action plan as developed. In 2010, we collaborated with John Nelson and Jean Watson to measure caring at the organizational level. In preparing for the study, we decided to offer the surveys in Spanish for both employees and patients because we serve a large Hispanic community.

METHODS

Surveys were e-mailed to a convenience sample of 3,790 staff members at SJHS in 162 units/departments within the Wayne and Paterson campuses. For those who did not have e-mails, an electronic link was provided on a computer in their unit/department. A sample of at least 400 responses was desired for comparison of up to 20 different groups (service lines or units), using a one-way ANOVA. This sample size would ensure a power of 0.87 and an effect size of 0.25, using an alpha of 0.05. To conduct Pearson's correlations between measures, a sample of at least 400 was necessary to ensure a power of 0.92 and a smaller effect size of 0.15 while using an alpha of 0.05. Finally, a sample of 400 using a stepwise regression of 10 variables would ensure a power of 0.99 and an even smaller effect size of 0.1 while using an alpha of 0.05.

Post hoc analyses were used to increase understanding of environmental factors, including examination of demographic data using t tests, correlations, and one- and two-way ANOVAs. An alpha of 0.05 was chosen to control for Type I errors (reporting a difference between demographic groupings when no difference occurred). Power of 0.80 was chosen to control for Type II errors (reporting no difference between demographic groupings when there actually was a difference). Post hoc power analyses and associated narrative are provided throughout the results section of this report for each respective statistical procedure.

Caring-at-the-Core Measures

Four surveys were used to understand the state of caring and the infrastructure where caring occurs. Caring measures included four psychometrically tested tools, including:

- **Caring Factor Survey–Caring for Self (CFS-CS).** Measures employees' level of self-care using Watson's theory of Caritas and described further in Chapter 4 by Lawrence and Kear.
- **Caring Factor Survey–Care Provider Version (CFS-CPV).** Measures employees' perceived execution of 10 caring behaviors as proposed by Watson's theory of Caritas and described by Johnson in Appendix G.
- **Caring Factor Survey (CFS).** Measures patients' perceptions of the 10 caring behaviors within Watson's theory of Caritas (DiNapoli, Nelson, Turkel, & Watson, 2010).
- **Healthcare Environment Survey (HES).** Used to evaluate essential health care environmental factors for RBC and described in more detail in Chapters 5 and 9. This measure is premised on sociotechnical systems (STS) theory and assesses both relational and technical aspects of the work environment. It is designed to be used by all employees who work in health care. It consistently predicts 66% of the variance of job satisfaction for employees who work in health care (personal communication with John Nelson, November 11, 2010).

A reflective practice approach was used for this study, incorporating quantitative and qualitative data in order to create action plans for process improvement at the unit/department level. This approach seeks to encourage collaboration of researchers and research participants with the common goal of establishing a meaningful understanding of the data. Situated and evaluated within the context of organizational processes, including the RBC initiative, such data facilitate dialogue focused on processes of caring and environmental improvement.

Scientific rigor is essential when conducting research, including meticulous evaluation of variables influencing data, such as differences in responses among demographic groupings. For example, responses may vary based on the unit the participant works in or the professional role of the participant.

Procedures

Staff received an e-mail on July 19, 2010, which introduced them to each of the three staff surveys. The HES was proposed to take approximately 20 minutes to complete, whereas the CFS-CS and CFS-CPV took 2 and

5 minutes, respectively, to complete. Each e-mail sent to each employee contained a link to his or her respective survey. Staff was asked to complete the survey by August 22, 2010. For those who did not have e-mails, kiosks were set up within SJHS for employees to access the survey portal. Once in the portal, they entered a unique access code that directed them to the survey. A total of 3,790 employees were invited to participate. An option for Spanish surveys was available for those staff who did not speak English well or at all.

Upon opening the survey via the Internet, respondents could view instructions for completing the surveys as well as an explanation of the intent of the study. The explanation included a statement of confidentiality assuring them that the final report would not link data to any individual participant—data would be provided only in aggregate form. In addition, contact information for the primary researcher and internal project coordinator within SJHS was provided so participants could contact him with questions if needed.

Participants were allowed as much time as desired to respond to each of the surveys and were able to save their responses if they wished to complete any one of the surveys at a later time. Upon completing each of the surveys, the staff member received instructions on how to submit them and, once submitted, was unable to access them again. Return of the survey was considered as a participant's consent to include their data in the study, as explained in the introductory page of the survey. Only the primary researcher—from an outside consulting organization in Minnesota—had access to the survey data. Two reminder e-mails were sent to those invited to participate. For patient surveys, 30 surveys were provided to each of the 33 patient care units. It was desired to secure 30 from each of the 33 units. Patients who elected not to respond to the survey informed the person collecting the data why they did not respond by selecting one of four options on the consent form. Nonresponders were not considered one of the 30 surveys, and units were to continue seeking responders until there were a total of 30 completed CFS.

RESULTS

Descriptive statistics and psychometric properties of the HES, the CFS, the CFS-CPV, and the CFS-CS are included within the review of the results. There is focus on the three services with the largest number of respondents, including ambulatory, operations, and patient care services. Response rates are described immediately below.

Healthcare Environment Survey (HES)

There were 758 of 3,790 staff who responded to the HES, representing a 20.2% response rate. The Wayne campus had a slightly higher response rate of 28.7% (196 of 682) when compared to the Paterson campus, which had a 18.1% response rate (562 of 3,108). Among the eight service lines, medical education and human resources had the highest response rates of 66.7% and 53.4%, respectively. The lowest response rate was in finance, with 0.03% responding.

Demographics

Nurses represented the largest group of respondents (n = 281, or 37.1%), followed by support staff (n = 255, or 33.6%) and leadership (n = 114, or 15.0%). Leadership was inclusive of advanced practice nurses, case management, managerial staff, or those in patient support roles with a master's or a doctoral degree. The remainder of the 12 role groupings was less than 20 in each respective grouping.

The largest age group among those who responded to the HES represented the 50–59 age grouping (n = 230), followed by 40–49 (n = 137). Responders were predominantly female (n = 614, or 80.9%). Just over 60% reported being married (n = 434) or domestically partnered (n = 22). Baccalaureate preparation was the most commonly reported highest level of education (n = 260, or 34.3%), followed by diploma (n = 208); master's/doctorate (n = 112); and, finally, associate's degree (n = 110).

Just over 55% reported working 36–40 hours per week (n = 427, or 56.3%) followed by those who work more than 40 hours per week (n = 233, or 30.7%). Almost 23% of the staff reported working more hours than they were scheduled (n = 173, or 22.8%). Ninety-one percent reported working only one shift (n = 692) in contrast to the 4% who stated they worked two different shifts (n = 28) and the 16 who reported working three or more different shifts.

Experience in the same unit was represented mostly by those with less than 5 years of experience (n = 302, or 39.8%), followed by 5–10 years (n = 302, or 26.6%). Hospital experience was most commonly reported to be less than 5 years as well (n = 263, or 34.7%), followed by 5–10 years (n = 189, or 24.9%). Professional years was most commonly reported to be less than 5 years (n = 155), followed by 5–10 years (n = 130, or 17.1%). It should be noted that there were 159 who had 26 or more years of experience in the same profession.

A demographic profile has been created for each of the large, responding service lines. This is important to understand the associated needs that accompany demographics. Over time these demographics may change, but these data provide a profile to understand needs and baseline description (Table 12.1).

Psychometrics of HES

Psychometrics for the HES total score and all 14 of the subscales demonstrated satisfactory performance, with Cronbach's alpha levels greater than 0.70. A subscale is a subset of items within an instrument (such as the HES) that measures a domain of interest. An example of a subscale

TABLE 12.1 Demographic Profile

DEMOGRAPHIC	PREDOMINATE GROUP %, AGGREGATE	PREDOMINATE GROUP %, AMBULATORY	PREDOMINATE GROUP %, OPERATIONS	PREDOMINATE GROUP %, PATIENT CARE
Age	50–59 (30%) 40–49 (23%)	50–59 (30%) 40–49 (21%)	50–59 (37%) 40–49 (19%)	50–59 (28%) 40–49 (26%)
Role	Nurse (37%) Support staff (34%)	Support staff (37%) Leadership (23%)	Support staff (55%) Leadership (20%)	Nurse (63%) Support staff (25%)
Gender	Female (81%)	Female (73%)	Female (67%)	Female (90%)
Partner status	Partnered (60%)	Partnered (73%)	Partnered (53%)	Partnered (60%)
Education	Baccalaureate (34%)	Master's (25%)	Diploma (47%)	Baccalaureate (44%)
Work over schedule	Work over schedule (23%)	Work over schedule (27%)	Work over schedule (15%)	Work over schedule (25%)
Professional experience	Less than 5 years (20%)	5–10 years (23%)	Less than 5 years (27%)	Less than 5 years (19%)
Hospital experience	Less than 5 years (35%)	Less than 5 years (34%)	Less than 5 years (41%)	Less than 5 years (31%)
Unit experience	Less than 5 years (40%)	Less than 5 years (41%)	Less than 5 years (45%)	Less than 5 years (35%)

would be a subset of the HES, which measures workload and addresses perceptions of tasks required within one's work. According to Polit (1996), relying on scales demonstrating Cronbach's alpha levels less than 0.70 is considered risky.

Descriptive of HES

When examining the responses to the environmental subscales, it is noted that the aggregate scores were all above the midpoint of 4.0 on the scale of 1–7. Recall that the midpoint indicates neutrality, and scores above 4.0 indicate greater satisfaction, whereas scores below 4.0 indicate more dissatisfaction. The variable receiving the highest score was job satisfaction with a mean aggregate score of 5.87. The lowest scoring variable was perception of workload with a mean score of 4.27. When examining the scores by role, all variables had mean scores above 4.0 for leadership and support staff. Only nurses had one variable below 4.0, which was perception of workload.

To identify environmental factors related to job satisfaction for each discipline, correlations for all variables were examined within a zero-order correlation table. A correlation between variables means that a relationship exists between the variables. The relationship can be positive or negative. A positive relationship means that two variables move in the same direction; therefore, if one variable increases, the paired variable also increases, or if one decreases, the other variable also decreases. Conversely, a negative relationship means that two variables move in opposite directions, so as one variable increases, the paired variable decreases. Examination of correlations for all variables in the aggregate data determined that every variable measured had a positive correlation with job satisfaction.

Examination of the correlation table separated by role determined that every variable correlated with job satisfaction for nurses and support staff. For leaders, every variable except professional patient care correlated positively with job satisfaction. All these correlations were found to be statistically significant at the 0.05 level (Table 12.2).

Differences Between Roles

Differences between role groupings were statistically significant using an alpha of 0.05 for 10 of the variables measured, including relationship with coworkers, relationship with physicians, relationship with nurses, workload, autonomy, distributive justice, professional patient care, pride in the organization, intent to stay, and job satisfaction. The differences were statistically significant between support staff and the two other roles of nurses and leadership for perception of professional patient care. Nurses were found to differ from both support staff and leadership when comparing perception of distributive justice, pride in

TABLE 12.2   Mean (Average) Scores All Variables (Aggregate, and by Role)

VARIABLE	AGGREGATE	LEADERSHIP	NURSES	SUPPORT STAFF
Job satisfaction	5.87	6.14	5.66	5.93
Pride in the organization	5.63	5.78	5.44	5.85
Participative management	5.62	5.70	5.55	5.68
Professional patient care	5.61	5.61	5.74	5.52
Relationship with coworkers	5.56	5.36	5.64	5.52
Relationship with nurses	5.47	5.36	5.68	5.32
Professional growth	5.40	5.54	5.41	4.52
Executive leadership	5.31	5.37	5.27	5.34
Relationship with physicians	5.30	5.09	5.33	5.48
HES total (subscales combined)	5.24	5.35	5.21	5.28
Staffing/scheduling	5.23	5.13	5.15	5.37
Autonomy	5.21	5.53	5.13	5.15
Intent to stay	5.17	5.52	5.07	5.10
Distributive justice	4.46	4.66	4.17	4.79
Workload	4.27	4.43	3.77	4.72

the organization, relationship with nurses, and job satisfaction. Leadership was found to differ in perception of relationship with coworkers, relationship with physicians, autonomy, and intent to stay. All roles differed from each other when comparing perception of workload.

These differences, using an alpha of 0.05, support a power of 0.88 and an effect size of 0.15. An effect size of 0.15 is very sensitive, created by the large sample size, and needs to be considered within interpretation and importance of differences. These differences are noted graphically in Figures 12.1 and 12.2.

Differences Between Service Lines

Data were examined for differences among the three largest service lines as well. Service lines included operations, rehabilitation services, and patient care services. A one-way ANOVA was used to examine differences. Identified differences are used to facilitate discussions with nurse managers for decision-making purposes related to resource allocation within the RBC initiative. Such use is consistent with a participative action research (PAR) method, using both data and dialogue to refine the work environment. Nine variables plus the total HES score were found to have differences when comparing service lines. Specific variables included job satisfaction, pride in the organization, participative management,

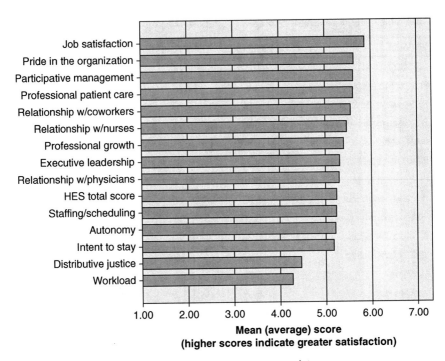

FIGURE 12.1   Variables in order of satisfaction, aggregate data.

professional patient care, relationship with coworkers, relationship with nurses, intent to stay, distributive justice, and workload. Ambulatory was more satisfied than operations and patient care services for perceptions of relationship with coworkers, intent to stay, and the total HES score. Operations was more satisfied than ambulatory care and patient care services when comparing relationship with nurses and professional patient care. Patient care services was more satisfied than operations and ambulatory care when comparing workload, distributive justice, and pride in the organization. Ambulatory and patient care services differed when comparing job satisfaction and participative management. Differences found were statistically significant at the 0.05 level. These differences are noted graphically in Figure 12.3.

Regression Equations of HES

To further illuminate aspects of employees' work environment, stepwise regression equations were used to examine key variables. There were three variables of interest:

   1. *Professional Patient Care (Primary Nursing).* This is the core product and consists of four elements: developing a relationship with the

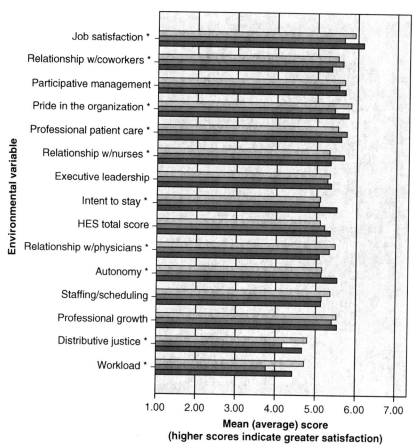

FIGURE 12.2   Variables of job satisfaction, comparing roles.

patient/family, care planning, collaborating with other disciplines, and providing continuity of care for the patient/family.

2. *Autonomy.* This variable addresses the care providers' ability to use their knowledge and experience to deliver the care appropriate for each individual patient/family. Inability to deliver care understood by the care provider to be important for the patient/family creates role strain, which increases depression and sick call and lowers productivity.

3. *Pride in the Organization.* This construct represents employees' enthusiasm in working for the organization and may result in bragging

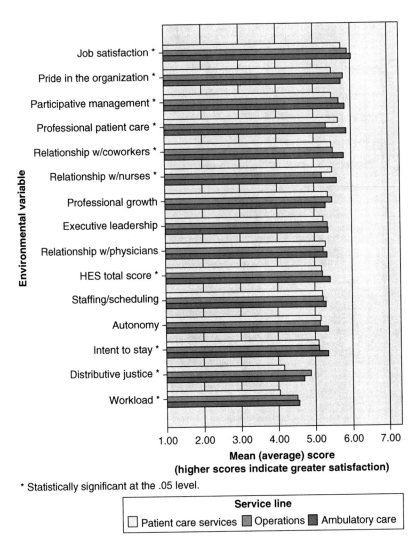

* Statistically significant at the .05 level.

Service line
☐ Patient care services ▨ Operations ■ Ambulatory care

FIGURE 12.3 All HES variables comparing service lines.

about the job they perform and/or the place where they work. This has implications for productivity and going the extra mile to ensure that quality work is provided.

Autonomy

Autonomy for support staff was predicted by participative management (22.7%), workload (7.1%), relationship with coworkers (3.8%), and staffing/scheduling (2.0%). Autonomy for nurses was predicted

TABLE 12.3   Predictors of Autonomy Within RBC, and Amount of Explained Variance

ROLE	EXPLAINED VARIANCE OF AUTONOMY (AS PERCENTAGE OF TOTAL EXPLAINED AUTONOMY)							
	PARTICIPATIVE MGMNT	WORK-LOAD	STAFF SCHED	PROF GROWTH	PROF PATIENT CARE	REL W/ CWKR	HOSP YRS	TOTAL VARIANCE EXPLAINED
Leadership	53.1%	5.5%	0	8.3%	0	0%	0	68.7%
Nurses	35.5%	10.8%	1.1%	0	5.8%	0%	1.0%	54.2%
Support staff	22.7%	7.1%	1.8%	0	0	3.8%	0	35.6%

by participative management (35.5%), workload (10.8%), professional patient care (5.8%), staffing/scheduling (1.1%), and number of years in current hospital (1.0%). Autonomy for leadership was predicted by participative management (53.1%), professional growth (8.3%), workload (5.5%), and staffing/scheduling (1.8%). These data are noted in Table 12.3.

Professional Patient Care

For support staff, professional patient care was predicted by professional growth (16.5%), staffing/scheduling (8.3%), and relationship with physicians (5.5%). Professional patient care for nurses was predicted by autonomy (28.0%), relationship with nurses (9.2%), professional growth (3.1%), level of education (1.2%), relationship with coworkers (1.1%), and executive leadership (0.09%). For leadership, professional patient care was predicted by relationship with nurses (15.3%) (Table 12.4).

Pride in the Organization

For support staff, pride in the organization was predicted by professional growth (39.2%), professional patient care (12.4%), relationship with co-workers (2.4%), and distributive justice (1.5%). Pride in the organization for nurses was predicted by professional growth (36.2%), professional patient

TABLE 12.4   Predictors of Professional Patient Care

ROLE	EXPLAINED VARIANCE OF PROFESSIONAL PATIENT CARE								
	REL W/ NURSES	PROF GRWTH	REL W/ MDS	AUTONOMY	STAFF/ SCHED	LEV EDUC	REL W/ CWRKER	EXEC LDRSP	TOTAL VAR EXPLAINED
Leadership	15.3%	0	0	0	0	0	0	0	15.3%
Nurses	9.2%	3.1%	7.1%	28.0%	0	1.2%	1.1%	0.09%	43.5%
Support staff	0	16.5%	5.5%	0	8.3%	0	0	0	30.3%

care (8.4%), workload (3.7%), executive leadership (2.1%), distributive justice (1.1%), and years in same profession (0.08%). For leadership, pride in the organization was predicted by professional growth (34.3%) (Table 12.5).

Qualitative Data of HES

Data were validated and idiosyncratic aspects of the organization identified by examining responses to open-ended statements. The following statements were presented for respondents to complete:

- The one aspect of my job that I enjoy the most is:
- The one aspect of my job that makes me want to stay with this organization is:
- The aspect of my job that creates the most stress for me within my work is:
- The one aspect of my job that makes me want to leave this organization is:

Comments were categorized and tallied. It is noted that the patient is what employees report they enjoy the most, followed by coworkers, and the work itself. Comments related to the patient included reports of taking care of the patient, just being with the patient, or being able to observe good patient outcomes. For coworkers, comments related to teamwork, having friends, or being able to teach or be taught by coworkers. For the work itself, comments related to a specific aspect of their job like balancing the books for accounting, or working in the intensive care unit (ICU) for ICU staff.

For a reason to stay, it is noted that coworkers were reported the most, followed by the patient and the work itself. There were about 50 employees who reported that they stay because of management and 40 employees who reported their current shift or hours as their reason to stay.

When inquiring about stress, it is noted that workload was the most common report by almost 300 employees. A distant second was "nothing."

TABLE 12.5 Predictors of Pride in the Organization

	EXPLAINED VARIANCE OF PRIDE (AS PERCENTAGE OF TOTAL EXPLAINED PRIDE)								
ROLE	PROF PATIENT CARE	EXEC LDRSHP	DISTRIB JUSTICE	PROF GRWTH	REL W/ CWRKR	PROF YEARS	STF/ SCHED	WORK-LOAD	TOTAL VAR EXPLAINED
Leadership	0	0	0	34.3%	0	0	0	0	55.6%
Nurses	8.4%	2.1%	1.1%	36.2%	0	0.08%	0	3.7%	52.3%
Supp staff	12.4%	0	1.5%	39.2%	2.4%	0	0	0	42.2%

This refers literally to nothing currently creating stress at the time of the survey.

Reports of reasons to leave were most commonly about coworkers. Thus, it becomes clear that employees do not view the same coworker relationship in the same way; whereas some stay because of coworkers, others want to leave because of coworkers. It is likely that this is biased by different units. Some units/departments likely are very successful at coworker relationships, whereas other units/departments have yet to identify how to achieve healthy teamwork (Figure 12.4).

Caring Surveys

This section reviews the results of caring behaviors as perceived by the employees and patients. It is premised on Watson's theory of Caritas (caring), which essentially asserts that when the 10 caring behaviors are demonstrated to self or others, there will be healing for the respective recipients of caring behaviors.

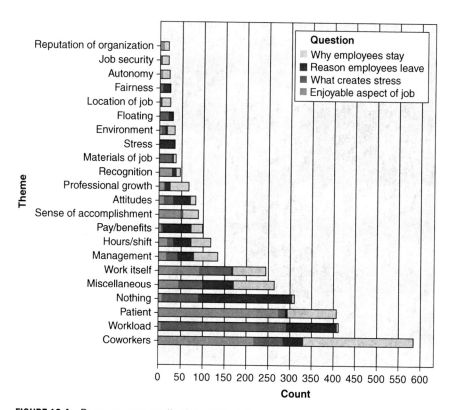

FIGURE 12.4   Responses to qualitative statements.

TABLE 12.6   Descriptive Statistics, CFS-CS

CARITAS CONCEPT	N	MINIMUM	MAXIMUM	MEAN	SD DEVIATION
Teaching and learning	426	1.00	7.00	6.3944	.98667
Helping and trusting relationship	425	1.00	7.00	6.3106	1.05621
Instill faith and hope	426	1.00	7.00	6.3075	1.09836
Miracles	399	1.00	7.00	6.1404	1.21769
Decision making	426	1.00	7.00	6.1009	1.11319
Healing environment	424	1.00	7.00	6.0825	1.13207
CFS-CS total	392	1.00	7.00	6.0740	.97503
Spiritual beliefs and practices	408	1.00	7.00	5.9877	1.32352
Promote expression of feelings	425	1.00	7.00	5.9741	1.23693
Holistic care	425	1.00	7.00	5.9506	1.31569
Practice loving kindness	426	1.00	7.00	5.6620	1.55020

Caring for Self

There were 427 employees of the 3,790 who responded to the CFS-CS, which represents an 11.3% response rate. It is noted that all caring factors were above 5.0 with teaching/learning for self being the highest score and loving kindness toward self as the lowest (Table 12.6 and Figure 12.5).

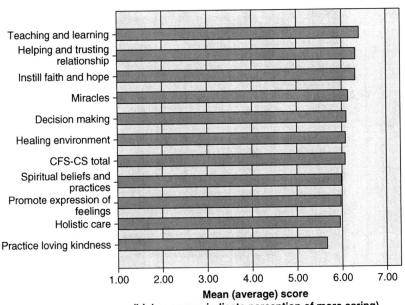

FIGURE 12.5   Rank order of caring factors from CFS-CS.

When looking at the differences between service lines, it was noted that there were three caring factors that had statistically significant differences, including loving kindness, decision making, and holistic care. These differences are noted in Figure 12.6.

When units were compared, there were differences that were statistically significant at the 0.05 level for loving kindness, decision making, holistic care, healing environment, the promoting of expression of both positive and negative feelings, allowing belief in miracles, and the total CFS-CS score. It is noted that the Regan 2 psych has the highest scores for 8 of the 10 caring factors (Figure 12.7).

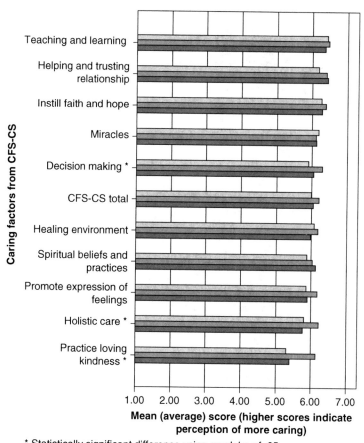

* Statistically significant difference using an alpha of .05.

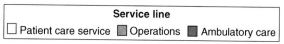

FIGURE 12.6 Caring factors for CFS-CS, comparing service lines.

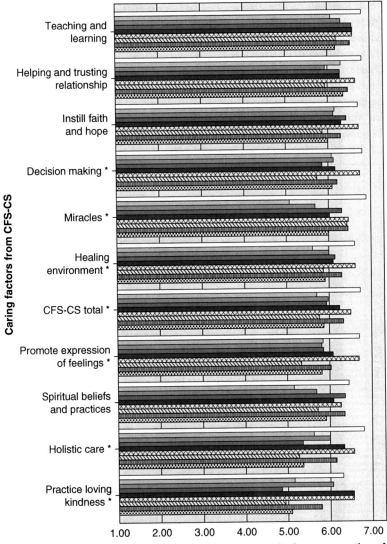

* Statistically significant difference using an alpha of .05.

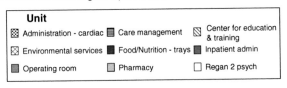

FIGURE 12.7 CFS-CS scores, comparing units with at least 10 respondents.

Caring Toward Patients as Perceived by Employees

There were 382 of the 3,790 staff who responded to the CFS-CPV, a 10.1% response rate. All employees were invited to respond because it was perceived that all employees interact with patients on some level and thus have an opportunity to create a caring moment. Some employees did contact the author of this report to inform that they did not have any contact with patients and thus did not respond to the survey. For the 382 who did respond, it is noted that all mean scores are above 6.0. Loving kindness was ranked as the most successful caring behavior and problem solving was the least. The rank order of all caring factors as operationalized by the employees and as perceived by the employees is noted in Table 12.7 and Figure 12.8.

Within the aggregate scores noted in Figure 12.8, there were 305 employees from the Paterson campus and 77 from the Wayne campus. When comparing campuses, there were no differences found that were statistically significant using an alpha of 0.05.

Examination of role revealed that there were 36 nurses, 127 from support staff, and 142 from the leadership staff who responded to the CFS-CPV. When comparing these groupings, it is noted that nurses reported the highest score for all caring factors and the total CFS-CPV score except for perception of problem solving. Support staff demonstrated better operationalization of problem solving. It is interesting to note for the factors in the CFS-CPV that problem solving is repeatedly found to be the lowest ranked factor in repeated studies conducted by the author of this report. The difference noted in this study for problem solving when comparing roles was statistically significant at the 0.05 level. Problem

TABLE 12.7   Descriptive Statistics of CFS-CPV, All Responders

CARITAS PROCESS	N	MINIMUM	MAXIMUM	MEAN	STD DEVIATION
Loving kindness	380	1.00	7.00	6.4671	.93006
Faith and hope	380	1.00	7.00	6.4171	.95497
Allow miracles	379	1.00	7.00	6.3219	.99033
Teach and learn	377	1.00	7.00	6.3156	1.05555
Holistic care	377	1.00	7.00	6.2997	.99417
Promote expression	379	1.00	7.00	6.2968	1.05140
Spiritual support	379	1.00	7.00	6.2889	1.00015
Total CFS-CPV	367	1.00	7.00	6.2602	.88609
Healing environment	377	1.00	7.00	6.1631	1.06281
Helping/trusting relationship	377	1.00	7.00	6.0796	1.05515
Problem solving	380	1.00	7.00	6.0697	1.10873

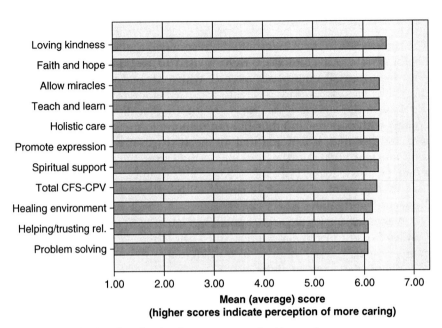

Mean (average) score
(higher scores indicate perception of more caring)

FIGURE 12.8   Rank order of caring factors, as perceived by employees.

solving was the only factor that had a difference that was statistically significant. It was leaders that differed from support staff (Figure 12.9).

When comparing service lines for the CFS-CPV, the only factor that was found to be statistically significant was perception of problem solving. No trends were noted among comparisons of service lines (Figure 12.10).

Caring Toward Patients as Perceived by Patients

A total of 455 CFS were distributed to patients and 419 were returned, a 92.1% response rate. Of the 36 who did not respond, 34 provided their reason and these reasons are noted in Table 12.8.

Descriptive statistics of the CFS revealed that helping/trusting relationship had the highest mean score of 6.41, with spiritual support reporting a mean score of 5.80. It is noted for the 421 patients who responded to the CFS that all scores were above 6.0, except perception of support for spiritual belief (Table 12.9 and Figure 12.11).

When examining the responses of patients, and patients' family members, the scores from the family members were consistently reported to be lower. There were 317 responders who identified themselves as family members ($n = 80$) or patient ($n = 237$). Using G-Power to identify power parameters, a t test revealed an alpha of 0.05, an effect size of 0.35, and power of 0.81. Using these parameters, it was identified that six of the caring factors plus the total CFS score had differences that were statistically significant. Variables with significant differences included decision making, holistic care, helping/trusting relationship, healing environment,

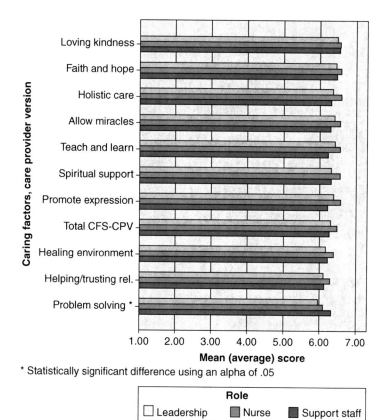

FIGURE 12.9   Caring factors within the CFS-CPV, comparing roles.

promoting of expression of feelings, allowing miracles, and the total CFS score (Figure 12.12).

When examining the differences between the Spanish-version CFS and the English-version CFS, it is noted that the English-version responses were higher for 8 of the 10 caring factors plus the total CFS score. Two of these differences were statistically significant, including perception of loving kindness and perception of care providers promoting expression of both positive and negative emotions/feelings (Figure 12.13).

When looking at the different races, it was noted that there were differences that were statistically significant for 3 of the 10 caring factors measured. There was also a trend for Whites reporting the highest caring scores for 7 of the 10 caring factors measured (Figure 12.14).

Correlations Between Measures

This section reviews the relationships that were found between caring and the work environment. It was hypothesized that the work environment would relate to the operations of caring for self and others.

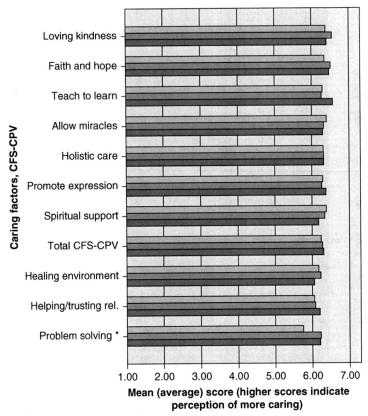

*Difference statistically significant at .05 level.

Service line		
☐ Patient care service	■ Operations	■ Ambulatory care

FIGURE 12.10 Caring factor scores, comparing service lines.

TABLE 12.8 Reasons for Not Participating in Study, Cited by Patients

REASON FOR REFUSAL	FREQUENCY
I am too sick or upset to respond to a survey	11
I do not want to spend my time responding to a survey	13
I do not like to give out information about myself	7
Other	3
Total nonrespondents with reason for refusal	34
Total nonrespondents who did not provide reason for refusal	2
Total respondents	419
Total respondents and nonrespondents	455

TABLE 12.9 Descriptive Statistics, CFS

CARITAS PROCESS	N	MINIMUM	MAXIMUM	MEAN	STD DEVIATION
Helping and trusting relationship	418	1	7	6.41	.971
Loving kindness	403	1	7	6.35	.933
Holistic care	416	1	7	6.31	1.094
Decision making	412	1	7	6.27	.980
Teach and learn	413	1	7	6.26	.958
CFS total	381	1	7	6.21	.886
Promote expression of feelings	417	1	7	6.20	1.074
Healing environment	414	1	7	6.17	1.103
Instill faith and hope	409	1	7	6.12	1.143
Allow miracles	403	1	7	6.02	1.217
Support spiritual belief	402	1	7	5.80	1.403
Valid N (listwise)	381				

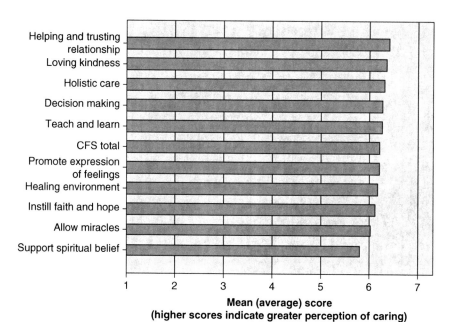

Mean (average) score
(higher scores indicate greater perception of caring)

FIGURE 12.11 Aggregate scores for the CFS ($n = 421$).

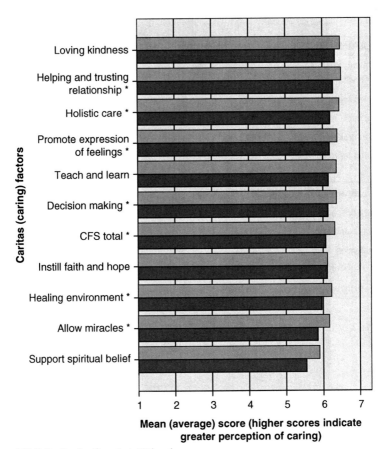

*Statistically significant at .05 level.

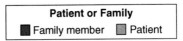

FIGURE 12.12   Differences between patients and family members.

Caring for Self and the Work Environment

It was hypothesized that self-care as measured by the CFS-CS would relate to perceptions of the work environment as measured by the HES. Findings revealed there was a positive relationship between self-care and relationships with nurses ($r = .142, p .024$) and relationships with physicians ($r = .125, p .046$). It is hypothesized that those who perform self-care understand more clearly their own gifts as well as limitations that they can offer to others. Such understanding is supported by self-care, which facilitates self-reflection, renewal, and greater access to frontal lobes due to increased release of healthy hormones like oxytocin. Further testing is warranted.

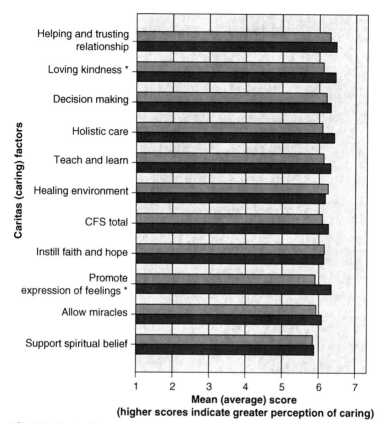

*Statistically significant at .05 level.

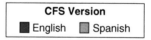

FIGURE 12.13 Differences between Spanish and English CFS.

Employee Perception of Caring for Others and the Work Environment

In examination of the perception of competence and personal operations of caring behaviors using the CFS-CPV, it was found that this related to the relationship with physicians ($r = .137, p .035$), the total HES score ($r = .161, p .027$), and hours worked ($r = .134, p .022$).

The relationship between competences in caring may relate to the relationship with the physician. This finding of the physician relating to caring is consistent with the findings in the regression equation for patient care where the relationship with the physician predicted 7.1% of the variance of patient care for nurses and 5.5% for support staff.

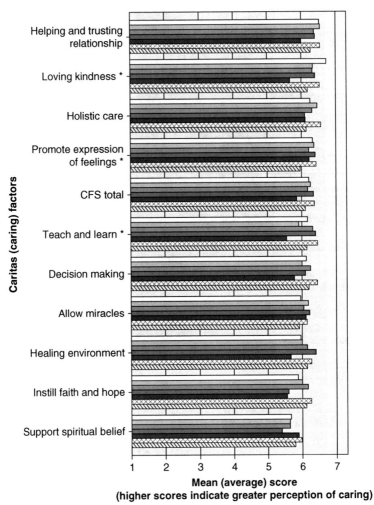

* Statistically significant using an alpha of .05.

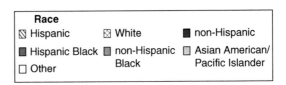

FIGURE 12.14   Comparing race.

The relationship between perceived operations of caring and the total HES scores suggests that there is an overall positive relationship between the work environment and being able to execute caring. This relationship is the accumulation of all the subscales and is something to consider as a whole, rather than each subscale and environment factor separately.

The relationship between perceived caring and actual hours worked infers that those who are there longer perceive greater ability to execute caring behaviors. Further testing is warranted.

Patient Perception of Caring and the Work Environment

Patients were not paired with employees, so the level of analysis that was required was the unit level. There were 20 patient care units that had enough responses from the HES to use for correlation analysis. It must be considered that using an alpha of 0.05 with a sample of 20 yields very low power. Using a large effect size of 0.4 with an alpha of 0.05 yields a power of 0.59. This should be considered a limitation of this study. When running a correlation analysis, the following variables from the HES were found to correlate with caring as reported by the patient using the CFS:

1. Staffing/scheduling, $r = .589, p .010$
2. Professional growth, $r = .584, p .007$
3. HES total score, $r = .44, p .020$
4. Distributive justice, $r .524, p .018$
5. Relationship with nurses, $r = .519, p .019$
6. Pride in the organization, $r = .459, p .042$

It is not clear if these environmental variables, as perceived by an employee, predict caring as perceived by the patient, but it is understood that these five environmental variables and the total HES score relate to the patient's perception of caring. Further testing with larger samples, along with theory to guide the questions, will be needed for further testing.

DISCUSSION

This baseline examination of the work environment, self-care of employees, and caring of patients as perceived by both employees and patients reveals that there is no "average" unit, relationship, or employee. This further exemplifies how caring needs to be tailored for that point in time and context (Watson, 2005). Data are currently being used at the unit, department, and hospital levels. It is also being examined at the individual level for self-care because caring begins with the care of self.

The process of using data in a reflective practice way, as in this baseline measure and presentation of data, is the first step in empirical refinement of the work environment. Data derived from the ongoing analysis will assist with understanding how self-care, care for others, and the work environment impact healing of employees and patients.

NEXT STEPS

As SJHS continues to roll out the Watson and RBC models and implement action plans developed by the departments and units, a longitudinal research study will be used to monitor the progress using the action plan tools. The first comparison of this baseline measure will be conducted in August 2011 to assess progress. One variable from this study of particular interest was the relationship between the nurses and the support staff, particularly within radiology and housekeeping. Their perceptions of the relationship with nursing scored lower than anticipated. The plan is to gather a task force with leadership and staff to drill further down using the TCAB problem-solving process, then use the August 2011 survey to measure level of successes.

A second, broader examination of workload will be conducted as well. The low score of workload was especially notable in nursing-care units that had high numbers of admissions, discharges, and transfers (ADTs). Midnight census is used at SJHS as the method for staffing nurse-to-patient ratios, and this method may not adequately capture the workload created by ADTs. A research group has been formed to examine this at the unit level. It is planned to create models of workload that are specified at the unit level. Once the models are generated by unit-specific staff, each participating unit will examine workload longitudinally to understand patterns of workload over time and for each nurse and associated demographic.

Finally, there are plans to examine the structure of the environment itself. Does the environment facilitate or impede self-care for staff? For example, it has been discussed with organization architects that the theory of architecture-proposed relationships are facilitated by cross sections in a building (e.g., intersecting hallways) and gathering spaces. This would in turn support the Caritas Process for self and others to take time for relationships and foster relationships. Thus, do units with cross sections and gathering spaces (e.g., break rooms, unit report rooms, conference rooms) have higher relationship scores in the CFS, CFS-CS, and CFS-CPV when compared to units without such gathering spaces? Or do units that have, or are in close proximity to, spiritual centers/rooms have higher scores for spiritual care on the CFS, CFS-CS, and CFS-CPV? Further inquiry is in the planning stage to understand how structure facilitates Caritas.

A higher participation rate is expected with the second time the Caring at the Core™ measures are used in 2011. It was fascinating to see staff who did not respond voice regret at not responding because they would have liked to have had their unit/department be more involved, but due to low response rate, were not able to. The authors of this study were informed that staff had not seen data used in such an intensive and purposeful way. Seeing the purposeful use of the data with staff participation appears to be a strong motivator for staff to not only respond, but to become empowered to action-plan and create their own change toward a more caring environment. This ongoing measure emphasizes the organization's commitment to creating and sustaining a culture of caring.

REFERENCES

DiNapoli, P., Nelson, J., Turkel, M., & Watson, J. (2010). Measuring the Caritas processes: Caring factor survey. *International Journal for Human Caring, 14*(3), 15–20.

Felgen, J. (2007). *I₂E₂; Leading lasting change.* Bloomington, IN: Creative Health Care Management.

Koloroutis, M. (Ed.). (2004). *Relationship-based care: A model for transforming practice.* Bloomington, IN: Creative Health Care Management.

Polit, D. F. (1996). *Data analysis and statistics for nursing research.* Stamford, CT: Appleton & Lange.

Watson, J. (2005). *Caring science as sacred science.* Philadelphia: F. A. Davis.

Watson, J. (2008). *Nursing; The philosophy and science of caring.* Boulder: University Press of Colorado.

13

"Partners in Care": Patient and Staff Responses to a New Model of Care Delivery

Dawn Julian and Marjorie J. Bott

At the beginning of 2009, the Patient Care Administration at a community hospital in Kansas asked the unit-based council (UBC) of a 28-bed medical/oncology nursing unit to develop a partnership model of care delivery for the unit. The purpose of the request was to increase patient satisfaction, improve patient outcomes, and retain staff. The unit had an average daily census of 25 patients with a shorter length of stay compared to similar units at comparable hospitals. Patient acuity had increased due to numerous factors including closure of the mental health unit, implementation of inpatient dialysis services, and an increase in cardiac interventions. The addition of several new physician specialties including nephrology and infectious disease, also had increased the number of patients with complex multisystem disorders.

A plan was initiated to use medical/oncology as the pilot unit with the intention of eventually implementing the care delivery system in other units in the hospital. The UBC for the medical/oncology unit was made up of staff whose members were asked to participate based on their experience, varied roles, and past record of participation in meetings. The UBC was made up of four registered nurses (RNs), two licensed practical nurses (LPNs), and one certified nursing assistant (CNA). The clinical coordinator (CC) attended the meetings as a management liaison. A staff development specialist attended to assist with literature searches for evidence-based practice.

Modified total patient care was the previous nursing-care delivery model. With modified total patient care, the nurse assigned to the patient is responsible for all of the care that the patient receives but is provided some assistance from a CNA. In reality, the majority of activities of daily living and vital signs are performed by CNAs. Staffing patterns usually resulted in a nurse-to-patient ratio of 1:4–5. The CNA-to-patient ratio was 1:8–14.

The UBC chose to name the new model "Partners in Care" and adopted Jean Watson's theory of human caring as the theoretical framework. The proposed model paired a nurse (RN or LPN) with a CNA who worked as a team to care for a group of five to six patients during the 7 a.m. to 7 p.m. day shift. The CNAs were assigned to fewer patients under the new model and reported to just one nurse for that shift. The unit continued to have a designated charge nurse with no patient assignments as well as a unit clerk who entered orders into the electronic medical record. The UBC also selected five caring behaviors (see Appendix 13.1 at the end of this chapter) as a guide for interacting with patients. Prior to implementation of the model, all unit staff received 4 hours of in-service on the partners-in-care model, that included information about Watson's theory of human caring, the five caring behaviors, leadership, and delegation. Education of new staff occurred during orientation, and Watson's theory of human caring and partners in care were discussed at bimonthly staff meetings and included in the unit newsletter.

PURPOSE

The purpose of this quality improvement project was to compare several indicators before and after implementation of the care delivery model including patient satisfaction, patient and caregiver perceptions of care, and the health care team's communication and teamwork. The survey was given to staff and patients prior to conducting the educational programs and the implementation of the partners-in-care model, and again 3 and 6 months after implementation.

BACKGROUND

Nursing Significance

Patient satisfaction is used as an indicator of quality care by health care institutions. It also is a contributing factor for financial success of a health care institution (Larrabee et al., 2004). Hospital administration uses patient-satisfaction reports to evaluate nursing services; consequently, it is important to monitor changes in patient satisfaction when implementing a new care-delivery model.

Literature Review

Guiding Studies

From the review of the patient-satisfaction literature, there was a study that served as a guide for this project because its purpose was "to evaluate the effect of implementing a *Caring Model* on patient satisfaction"

(Dingman, Williams, Fosbinder, & Warnick, 1999, p. 1). Because the UBC had just selected a caring theory, this was very relevant to the practice setting and the project.

Dingman et al. (1999) looked at implementation of the model and the impact on patient-satisfaction scores for the unit. The setting was a community hospital that was part of a multihospital corporation, whereas my practice setting is part of a larger management organization. Dingman et al. (1999) selected five caring behaviors to include in the care-delivery model: (a) introduce yourself to patients and explain your role in their care that day; (b) call the patient by his or her preferred name; (c) sit at the patient's bedside for at least 5 minutes per shift to plan and review the patient's care; (d) use a handshake or a touch of the arm; and (e) use the mission, vision, and value statements in planning your care (see Appendix 13.1 at the end of this chapter). The article described reviews done before implementation of the model along with methods such as education programs, inclusion in monthly staff meetings, adding competencies to job descriptions and performance reviews, and of in-servicing nurses to the caring model.

A widely accepted, reliable survey tool, developed by the Gallup Organization, was used in the Dingman study (1999), a good indicator of patient satisfaction that also was used for several years at the facility. Postimplementation of the model, analysis of variance (ANOVA), and leverage analysis were performed on 8 of the 16 attributes that were related to patient satisfaction and that were obtained from the Gallup survey data: overall nursing care, staff showed concern, nurse anticipated needs, nurses explained procedures, nurses demonstrated skill in providing care, nurses helped calm fears, staff communicated effectively, and nurse/staff responded to requests (Dingman et al., 1999).

Analysis results showed an improvement in patient satisfaction at 3 and 6 months; the positive trend continued but it was not as significant. Dingman and colleagues (1999) suggested the need for ongoing education or a reward system based on continued improvement in patient satisfaction. Having a nurse sit with the patient for 5 or more minutes during the shift to discuss the plan of care was very similar to a recommended, but not usually done, intervention at my practice setting. The study found this to be an important patient satisfier. According to Dingman and colleagues, patients can contribute to their care, giving them a sense of control, and, ultimately, this impacts their outcomes. To promote this, nurses use caring interventions, that is, (a) introduce themselves to the patients when they enter the room, (b) call the patients by their preferred name, and (c) always explain to the patients what they are doing. This reassures the patients and makes them feel that the nurse has a personal interest in them and that they contribute to their own plan of care. Recommendations included the need for ongoing reminders, incorporating caring into the culture, sharing of patient-satisfaction data, and the need for nursing leadership to understand the impact that patient satisfaction has on the financial performance of the organization.

Another study by Birk (2007) described a hospital that chose Jean Watson's caring theory and integrated it into nursing services; the approved pilot study showed a positive effect. The many ways that the theory was incorporated into nursing services were presented. The goals were to translate caring concepts to a wide range of employees, provide cohesion across hospital processes, and support evidence-based practice.

Other Relevant Studies

Motivated by the findings and information from the Dingman and Birk studies and possible application to my practice setting, a literature review of nurse caring (initially focusing on Watson's theory) and patient satisfaction was completed.

A descriptive, correlation research design was used in a 500-bed hospital by Duffy and Gaut (1992) to measure the relationships between nurse caring and several outcomes, including patient satisfaction, with Watson's theory on caring used as the framework. One hypothesis was that there would be a positive relationship between nurse caring and patient satisfaction for patients hospitalized in medical or surgical units. The study also used a quantitative approach to examine relationships between nurse-caring behaviors and four variables: patient satisfaction, health status, length of stay, and cost of nursing care. Data were collected from a purposeful sample of 86 selected medical/surgical patients who had been hospitalized 48 hours. Confused and critically ill patients were excluded. The study found that nurse-caring behaviors were related to patient satisfaction, but nurse caring was not related to the other variables in the study.

Duffy (2003) expanded on the quality-caring model and focused on the phases of caring. The nursing model was created as a guide for practice and as a research foundation. The authors of another study (Duffy & Hoskins, 2003) discussed the positive relationship between nurse caring and patient outcomes, especially in regard to professional nursing care. The pilot implementation plan looked at patient satisfaction as an outcome indicator. A component of the plan was staff schedules that included either three consecutive 8-hour shifts or two consecutive 12-hour shifts for continuity of care, as well as the ability to access nursing literature on the nursing unit to allow for evidence-based practice (Duffy, Baldwin, & Mastorovich, 2007).

Greeneich (1993) delineated a patient-satisfaction model, and reported that "the match between patient expectations and nursing care and the care actually received is expressed as patient satisfaction" (p. 64). Thus, new and return business for a hospital has been linked to quality care identified through patient satisfaction. Long and Greeneich (1994) also identified that it is important that the family views the nurse as caring in order to feel satisfied in the care that the nurse provides for their family member. Several techniques that help to increase family satisfaction by meeting their expectations or by helping them adjust their expectations were discussed.

Williams (1998) used the Holistic Caring Inventory (HCI) to look at what dimensions of nurse caring influenced the patient's perception of quality and of caring behaviors by the nurse. The inventory defines four dimensions of caring including physical caring, spiritual caring, interpretive caring, and sensitivity to individual needs and feelings. Inpatients ($n = 94$) and outpatients ($n = 165$) who were receiving intravenous (IV) therapy for cancer completed the survey. The patients viewed quality care as more related to caring and interpersonal interactions than competent nursing care. The patients perceived that they received more physical and sensitive care and less spiritual and interpretive caring from nurses.

An emergency department (ED) setting was used in Iceland to conduct a study (Baldursdottir & Jonsdottir, 2002) designed to identify what nurse-caring behaviors the patients thought were indicators of caring, using Watson's caring theory. The survey was mailed to a sample of 300 patients with a 60.7% response rate. The survey instrument was a 61-item questionnaire based on Croin and Harrison's Caring Behaviors Assessment tool. Patient responses indicated that nurses' competencies, such as knowing what they were doing, knowing when to call the physician, knowing how to give shots and start IVs, and knowing how to handle equipment, were the most important behaviors related to caring.

Another study (Boykin, Schoenhofer, Smith, St. Jean, & Aleman, 2003) was published describing a 2-year research project that examined a nursing practice model of caring. Because a Press Ganey patient-satisfaction tool was used to measure outcomes in one pilot unit, application and generalizability may be limited. However, the findings did reveal a significant improvement in patient satisfaction following the implementation of a practice model of caring.

The hypothesis of a study by Larrabee et al. (2004) was that the patient's perception of nurse caring would predict patient satisfaction. The predictive, nonexperimental study used convenience samples of 362 patients and 90 RNs from an academic medical center. Other variables investigated were RN job satisfaction, patient characteristics, and the context and structure of care. Findings indicated that patient-perceived nurse caring predicted patient satisfaction. RN and medical doctor (MD) collaboration also was seen as a direct predictor of patient satisfaction. The other variables were not significant predictors of patient satisfaction.

Ryan (2005) described a research study that hypothesized that the patients' perceptions of caring behaviors would increase after implementation of a strategic action plan that integrated Watson's theory into the plan. The author felt that it would be important for nurses to realize that their role in health care is unique and essential. The anticipated barriers included the fast pace of the health care environment and the diversity of the nursing staff.

A study by Persky, Nelson, Watson, and Bent (2008) that examined the characteristics of the "Caritas" nurse (from Jean Watson's theory) was done in a large acute care hospital with 85 nurses and 85 patients using the Caring Factor Survey and Healthcare Environment Survey. The purpose of the study was to measure the impact of caring on operational and patient outcomes. Both quantitative and qualitative data were collected. This study looked at nurse characteristics but did not examine effects on patient satisfaction. Future studies were recommended to compare caring with patient outcomes. A surprise finding was the negative correlation between nursing caring and frustration with the work environment.

Marckx (1995) presented a model based on Watson's caring theory. The proposed outcome was that the quality of resident care in a dementia unit will be enhanced when caring is evident. Ideas about how to integrate Watson's caring theory into clinical practice in a nursing unit also were discussed by McCance, McKenna, and Boore (1999). They compared four caring theories in nursing and concluded with the discussion of the use of caring theories in nursing practice and stated that "the development of specific theories focusing on caring in nursing is indicative of the increasing recognition being given to caring as a central concept within the discipline" (p. 1394).

Felgen (2003) shared two exemplar stories from a critical care setting and discussed Jean Watson's caring model in association with Dingman's five intentional interventions: (a) asking the patient/family their preferred name, (b) introducing self and explaining their role in care, (c) sitting for 5 minutes with patient and family to plan care, (d) using appropriate touch as defined by the patient, and (e) connecting the organization's mission statement with the patient's plan of care. He reported that evidence suggested that caring behaviors in a caring, healing culture promote patient, family, and staff satisfaction.

Dorn (2004) presented a caring, healing model of inquiry that could be used for research and performance-improvement activities. The author stated that nurses were able to integrate the theory with evidence-based practice, but there was no evidence supporting the assumption. Caring theory often has been used as a conceptual framework for research and as a way for nurses to describe their contributions to health care.

Smith (2004) reviewed studies based on Jean Watson's theory of caring. Findings suggested that patients include technical competence as a nurse-caring behavior, whereas nurses do not. Smith identified four categories of research related to Watson's theory: (a) the nature of nurse caring, (b) nurse-caring behaviors as seen by nurses and clients, (c) human experiences and caring needs, and (d) evaluating outcomes of caring in education and practice. Smith stated that one of the limitations was that many studies were qualitative, and with some it was difficult to see the connection with Watson's theory.

Warelow, Edward, and Vinek (2008) discussed problems in the work environment that limit the nurse's ability to practice in a caring manner. Problems such as time and workload pressures, frequent interruptions, and no predictability in the workplace affected the nurse's ability to form caring relationships with patients and families.

Review of Assessment Tools

Koloroutis (2004) provided additional information about Dingman's "The Caring Model" as well as a chapter authored by Dingman on outcomes measurement. Additionally, Dingman et al. (1999) mentioned another hospital only 60 miles away from my location that had used "The Caring Model" to "recapture" the essence of nursing. A generic outcomes grid with patient satisfaction with care was presented along with information about data-collection tools, evaluation and tracking, and a celebration to recognize improvements.

Wolf, Giardino, Osborne, and Ambrose (1994) conducted a study to validate the caring-behaviors inventory. The findings reported by nurses ($n = 278$) and patients ($n = 263$) suggested a relationship between nurse caring and Jean Watson's theory of caring. A later study by Wolf et al. (1998) reviewed nurse caring as reported by the patients ($N = 335$) about their satisfaction with the care. Two instruments, the caring-behaviors inventory and a patient-satisfaction instrument, were given to patients in the hospital or mailed to them within 1 year. Nurse caring and patient satisfaction were found to have a strong positive correlation.

Watson (2009) was reviewed as a source for tools to use in the evaluation of the partners-in-care intervention. She promoted the use of evidence-based practice and the measurement of outcomes that assist in the assessment of the caring role and its influence on the care outcomes that contribute to best care practices. Watson presented research studies that demonstrated the validity of several simple measurement tools to evaluate the effectiveness of new models of care delivery. In her book Watson describes the Caring Factor Survey for patients (CFS) and the Caring Factor Survey–Care Provider Version (CFS-CPV), which were selected to be used in this study.

A national effort by the Robert Wood Johnson Foundation and the Institute for Healthcare Improvement (IHI) published a guide to "transform care at the bedside" (Lee, Shannon Rutherford & Peck, 2008). The guide has a tested and validated tool, called the Healthcare Team Vitality Instrument (HTVI), to measure the functioning of unit staff. The tool generates data about the unit work environment, engagement and empowerment, handoffs and care transitions, and team communications.

Summary

Evidence-based studies should be the standard for determining inpatient nursing care models. The partners-in-care model was derived using caring theory as the framework. Caring has been shown to influence inpatient care and outcomes. In order to evaluate quality of care, measurement of outcomes was needed, and in order to evaluate the effects of the implementation of "Partners in Care," it was necessary to identify validated instruments. Research studies have demonstrated the validity of several simple measurement tools to evaluate the effectiveness of a partners-in-care delivery model. For the purposes of this project, Watson's (2009) work was used as a source for determining the measurement tools necessary for this evaluation.

METHODS

The goal of the proposed project was to improve care by changing the model of care delivery based on the adoption of Watson's theory of human caring, and to determine if implementation could lead to better outcomes in a particular nursing unit that was facing challenges in the present health care climate. The aim of the quality improvement activity was to answer the following four clinical questions: (a) Does patient satisfaction increase after implementation of a new care-delivery model based on Watson's theory of human caring? (b) Do the patients' perceptions of the care change after implementation of a new care-delivery model based on Watson's theory of human caring? (c) Do the caregivers' (RNs, LPNs, CNAs) perceptions of care change after implementation of a new care-delivery model based on Watson's theory of human caring and practice? (d) Does staff communication and teamwork change after implemetation of a new care-delivery model?

Design

The quality-improvement study used surveys prior to the intervention, and 3 and 6 months after the intervention, the partners-in-care nursing care-delivery model. The study used a nonexperimental survey design examining scores for satisfaction, teamwork, and caring before and after the new model of care delivery was implemented. The surveys were for nursing-care providers (nurses, CNAs, and unit clerks) and for patients.

Sample and Setting

The setting was a 28-bed medical/oncology inpatient unit in a 130-bed community acute care hospital in the Midwest. Separate groups of 50 eligible, discharged patients who were older than 18 years of age, with varied medical or oncology diagnoses, were mailed the Press Ganey surveys at preintervention and at 3- and 6-month postintervention time points. No exclusion criteria were applied because a family member also could complete the survey. Approximately 80 staff (RNs, LPNs, CNAs, and unit secretaries), who worked in the medical/oncology unit, were eligible to participate in the study.

Fifty patients received the CFS, a 10-item instrument developed to reflect Watson's theory of Caritas, prior to staff education sessions; another sample of 50 patients completed the CFS 3 months later. All nursing staff (approximately 80: RNs, LPNs, CNAs, and unit secretaries) in the medical unit were asked to complete a CFS-CPV prior to receiving education on Watson's theory of human caring with 3- and 6-month follow-up data collections.

Intervention

The partners-in-care model was introduced to staff during 4-hour in-services. The in-services were offered numerous times over a 2-week period so that all staff would be able to attend. The sessions covered delegation, teamwork, and Jean Watson's theory of human caring. The five caring behaviors (see Appendix 13.1 at the end of this chapter) were emphasized. Following the staff education sessions, the unit staffing patterns were changed so that a nurse was paired with a CNA to provide care for five to six patients; thus, the model: partners in care.

Measures

Four tested and validated instruments were used to measure changes. These included the Press Ganey surveys, CFS, CFS-CPV (Watson, 2009), and HTVI (Lee et al., 2008).

Press Ganey Survey

Press Ganey collects information for hospitals regarding level of satisfaction with the patient's most recent hospital stay (Press Ganey Associates, Inc., 2010). The goal of the survey is to collect data that will provide useful information that might lead to improved care. Items are related to the admission process, room, nurses, test and treatments, visitors and family, and meals. For the purposes of this project, scores for nurse categories include: friendliness/courtesy of the nurses, prompt response to call, nurses' attitude toward request, attention to special/personal needs, nurses keeping you informed, and skill of the nurses. Personal issues categories include: staff concern for your privacy, how well your pain was controlled, staff addressing emotional needs, response concerns/complaints, staff including decisions regarding treatment, and staff providing care in a safe manner.

CFS and CFS-CPV

The CFS is a 10-item instrument (see Appendix 13.2) and the CFS-CPV is a 20-item instrument (see Appendix 13.3). The CFS and CFS-CPV were developed in conjunction with Watson (2009), nursing theorist who developed the theory of human caring, and John Nelson. Reliability and validity information has been published in Jean Watson's book, *Assessing and Measuring Caring in Nursing and Health Sciences*. Reliability using Cronbach's alpha was 0.97 and 0.98 for the two surveys, respectively. Content validity was established by a panel of four experts. CAT-II was used to establish criterion validity. Predictive validity was established in a study implementing caring intervention.

Healthcare Team Vitality Instrument (HTVI)

The HTVI is part of the "Transforming Care at the Bedside" initiative of the Institute for Healthcare Improvement (IHI) and the Robert Wood Johnson Foundation that measures functioning of unit staff. The tool generates data about the unit work environment, engagement and empowerment, handoffs and care transitions, and team communications. Responses for the 19 items on the Likert scale range from 1 to 5 (1 = *strongly disagree*, 2 = *disagree*, 3 = *neutral*, 4 = *agree*, and 5 = *strongly agree*). Key findings reported by the Robert Wood Foundation (2008) were that the HTVI survey measured what it was designed to measure (team vitality) and that the participants had a consistent understanding of the meaning of items in the survey. Upenieks, Lee, Flanagan, and Doebbeling (2010) studied the HTVI to refine, shorten, and validate it. They reported the validity of the HTVI and stated that it was a useful tool for bedside nurses to track progress in organizational change by assessing support structures, engagement/empowerment, patient-care transitions, and team communication.

Procedures

Approval to conduct the project was obtained from the hospital research review committee. Also, human subject approval was obtained from the human subject committee of the academic medical center where the project leader was enrolled in doctoral course work.

Patients

The CFS, along with a survey cover letter that stated that participation in the survey implied patient consent, was given to the inpatients of the 28-bed medical/oncology unit by the project leader on director rounds. The surveys were distributed within a 3- to 5-day time frame, depending on patient turnover, and were to be returned by the patients in a drop box in the family waiting room. There was no identifying information on the patient surveys. The patient surveys were distributed prior to the partners-in-caring model implementation and 3 months after implementation.

The second instrument for patients was the Press Ganey questionnaire that was mailed by an outside company (Press Ganey) to all inpatients after discharge. The surveys were returned to Press Ganey, and the results were available for all the items on a weekly basis. Reports could be run that provided: (a) data based on the unit where the patient was located, (b) group answers to specified questions, and (c) statistical analysis based on specified criteria. Data that were collected from patients at preintervention and at 3 and 6 months postintervention were used.

Staff

All of the medical/oncology unit nursing staff received a staff information letter (implied consent form) prior to receiving the two staff surveys. Participation was anonymous and voluntary. Surveys for the HTVI and the CFS-CPV were returned by staff to a sealed box in the meeting room prior to the educational in-service on the intervention. The staff members were given the CFS-CPV at a staff meeting at 3 and 6 months postimplementation. Data on the HTVI were collected at 3 months postimplementation, only. The only demographic question asked was, "What is your role on the unit (nurse, CNA, or unit secretary)?"

Data Analysis

A software program from Healthcare Environment, Inc,. was used for the CFS results. Press Ganey patient-satisfaction scores and HTVI mean scores were analyzed looking for significant ($p < .05$) changes. The analysis of the HTVI, CFS, and the CFS-CPV included comparing mean scores of individual items with those of the entire survey before and after implementation at 3 and 6 months. Using t tests and ANOVA, changes in mean scores were used to analyze how nurse-caring behaviors and the new model of care delivery affected patient satisfaction on the Press Ganey and HTVI scores.

RESULTS

Of the 61 staff participants who responded to the surveys, 32 were RNs, 8 were LPNs, 15 were CNAs, and 5 were unit clerks. One survey was returned completed with no role indicated. At the 3-month postimplementation of partners in care, about 25% of the staff attended the "mandatory" staff meeting. Nineteen participants responded to the surveys: 12 RNs, 1 LPNs, and 5 CNAs. Again, one survey was completed with no role indicated.

Mean Total Score for the HTVI Survey

The overall mean score for all the items on the HTVI survey was 3.82 (see Table 13.1). The items with the lowest average scores were: (a) My ideas really count on this unit (M = 3.39); (b) care-team members on this unit feel free to question the decisions or actions of those with more authority (M = 3.39); and (c) essential patient-care equipment is in good working condition on this unit (M = 3.46). The items with the highest preimplementation average scores were: (a) I speak up if I have a patient safety concern (M = 4.34); (b) the work environment on this unit promotes patient safety (M = 4.11); and (c) the support services to this unit respond in a timely manner (M = 4.10).

At 3 months postimplementation the mean total score for the HTVI survey was 3.90 (see Table 13.1). The items with the lowest scores were: (a) the work environment on this unit is well organized (M = 4.00); (b) staff members on this unit treat each other with respect (M = 3.63); and (c) essential patient-care equipment is in good working condition on this unit (M = 3.63). The items with the highest average scores were: (a) I speak up if I have a patient safety concern (M = 4.63); (b) I can discuss challenging issues with care team members on this unit (M = 4.21); and (c) I feel a sense of accomplishment and pride after I have completed my work on this unit (M = 4.18). All of the items with the lowest average scores increased on the postintervention survey.

TABLE 13.1 Healthcare Team Vitality Instrument Scores, Descriptive Statistics at Preimplementation and at 3 Months Postimplementation and T Tests*

IMPLEMENTATION ITEMS	PRE- (N = 61) M (SD)	POST-3 (N = 19) M (SD)	P
I have easy access to the supplies and equipment I need to do my work on this unit.	4.07 (0.79)	4.00 (0.47)	.62
Care-team members on this unit feel free to make important decisions about patient care.	3.99 (0.67)	3.97 (0.63)	.92
The work environment on this unit promotes patient safety.	4.11 (0.77)	4.00 (0.82)	.58
The support services to this unit respond in a timely manner.	4.10 (0.73)	3.89 (0.74)	.29
I can discuss challenging issues with care-team members on this unit.	4.08 (0.81)	4.21 (0.85)	.55
There is good cooperation among different hospital departments.	3.70 (0.70)	3.68 (0.75)	.91

(continued)

TABLE 13.1   *(continued)*

IMPLEMENTATION	PRE- (*N* = 61)	POST-3 (*N* = 19)	
ITEMS	*M* (SD)	*M* (SD)	*P*
My ideas really seem to count on this unit.	3.39 (0.80)	3.79 (0.63)	.04
I feel a sense of accomplishment and pride after I have completed my work on this unit.	3.95 (0.84)	4.18 (0.61)	.29
Nurses, physicians, and other staff on this unit work as a high-functioning team.	3.84 (0.69)	3.97 (0.54)	.43
I speak up if I have a patient safety concern.	4.34 (0.88)	4.63 (0.50)	.18
Care-team members on this unit feel free to question the decisions or actions of those with more authority.	3.39 (0.85)	3.79 (0.79)	.07
Important patient care information is exchanged during shift changes.	4.02 (0.69)	3.95 (1.03)	.77
The work environment on this unit is well organized.	3.64 (0.80)	3.58 (0.61)	.76
If I have an idea about how to make things better on this unit, the manager and other staff are willing to try it.	3.52 (0.85)	3.89 (0.81)	.10
Care professionals communicate complete patient information during handoffs.	3.66 (0.90)	3.67 (0.79)	.96
Staff members on this unit treat one another with respect.	3.54 (0.93)	3.63 (0.60)	.69
Essential patient-care equipment is in good working condition on this unit.	3.46 (1.03)	3.63 (0.60)	.37
There are enough experienced registered nurses to care for the patients on this unit.	3.85 (0.99)	3.84 (0.76)	.97
I am part of an effective work team that continuously strives for excellence even when the conditions are less than optimal.	3.98 (0.91)	3.97 (0.63)	.96
Total items	3.82	3.90	.57

Note: *HTVI data were collected at preimplementation and at 3 months postimplementation.

Press Ganey Patient Satisfaction

The Press Ganey scores were reviewed for patients during the month prior to the implementation of the partners-in-care model of care delivery and during the third month and after the sixth month postimplementation. The score (*M* = 89.5) on the medical/oncology unit for the entire survey was higher at preimplementation than during the third month postimplementation follow-up (*M* =88.6) and during the sixth month postimplementation (M = 84.4); however, none were statistically different (p > .05). Table 13.2 provides data about the categories. Six items about nursing were reviewed. These items evaluated: (a) friendliness/courtesy of the nurses; (b) promptness of response to call; (c) nurses' attitudes toward requests; (d) attention to special/personal needs; (e) nurses keeping you informed; and (f) skill of the nurses. Again the score (M = 90.1) was higher at preimplementation than at 6 months postimplementation (M = 87.5). Another section of items included: (a) staff concern for your privacy; (b) how well your pain was controlled; (c) staff addressing emotional needs; (d) response concerns/complaints, (e) staff including decisions regarding treatment; and (f) staff providing care in a safe manner. The score was higher at preimplementation (M = 91.0) than at postimplementation (M = 84.1).

TABLE 13.2 Press Ganey Categories and Scores at Preimplementation and at 3 and 6 Months Postimplementation

CATEGORIES	PRE- (T1) M (SD) $N = 24$	3 MONTHS POST (T2) M (SD) $N = 32$	6 MONTHS POST (T3) M (SD) $N = 36$	F VALUE* T1–T2 T1–T3
Overall nurses category	90.1 (17.8)	90.9 (13.5)	87.5 (14.5)	−0.18 1.68
Friendliness/courtesy of the nurses	93.8	91.5	90.7	–
Promptness of response to call	86.9	83.3	85.3	–
Nurses' attitudes toward requests	90.2	87.8	87.9	–
Attention to special/personal needs	88.6	84.6	84.6	–
Nurses kept you informed	88.0	82.9	84.3	–
Skill of the nurses	91.7	85.5	91.2	–
Overall personal needs	91.0 (12.5)	87.9 (14.5)	84.1 (17.9)	0.85 1.74
Staff concern for your privacy	93.5	84.3	87.1	–
How well your pain was controlled	90.5	84.4	80.2	–
Staff addressed emotional needs	90.3	80.7	81.7	–
Response concerns/complaints	93.1	76.8	81.9	–
Staff include decisions regarding treatment	88.8	80.0	82.5	–
Staff provide care in safe manner	90.2	78.5	84.3	–
Total	89.5 (11.9)	88.6 (9.3)	84.4 (14.2)	0.26 1.24

Note: *Significant F value = ±1.96.

CARING FACTOR SURVEY–CARE PROVIDER VERSION (CFS-CPV)

Table 13.3 provides the means and standard deviations for the items from the CFS-CPV for preimplementation and for those at 3 and 6 months postimplementation of the model. Comparing the preimplementation score to the postimplementation score at 3 and 6 months, the mean for the total survey decreased from 6.46 to 6.25 and 6.30 at 3 and 6 months, respectively. None of the scores showed improvement; however, with the exception of the support-of-spiritual-belief score none of these scores were statistically different (Figure 13.1). The support-of-spiritual-belief score score was statistically lower at 6 months postimplementation (M = 6.33) from preimplementation (M = 6.72).

TABLE 13.3   Caring Factor Survey–Care Provider Version (CFS-CPV), Descriptive Statistics at Preimplementation, at 3 and 6 Months Postimplementation, and ANOVA Results

SUBSCALE	PRE- OR POST-	N	MEAN	SD	ERROR MEAN	P
Loving kindness	Pre-	52	6.62	.56	.08	.29
	Post-3	19	6.37	.76	.17	
	Post-6	23	6.63	.63	.13	
Problem solving	Pre-	52	5.79	.85	.12	.84
	Post-3	18	5.67	.73	.17	
	Post-6	23	5.76	.62	.13	
Faith and hope	Pre-	52	6.60	.62	.09	.39
	Post-3	19	6.61	.68	.16	
	Post-6	23	6.39	.60	.13	
Teach in a way I understand	Pre-	49	6.49	.74	.11	.26
	Post-3	19	6.26	.81	.18	
	Post-6	23	6.22	.62	.13	
Support spiritual beliefs	Pre-	51	6.72	.56	.08	.01[a]
	Post-3	19	6.29	.82	.19	
	Post-6	23	6.33	.60	12	
Healing environment	Pre-	52	6.50	.63	.09	.09
	Post-3	19	6.16	.82	.19	
	Post-6	23	6.22	.62	.13	
Helping and trust-ing relationship	Pre-	50	6.16	.84	.12	.83
	Post-3	19	6.05	.57	.13	
	Post-6	23	6.09	.54	.11	

(continued)

TABLE 13.3 *(continued)*

SUBSCALE	PRE- OR POST-	N	MEAN	SD	ERROR MEAN	P
Holistic care	Pre-	52	6.56	.62	.09	.55
	Post-3	19	6.50	.55	.13	
	Post-6	23	6.39	.62	.13	
Promote expression	Pre-	52	6.60	.71	.10	.35
	Post-3	19	6.34	1.21	.28	
	Post-6	22	6.34	.70	.15	
Allow miracles	Pre-	52	6.66	.68	.09	.42
	Post-3	19	6.42	.95	.23	
	Post-6	22	6.50	.74	.16	
Total CFS-CPV	Pre-	49	6.46	.52	.07	.25
	Post-3	18	6.25	.52	.12	
	Post-6	22	6.30	.52	.11	

Note: [a]Preimplementation scores were significantly higher than 6-month postimplementation scores.

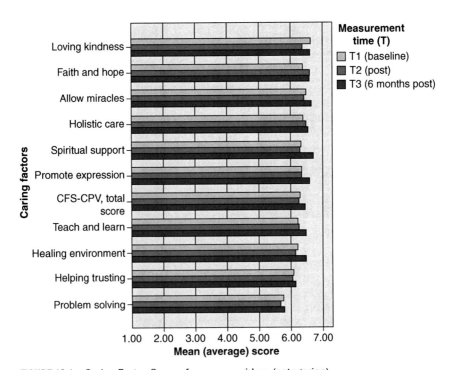

FIGURE 13.1 Caring Factor Survey for care providers (categories).

Caring Factor Survey (CFS)

The CFS total mean scores ($p < .05$) increased significantly from 5.49 (preimplementation) to 6.46 (3 months postimplementation (Table 13.4). The support-of-spiritual-belief score had a statistically

TABLE 13.4 Caring Factor Survey for Patients Descriptive Statistics at Preimplementation and at 3 Months Postimplementation

ITEMS		N	M	SD	STD ERROR	T TEST
Every day I am here, I see that the care is provided with loving kindness.	Pre-	9	6.11	.78	.26	−2.02
	Post-3	8	6.75	.46	.16	
As a team, my caregivers are good at creative problem solving to meet my individual needs and requests.	Pre-	8	5.75	1.16	.41	−2.26
	Post-3	8	6.75	.46	.16	
The care providers honored my own faith, helped instill hope, and respected my belief system as part of my care.	Pre-	8	5.50	1.20	.42	−1.09
	Post-3	7	6.14	1.07	.40	
When my caregivers teach me something new, they teach me in a way I can understand.	Pre-	9	6.11	1.17	.39	−.58
	Post-3	7	6.43	.98	.37	
My caregivers encouraged me to practice my own, individual, spiritual beliefs as part of my self-caring and healing.	Pre-	8	4.50	1.07	.38	−3.17*
	Post-3	7	6.29	1.11	.42	
My caregivers have responded to me as a whole person, helping to take care of all my needs and concerns.	Pre-	9	6.00	1.12	.37	−1.84
	Post-3	8	6.75	.46	.16	
My caregivers have established a helping and trusting relationship with me during my time here.	Pre-	9	6.00	1.12	.37	−1.84
	Post-3	8	6.75	.46	.16	
My health care team has created a healing environment that recognizes the connection between my body, mind, and spirit.	Pre-	8	5.13	1.64	.58	−1.40
	Post-3	7	6.14	1.07	.40	
I feel like I can talk openly and honestly about what I am thinking, because those who are caring for me embrace my feelings, no matter what they are.	Pre-	8	6.00	.93	.33	−1.32
	Post-3	8	6.50	.53	.19	
My caregivers are accepting and supportive of my beliefs regarding a higher power, which allows for the possibility of me and my family to heal.	Pre-	8	5.38	1.19	.42	−1.53
	Post-3	7	6.29	1.11	.42	
CFS total	Pre-	7	5.49	.89	.30	−2.472*
	Post-3	7	6.46	.66	.25	

Note: *$p < .05$.

significant ($p < .05$) increase from preimplementation ($M = 4.50$) to 3 months postimplementation ($M = 6.29$).

DISCUSSION

The findings were mixed from the four different survey tools from patients and staff in the evaluation of the partners-in-care model of care delivery. The Press Ganey patient satisfaction scores and the CFS-CPV scores were lower. The HTVI mean score increased. There was a statistically significant increase in the CFS.

Introduction of Jean Watson's theory of human caring was done during a 4-hour educational offering in August after the initial staff surveys were completed. The model of care delivery implemented was partners in care. The staffing ratios changed; however, the CNAs did not begin training until after the postimplementation survey. Therefore, the day shift nurses were assigned an additional one or two patients and were partnered with a CNA, but the CNA was not yet able to perform additional functions such as removing intermittent IV needles and Foley catheters, changing dressings and ostomy pouches, entering orders for specimen collection, or disconnecting nasogastric (NG) tubes for ambulation. The nurses expressed dissatisfaction at unit meetings about the difficulty in providing nursing care to an additional patient.

The Press Ganey patient satisfaction scores did not increase as reported in the study by Dingman et al. (1999). The expectation by the researcher was that all the surveys would show higher scores at postimplementation, indicating higher staff and patient satisfaction. Although there was an initial decrease in call lights ringing immediately after implementation of the model, there appeared to be a reversion to earlier call-light usage during the study period.

There were many confounding factors to consider when reviewing the findings in order to improve staff and patient satisfaction. These confounders include: (a) increased turnover of nurses during the study period; (b) several nurses orienting to nursing unit; (c) decreased CNA turnover; (d) implementation of walking rounds; (e) lack of student nurses in the summer (during November, RN and LPN students from two nursing programs were training to provide care for patients several days per week); (f) continued financial concerns for the hospital; (g) significant change in the employee benefits package announced prior to the 3-month postimplementation test; (h) the partners-in-care model implemented only on day shift; and (i) change in staffing ratios. There also was the possibility that the unit is still reacting to the changes and not enough time has evolved to see a positive impact from the change.

Shortly after the 3-month postimplementation data were obtained, a decision was made to continue the partners-in-care model of nursing care delivery, but to staff the unit so each nurse and CNA partner pair were assigned up to five patients instead of six. The CFS-CPV was offered to staff again 6 months after implementation. Despite the modification, the preimplementation test scores were significantly higher than the post-6 scores as well as the post-3 scores. The expected increase in scores did not occur even with the patient care technician (PCT) role established and the staffing ratios improved. Fifty surveys had been distributed to patients at preimplementation and at 3 months postimplementation. Less than 20% were returned. Many of the patients on the medical/oncology unit were elderly and very ill.

The initial response rate for the staff surveys was high because all staff attended an educational program. The postimplementation surveys were offered at a staff meeting in which only 20% of the staff attended (although staff meetings are mandatory). Even though the surveys were placed in the report room so that staff who did not attend the staff meeting could participate, no additional staff completed the surveys. A higher staff response rate would make the findings more valid. It is possible that the subgroup of staff who attended the staff meeting responded differently than what the entire unit staff would have responded. Using two different surveys for staff was time consuming and may have contributed to resistance in completing the survey. It may have been more effective to choose one staff survey.

Initially, we saw decreases (although not statistically different) in the satisfaction of both patients and staff. Changes that impact the daily delivery of care take time to be assimilated into daily routines, and that change by itself could result in lower satisfaction. In reviewing the findings, it is not possible to see what impact the adoption of Jean Watson's theory of human caring had on the unit. Although initial teaching of the theory with reinforcement with a poster and information in the newsletter was done, it was possible that in this short time the theory had not become integrated into the unit culture. If the entire division of Patient Care Services adopted the theory there would be more assimilation into the culture of the organization and information could be presented at clinical orientation. When the CFS-CPV survey was repeated by 22 staff 6 months postimplementation, the scores had increased from those obtained at post-3 but were still lower than the preimplementation scores, again possibly indicating that inadequate time had elapsed for there to be positive outcomes from the changes in the care-delivery model.

The findings from this study did not demonstrate the expected increase in patient satisfaction that was anticipated based on the findings of the Dingman et al. (1999) study. Although there was a significant increase in caring as measured by the patient surveys at 3 months postimplementation, the caregiver caring scores had decreased at the data-collection time period. The caregiver caring scores were higher at 6 months postimplementation but were still less than those at preimplementation. The HTVI scores had increased slightly at 3 months postimplementation.

LIMITATIONS

Several factors need to be considered when evaluating for limitations, including staff turnover, which was approximately 30% during this period. Because the caregiver surveys were anonymous, no demographic information was available about the staff other than their role on the unit. There is a possibility that the same patient could complete the initial survey and a follow-up survey, thus creating some dependency in the data. Other unit factors, in addition to the new model of care delivery, could influence the findings. The partners-in-care model was studied only on one unit in the hospital, thus limiting the generalizability of the findings.

FUTURE EVALUATION

The HTVI will be used in the future to monitor teamwork on the unit. Based on the staff responses to the survey to improve teamwork, an action plan needs to be developed. There also is a need to examine staff engagement on the unit. A literature search has been initiated to determine if there are interventions with staff that might improve engagement. Financial concerns have affected the feasibility of having a CNA assigned to only five patients. Patient-care administration is considering again modifying the model by assigning each CNA/PCT to work with two nurses to care for eight to ten patients on the day shift. The data obtained before and after implementation have been very useful in evaluating the impact of the changes. The findings from the surveys were used during the unit's annual budget meeting with finance and the chief executive officer to show the effects the change in model-of-care delivery had on patient satisfaction, perception of caring, and teamwork.

REFERENCES

Baldursdottir, G., & Jonsdottir, H. (2002). The importance of nurse caring behaviors as perceived by patients receiving care at an emergency department. *Heart & Lung: The Journal of Acute and Critical Care, 31*(1), 67–75.

Birk, L. K. (2007). The magnetism of theory: Resonance to radiance. *Journal of Nursing Administration, 37*(3), 144–149.

Boykin, A., Schoenhofer, S. O., Smith, N., St. Jean, J., & Aleman, D. (2003). Transforming practice using a caring-based nursing model. *Nursing Administration Quarterly, 27*(3), 223–230.

Dingman, S. K., Williams, M., Fosbinder, D., & Warnick, M. (1999). Implementing a caring model to improve patient satisfaction. *Journal of Nursing Administration, 29*(12), 30–37.

Dorn, K. (2004). Caring–healing inquiry for holistic nursing practice: Model for research and evidence-based practice. *Topics in Advanced Practice Nursing, 4*(4), 1.

Duffy, J. R. (2003). Caring relationships and evidence-based practice: Can they coexist? *International Journal for Human Caring, 7*(3), 45–50.

Duffy, J. R., Baldwin, J., & Mastorovich, M. J. (2007). Using the quality-caring model to organize patient care delivery. *Journal of Nursing Administration, 37*(12), 546–551.

Duffy, J. R., & Gaut, D. A. (1992). The impact of nurse caring on patient outcomes. In D. Gaut (Ed.), *The presence of caring in nursing* (pp. 113–136). New York, NY: National League for Nursing.

Duffy, J. R., & Hoskins, L. M. (2003). The quality-caring model: Blending dual paradigms. *Advances in Nursing Science, 26*(1), 77–88.

Felgen, J. A. (2003). Caring: Core value, currency, and commodity...is it time to get tough about "soft"? *Nursing Administration Quarterly, 27*(3), 208–214.

Greeneich, D. (1993). The link between new and return business and quality of care: Patient satisfaction. *Advances in Nursing Science, 16*(1), 62–72.

Koloroutis, M. (Ed.). (2004). *Relationship-based care: A model for transforming practice.* Minneapolis, MN: Creative Health Care Management.

Larrabee, J. H., Ostrow, C. L., Withrow, M. L., Janney, M. A., Hobbs, G. R., Jr., & Burant, C. (2004). Predictors of patient satisfaction with inpatient hospital nursing care. *Research in Nursing & Health, 27*(4), 254–268.

Lee, B., Shannon, D., Rutherford, P., & Peck. C. (2008). *Transforming care at the bedside how-to guide: Optimizing communication and teamwork.* Cambridge, MA: Institute for Healthcare Improvement. Retrieved from http://www.IHI.org

Long, C. O., & Greeneich, D. S. (1994). Family satisfaction techniques: Meeting family expectations. *Dimensions of Critical Care Nursing, 13*(2), 104–111.

Marckx, B. B. (1995). Watson's theory of caring: A model for implementation in practice. *Journal of Nursing Care Quality, 9*(4), 43–54.

McCance, T. V., McKenna, H. P., & Boore, J. R. P. (1999). Caring: Theoretical perspectives of relevance to nursing. *Journal of Advanced Nursing, 30*(6), 1388–1395.

Persky, G. J., Nelson, J. W., Watson, J., & Bent, K. (2008). Creating a profile of a nurse effective in caring. *Nursing Administration Quarterly, 32*(1), 15–20.

Press Ganey Associates. (2010). Re: Press Ganey survey development. Retrieved from http://www.pressganey.com/cs/surveys_and_reports/survey_development

Robert Wood Foundation. (2008). *A new nursing survey tool.* Retrieved from http://www.rwjf.org/reports/grr/058123.htm

Ryan, L. A. (2005). The journey to integrate Watson's caring theory with clinical practice. *International Journal for Human Caring, 9*(3), 26–30.

Smith, M. (2004). Review of research related to Watson's theory of caring. *Nursing Science Quarterly, 17*(1), 13–25.

Upenieks, V., Lee, E., Flanagan, M., & Doebbeling, B. (2010). Health care team vitality instrument (HTVI): Developing a tool assessing health care team functioning. *Journal of Advanced Nursing, 66*(1), 168–176.

Warelow, P., Edward, K., & Vinek, J. (2008). Care: What nurses say and what nurses do. *Holistic Nursing Practice, 22*(3), 146–153.

Watson, J. (2009). *Assessing and measuring caring in nursing and health sciences.* New York, NY: Springer.

Williams, S. A. (1998). Quality and care: Patients' perceptions. *Journal of Nursing Care Quality, 12*(6), 18.

Wolf, Z. R., Colahan, M., Costello, A., Warwick, F., Ambrose, M. S., & Giardino, E. R. (1998). Research utilization. Relationship between nurse caring and patient satisfaction. *MEDSURG Nursing, 7*(2), 99–105.

Wolf, Z. R., Giardino, E. R., Osborne, P. A., & Ambrose, M. S. (1994). Dimensions of nurse caring. *Image: Journal of Nursing Scholarship, 26*(2), 107–111.

APPENDIX 13.1

Five Caring Behaviors Adopted by Unit-Based Council

1. Introduce yourself to patients and explain your role in their care that day.
2. Sit/stand at the patient's bedside for at least 5 minutes per shift to plan and review the patient's needs and goals.
3. Work as a team to meet the patients' needs and requests.
4. Provide assistance to patients when they use their call light as soon as they want it.
5. When leaving a patient's room, ask, "Is there anything else I can do for you?"

APPENDIX 13.2

Caring Factor Survey Items

1. Every day I am here, I see that the care is provided with loving kindness.
2. As a team, my caregivers are good at creative problem solving to meet my individual needs and requests.
3. The care providers honored my own faith, helped instill hope, and respected my belief system as part of my care.
4. When my caregivers teach me something new, they teach me in a way I can understand.
5. My caregivers encouraged me to practice my own, individual, spiritual beliefs as part of my self-caring and healing.
6. My caregivers have responded to me as a whole person, helping to take care of all my needs and concerns.
7. My caregivers have established a helping and trusting relationship with me during my time here.
8. My health care team has created a healing environment that recognizes the connection between my body, mind, and spirit.
9. I feel like I can talk openly and honestly about what I am thinking, because those who are caring for me embrace my feelings no matter what they are.
10. My caregivers are accepting and supportive of my beliefs regarding a higher power, which allows for the possibility that I and my family will heal.

APPENDIX 13.3

Caring Factor Survey–Care Providers Version Items

1. Overall, the care I give is provided with loving kindness.
2. I believe the health care team that I am currently working with solves unexpected problems really well.
3. Every day that I provide patient care, I do so with loving kindness.
4. As a team, my colleagues and I are good at creative problem solving to meet the individual needs and requests of our patients.
5. The care I provide honors the patients' faith, instills hope, and respects the patients' belief system.
6. When I teach patients something new, I teach in a way that they can understand.
7. I help support the hope and faith of the patients I care for.
8. I am responsive to my patients' readiness to learn when I teach them something new.
9. I am very respectful of my patients' individual spiritual beliefs and practices.
10. I create an environment for the patients I care for that helps them heal physically and spiritually.
11. I encourage patients to practice their own, individual, spiritual beliefs as part of self-caring and healing.
12. I work to create a healing environment that recognizes the patients' connection between body, mind, and spirit.
13. I am able to establish a helping-trusting relationship with the patients I care for during their stay here.
14. I work to meet the physical needs as well as the emotional or spiritual needs of the patients I care for.
15. Everybody on the health care team values relationships that are helpful and trusting.
16. I respond to each patient as a whole person, helping to take care of all of their needs and concerns.
17. I encourage patients to speak honestly about their feelings no matter what those feelings are.
18. If a patient told me that he or she believed in miracles, I would support the patient in this belief.
19. Patients I care for can talk openly and honestly with me about their thoughts because I embrace their feelings no matter what those feelings are.
20. I am accepting and supportive of patients' beliefs regarding a higher power if they believe it allows for healing.

14

The Caring Moment and Participative Action Research (PAR) in Outcomes Management

Joyce Turner and Linda Toomer

In 2007, in our new shared governance environment, the nurse executive committee (NEC) voted to expand our care-delivery model to incorporate patient/family-centered care as a core value. The concept of caring theory was not new to the organization because Jean Watson's theory of caring had been the basis of our philosophy of nursing as far back as 1995. The challenge we faced was to make caring a more tangible and ongoing process. We believed that patient-focused care and the patient/family–nurse relationship was essential and critical to the development of our professional practice model. Therefore, to foster caring with concrete actions, Jean Watson's "caring moment" was instituted into nursing practice at the Grady Health System on September 1, 2009. We believed that through tangible caring, our patient/family relationships would be strengthened.

BACKGROUND/REVIEW OF LITERATURE

Watson's (2008) philosophy of transpersonal caring was originally based on 10 Carative Factors that provide an understanding of where human caring lies without giving distinct guidelines. The Carative Factors are abstract interventions that can be used to form nurse–patient caring relationships. Their goal is to permit the patient and nurse to connect through caring transactions. However, both the patient and the nurse must be engaged in order for this authentic connection to take place. Watson's Carative Factors (the concepts) are:
1. Formation of a humanistic-altruistic system of values
2. Instillations of faith and hope
3. Cultivation of sensitivity to one's self and others

4. Development of a helping, trusting, human caring relationship
5. Promotion and acceptance of the expression of positive and negative feelings
6. Systematic use of a creative problem-solving caring
7. Promotion of a transpersonal teaching and learning
8. Provision for a supportive, protective, and/or corrective mental, physical, societal, and spiritual environment
9. Assistance with gratification of human needs
10. Allowance for existential-phenomenological-spiritual forces

However, as Watson's theory evolved, the Carative Factors also evolved from "factors" into more dynamic "processes" rooted in the spiritual dimension. The evolution is clear:

1. Formation of humanistic-altruistic system of values becomes: "Practice of loving kindness and equanimity within context of caring consciousness."
2. Instillation of faith and hope becomes: "Being authentically present, and enabling and sustaining the deep belief system and subjective life world of self and the one being cared for."
3. Cultivation of sensitivity to one's self and to other becomes: "Cultivation of one's own spiritual practices and transpersonal self, going beyond the ego self."
4. Development of a helping, trusting, human caring relationship becomes: "Developing and sustaining a helping, trusting, authentic caring relationship."
5. Promotion and acceptance of the expression of positive and negative feelings becomes: "Being present to, and supportive of, the expression of positive and negative feelings as a connection with a deeper spirit of self and the one being cared for."
6. Systematic use of a creative problem-solving, caring process becomes: "Creative use of self and all ways of knowing as part of the caring process; to engage in artistry of caring–healing practices."
7. Promotion of transpersonal teaching-learning becomes: "Engaging in genuine teaching-learning experience that attends to unity of being and meaning attempting to stay within the other's frame of reference."
8. Provision for a supportive, protective, and/or corrective mental, physical, societal, and spiritual environment becomes: "Creating a healing environment at all levels (physical as well as a nonphysical, subtle environment of energy and consciousness), whereby wholeness, beauty, comfort, dignity, and peace are potentiated."
9. Assistance with gratification of human needs becomes: "Assisting with basic needs, with an intentional caring consciousness, administering 'human care essentials,' which potentiate alignment of

mind-body-spirit, wholeness, and unity of being in all aspects of care"; tending to both embodied spirit and evolving spiritual emergence.
10. Allowance for existential-phenomenological-spiritual forces, becomes: "Opening and attending to spiritual, mysterious, and existential dimensions of one's own life-death"; soul care for self and the one being cared for.

In the patient–nurse interaction, concepts of any one or more Carative Factors may be involved. Watson's caring moment, using her Carative Factors and Caritas Processes, becomes a focal point in time and space for the patient and nurse on an existential level. Both the patient/family and nurse transcend when this transaction takes place, but the patient benefits more because healing processes take place.

The literature review identified many articles on translating Watson's theory into practice. Gallagher-Lepak and Kubsch (2009) and Zraigat (2007) sought to integrate Watson's theory into practice. Gallager-Lepak and Kubsch (2009) did a qualitative study with Registered Nurse-Bachelor of Science in Nursing (RN-BSN) students, who were instructed to provide stories of human caring using Watson's Carative Factors. The purpose was to develop a guideline to operationalize Watson's theory. Through rich stories told by the students, they were able to develop a guideline for the transpersonal caring intervention; however, the guideline needs to be validated to demonstrate that holistic care, unity, harmony, and balance are truly taking place. Zraigat (2007) applied Watson's theory, using the Carative Factors, to a family that resulted in an authentic relationship, fostering healing and promoting quality of care for the patient. Norman, Rutledge, Keefer-Lynch, and Albeg (2008) did an exploratory, descriptive study seeking to identify whether narratives differed in experienced nurses versus less experienced nurses. They found examples of all of Watson's Caritas Processes (the actions) in the narrative; however, they noted that the experienced nurses showed less caring than the nurses who were less experienced. They hypothesized that competing life priorities could have reflected on their motivation for work. Dingman (2008) did a descriptive design study to evaluate differences in patient satisfaction before and after implementing "The Caring Model" into practice at her hospital. She found that two attributes of patient satisfaction improved significantly postintervention.

OVERVIEW OF THE PROJECT

The foundation of the project was built on strong support for nursing implementation of transpersonal caring that would result in positive outcomes for both the patient and the nurse and Grady Health System's continuous search for ways to improve caring. We decided to take a quality improvement (QI) approach to develop and try a new nursing intervention: "the caring moment." The long-term goal of the project was to test the intervention throughout the hospital. The short-term goal was to determine if there would be a positive change in patients' self-reports of holistic care when compared before and after the RN staff was educated on the caring moment. Our hypothesis was that patients who were cared for by nurses who participated in the caring moment education would report a higher score on the Caring Factor Survey (CFS) than patients who were cared for by nurses prior to delivery of education on the caring moment.

The QI project was implemented in a 958-bed, public, teaching hospital in the Southeast in August 2009. All patients were English- or Spanish-speaking adults 18 years or older in medical-surgical and critical care units. Perinatal and pediatric patients, prisoners, the emergency department, and the psychiatry units were excluded from this work.

Nurses trained to collect survey data were asked to approach patients in medical-surgical and critical care units to ask them to complete a 20-item CFS. The survey was available in English and Spanish. A Health Insurance Portability and Accountability Act waiver was not requested because identifying patient data were not accessed. Patients were not asked to sign their names, nor were they given an identification number in order to provide anonymity. Although the survey was written at the eighth-grade level, there were no problems with completion of the survey in the preliminary QI work.

THE SURVEY INSTRUMENT

The 10-item CFS is based on Jean Watson's 10 Caritas Processes with two questions for each Caritas Process. The stem of the items is seeking caring behaviors derived from the Caritas Processes. The CFS instrument was developed in 2006 by John Nelson and others of Healthcare Environment, Inc., in collaboration with Jean Watson (Watson, 2009). The CFS is a 10-item modification of the original 20-item CFS that assesses "subjects' perception of the degree to which the goals of the Caritas Processes have been met" on a Likert scale of 1–7. A scale of 1–3 indicates levels of disagreement, 7 includes the highest level of agreement, and 4 equals neutrality. Total score is derived from adding all 10 items and then dividing by 10. Face validity was determined by Watson, and Watson and other experts on the Caritas Processes established content validity (Watson, 2009). Criterion validity was measured against the CAT-11, a well-validated caring tool (Duffy, 1990); Pearson correlation was $r = .69$, $p = .06$. Cronbach's alpha for the 10-item CFS was .95. All items are phrased in positive language.

PROCEDURE

After the CFS was completed, an educational program was developed for the nurses. All nurses were required to attend the educational program on the caring moment. The educational program included a 30-minute lecture on Jean Watson's Carative Factors and Caritas Processes and how to integrate them into daily practice. A practical example was given for each of the Carative Factors. Following the lecture, the nurses were given badge cards with examples of caring behaviors and were asked to sign a commitment statement to perform at least two caring behavior interventions per shift of work. The priority intervention was to sit at bedside for 5 minutes, giving undivided attention to the patient. Lastly, the nurses were introduced to a caring-moment chime that would be played at 9 a.m., 4 p.m., and 9 p.m. every day as a reminder to do their caring moment for that day. The nurses who did not attend the live educational program were required to go to the intranet and view the PowerPoint presentation and print the badge card and commitment statement. The commitment statement was to be returned to the nurses' unit director. A sound of the chime was also provided on the Gradynet. New nurses who came after the educational program had commenced were introduced to it during orientation. They also were given the badge card and commitment statement and were introduced to the caring-moment chime. All nurses had access to the live educational program or the Gradynet.

Nurses who were trained to collect survey data approached patients in medical-surgical and critical care units. If a patient or family agreed to participate in the survey, this was considered oral informed consent. The surveys took 10–15 minutes to complete. The nurses were given the option to read the survey to the patient or family and could then wait to retrieve the survey or go back within 30 minutes if needed. After completion, the surveys were returned to the coordinator of the project. The surveys were placed in a locked drawer in the coordinator's office until data were analyzed. There were no risks to a subject's participation and there were no direct benefits. However, we believe that patients and families received more holistic care as a result of the project.

DATA ANALYSIS

There were 54 responses in measurement time 1 and 75 in time 2, with 26 units being listed by respondents. For respondents who provided information if they were the patient or family, 63 reported being the patient and 13 reported being a family member of a patient. Family members were allowed to respond for the patient if the patient was too sick to respond. Repeat studies have shown that there have been no differences between the responses of patients and family members. The 129 respondents' races included: Hispanic Black (n = 3), non-Hispanic Black (n = 49), White (n = 8), Alaska Native/American Indian (n = 1), and "other" (n = 11). Several respondents did not report their race.

There were 129 respondents in the dataset. For an independent t test, the power analysis revealed a power of .82 and an effect size of .25 using an alpha of .05.

The Cronbach alpha for the CFS was .77, notably lower than those in other CFS studies where it is most common to have a Cronbach alpha greater than .90. If the item relating to spiritual beliefs was deleted, the Cronbach alpha increased to .92.

No statistically significant differences using an alpha of .05 were found. There were three caring factors that improved from pre- to post implementation, including promotion of expression of feeling, creation of a healing environment, and allowing patients to believe in miracles. The remaining caring factors plus the total CFS score, which included all variables, combined all declines. These findings are noted in Figure 14.1.

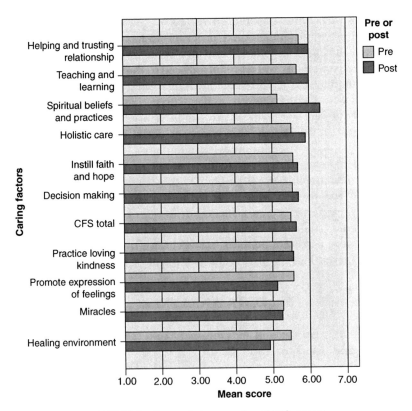

FIGURE 14.1 Comparing pre- and post-CFS scores.

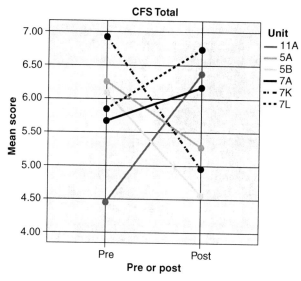

FIGURE 14.2   Interaction effect of unit and time for CFS total score.

INTERACTION OF NURSING UNITS

A general linear model procedure was used to determine if there was an interaction effect of a unit for the six nursing units that had patients who responded in both preimplementation (n = 25) and postimplementation (n = 34). Results revealed a statistically significant interaction of unit and time for the total CFS score, which is all 10 caring factors combined (Figure 14.2).

DISCUSSION

It is interesting to note that the item from the CFS that was not understood related to patients' perceptions of feeling supported spiritually. It also is interesting to note the dramatic decline in scores for some units with a concomitant increase in scores on other units. Although we are unable to substantiate a causal relationship because a convenience sample was used for this project, it is possible that one or more of the following factors could have had an impact:

1. Differences in nurses used to administer the survey (personal attributes, patient approach)
2. Differences in the nurses caring for the patients
3. A change in the physical condition of the patient

4. A disconnect between patient and nurse secondary to cultural differences
5. Conflicting or opposing views on spirituality
6. No assessment of the patients' understanding of the survey at the time of completion
7. General communication barriers

CONSIDERATIONS/NEXT STEPS

Evaluate, with direct care providers and patients, why the item related to spiritual care was not well understood by patients and evaluate the operational effectiveness of the caring intervention on units with declined caring scores. In addition, evaluate retention and acceptance of the critical elements provided during staff nurse training and hardwire the caring processes through existing communication loops such as corporate and departmental orientations, nursing grand rounds, and annual competency validation. Lastly, we will continue to make quality rounds to validate caring processes with patients and nursing staff.

REFERENCES

Dingman, S. K. (2008). *The caring model—A practical application to improve patient satisfaction.* Retrieved July 2, 2009, from http://www.chcm.com

Duffy, J. R. (1990). *An analysis of the relationship among nurse caring behaviors and selected outcomes of care in hospitalized medical and/or surgical patient.* (Doctoral dissertation, Catholic University of America, Anne Arbor, MI, 1990). *University Microfilm* (1992137361).

Gallagher-Lepak, S., & Kubsch, S. (2009). Transpersonal caring: A nursing practice guideline. *Holistic Nursing Practice, 23*(3), 171–182.

Norman, V., Rutledge, D. N., Keefer-Lynch, A., & Albeg, G. (2008). Uncovering and recognizing nurse caring from clinical narratives. *Holistic Nursing Practice, 22*(6), 324–335.

Watson, J. (2008). *The philosophy and science of caring.* Boulder, CO: University Press of Colorado.

Watson, J. (2009). *Assessing and measuring caring in nursing and health sciences.* Retrieved June 18, 2010, from http://books.google.com/books

Zraigat, H. (2007). *Integration of Watson's theory within nursing practice.* Retrieved July 2, from http://www.scribd.com/doc/2060405/Watson-Theory-Application-into-Nursing-Practice

15

Therapeutic Music Pilot in the Context of Human Caring Theory

Shannon S. Spies Ingersoll and Ana M. Schaper

ROLE OF THE DOCTORATE OF NURSING PRACTICE

I (Shannon Ingersoll) always knew that I wanted to continue my education after obtaining my Master of Science in anesthesia. Having a renewed desire to achieve this goal, I searched the various doctoral education programs available. Doctorate of Nursing Practice (DNP) programs were just beginning to make their way into the path of nursing practice. Because I have always loved my advanced practice in anesthesia, obtaining a nursing practice degree at the doctoral level was the perfect choice for me. My journey became a walking spiritual pilgrimage, which I shared with my colleague, mentor, and coauthor (Ana Schaper). Being open to "way-markers" influenced this journey and continues to guide us on new pathways in our lives (Watson, 2006, p. 293).

The DNP is a new academic degree formally approved by the American Association of Colleges of Nursing (AACN) in October 2004 (Edwardson, 2011). Factors propelling the creation of the practice degree included the increasing complexity of health care, rapid change occurring in health care delivery, and the need for scientific evidence to underpin nursing practice. The role of nurses with the DNP degree is complex and focuses on translating research to practice, thereby improving care for individuals, families, systems, and populations. Nurses with a DNP will enhance system improvement based on scientific evidence and affect health policy at all levels. At the core, nurses with a DNP will lead the nursing profession through evidence-based practice to ensure high-quality patient outcomes.

Preparation for the DNP degree culminates in a scholarly project. In planning for my DNP project, I connected with my coauthor, Ana Schaper, a PhD-prepared nurse scientist guiding evidence-based nursing practice in my work setting. Over the course of the project, we created a working relationship that reflected the complementary roles of the DNP and PhD in a clinical practice setting. After we explored several options for projects, I approached the manager of the hematology–oncology outpatient unit to discuss the value of music listening in this setting. My grandmother had received cancer treatment on this unit, and I had noticed limited options for helping patients relax during treatments. From my background in anesthesia, I was aware of the role music could play in relaxation. Coincidentally, nurses working on this unit had recently identified music as a complementary care alternative that could facilitate patients' relaxation and decrease their distress during treatment. The alignment of these circumstantial way-markers led to a plan negotiated with administration and supported by staff nurses to conduct an evidence-based pilot project focusing on music listening. As the project moved forward, two unit staff nurses joined our team. They became the "nurse champions" promoting the change. Working together, our project incorporated not only an evaluation component, but also strategies for sustaining the new practice.

Surprisingly, soon after the plan was under way, Dr. Jean Watson presented at our health care organization. She discussed her human caring theory and her book, *Nursing: The Philosophy and Science of Caring* (2008), which focuses on the 10 Caritas Processes. Watson shared her work and its relevance for a new "awakening" among nurses and the profession in the 21st century. The choice of Watson's theory as the framework to guide the project was an unexpected way marker in my journey. After meeting Dr. Watson and learning about her theory, I designed my DNP scholarly project to evaluate the use of music listening as a caring–healing modality in the context of the nurse–patient interaction. Two questions were the focus for the project: (1) In the context of a human caring nurse–patient interaction with adult patients receiving chemotherapy treatment, will listening to music increase patients' sense of the nurse's effectiveness in caring? and (2) Will implementation of a music-listening pilot project within the context of human caring influence: (a) nurses' insights into and experiences with music and (b) nurses' sense of effectiveness in caring for their patient(s)?

BACKGROUND

Review of the Literature

A computerized database search was conducted to identify studies evaluating the effectiveness of music as an intervention with patients receiving chemotherapy treatment. Of 1,622 sources initially identified, 82 were retrieved for review from nursing and music therapy journals. Very few studies were conducted with patients with cancer, and the quality of many studies was poor. The final sources of scientific evidence underpinning this project consisted of 10 single studies, two systematic reviews, and a meta-analysis.

The majority of the studies addressed the physiological benefits of music (Evans, 2002; Richards, Johnson, Sparks, & Emerson, 2007). Focusing on music listening as a healing modality in music therapist–patient interactions, four studies cited by Pothoulaki, MacDonald, and Flowers (2005) supported the effect of music in enhancing positive experiences and feelings as well as improvement in well-being and quality of life. A small body of qualitative work has shown that music therapy can foster a sense of identity, expressions of joy and release from negative emotions, experiences of creativity, and feelings of freedom and release "to let go" in adult patients with cancer (Daykin, McClean, & Bunt, 2007; O'Callaghan, 2001). In addition, music therapy can facilitate communication, self-reflection, self-expression, and creativity in children (O'Callaghan, Sexton, & Wheeler, 2007). It is possible that the anxiety-reducing effects of music demonstrated by the quantitative studies (Ferrer, 2007; Pothoulaki et al., 2005; Weber, Nuessler, & Wilmanns, 1997) will promote the psychological benefit of music interventions in patients with cancer, such as creatively expressing issues that are important to them (Daykin et al., 2007; O'Callaghan, 2001; O'Callaghan et al., 2007).

The evidence from the qualitative studies is consistent: Music interventions within the context of an interaction promote psychological benefits of individual meaning and self-expression for adults and children with cancer. Using a qualitative approach, Daykin et al. (2007) found seven key themes expressed by participants with cancer who had participated in group music therapy in a 3-month period: choice and enrichment; power, freedom and release; music and healing; balance; individuation; and creativity and loss. The importance of identity and the role of creativity in the processes of individuation of patients with cancer using music therapy was evident in the study. In a study by Weber et al. (1997), patients with cancer reported high satisfaction with music listening and requested music during future chemotherapy treatments. Limitations of the research methodology included small study samples, predominantly female gender, and consistency of the studies.

No studies were found that demonstrated the use of music as a caring–healing modality for nurse–patient interactions. However, three studies demonstrated that a therapeutic interaction with a music therapist enabled self-reflection, alternate ways of "being," and a deeper human connection (Daykin et al., 2007; O'Callaghan, 2001; O'Callaghan et al., 2007).

MOVING FORWARD IN THE JOURNEY: CONDUCTING AN EVIDENCE-BASED-PRACTICE PILOT PROJECT

In this project, our team worked with the chemotherapy treatment nurses using the 10 Caritas Processes to increase the nurses' sense of effectiveness in caring for their patients. We began with the intent of working with the nurses to support their deeper connection with patients undergoing chemotherapy treatment through the use of music as a caring–healing modality. As nurses develop and sustain "deeper" human-to-human connections with their patients using music, they practice the core philosophy and framework of our profession. Nurses who incorporate caring–healing values and beliefs into their practice promote health and well-being for their patients and themselves (Watson, 2001). Integration of caring–healing practice into nursing care delivery is one pathway for nurses to take ownership of their profession. Watson (1999) states the caring–healing modalities: "potentiate wholeness, harmony, integrity and beauty, and preserve dignity and humanity with every act" (p. 205). Through the use of music, we proposed that nurses would be more in touch with who they are and the care they deliver. In addition, patients would gain self-knowledge, self-control, and self-healing knowledge (Watson, 2001).

Human Caring Theory Operationalized

Watson's human caring theory was operationalized through the processes and tools that were used in preparing the nurses for the intervention: educational sessions, a nurse and patient interaction script, role-playing, role modeling, and the use of intentionality. The theory was also operationalized in measuring the patient (Caring Factor Survey [CFS]) and nurse (Caring Factor Survey-Care Provider Version [CFS-CPV]) outcomes (J. Watson, personal communication, April 25, 2008).

Educational Sessions

Three educational sessions were offered to engage the nurses in understanding Watson's human caring theory and using music as a caring–healing modality. The first session covered the scientific evidence supporting music as a healing modality and Watson's human caring theory including the 10 Caritas Processes. The second session focused on nurse–patient interactions delivering care through the 10 Caritas Processes. The final educational session focused on use of intentionality (Watson, 2002). Intentionality is placing consciousness on music listening as a caring–healing modality. Setting intention serves to remind the nurse of what is important in this action and provides the nurse the opportunity to be mindfully present. Intentionality was demonstrated through role-playing and modeling the nurse–patient interactions. The Nurse and Patient Interaction Script, designed as a guide to support intentionality, consisted of open-ended items that addressed music listening and the 10 Caritas Processes. Examples of these items were: "What are you listening to today?" and "Tell me what you think of when you listen to this music (story)." Acts of caring were displayed toward the nurses during the sessions and included playing music, providing treats, giving small tokens of appreciation, and verbalizing positive reinforcement.

PILOT STUDY METHODOLOGY

Design

A dual-focus implementation strategy (patient focus and nurse focus) was selected to enhance the success of the change efforts to incorporate music and to support the caring–healing relationship between nurse and patient. Quinn, Smith, Ritenbaugh, Swanson, and Watson (2003) state that research on healing modalities delivered by nurses must take into account the patient–nurse relationship, because the healing relationship involves "(at least) two individuals engaged in a mutual, simultaneous process" (p. A70). Limiting the focus of the pilot project to the impact of the caring–healing relationship on the patient only is conceptually incomplete. The health and well-being of the nurse is as legitimate a concern for research on the impact of the caring–healing relationship as that of the patient (Quinn et al., 2003). Thus, we focused on implementation and evaluation strategies for both the patient and the nurse. Institutional review board approval was obtained and informed consent was received from both patients and nurses.

Patient Focus

For this project, the patient's role was to evaluate the effectiveness of using music listening as a caring–healing modality. A convenience sample of patients from an adult chemotherapy unit was recruited during a 2-month period. The sample consisted of nine Caucasian females and five Caucasian males with ages ranging from 20 years to greater than 50 years. Thirteen of the participants were married. The types of cancer the participants had varied. Inclusion criteria were: (a) age 21 or older; (b) able to speak and read English; and (c) undergoing a regimen requiring chemotherapy for cancer at least one time per week for a minimum of three cycles. Patients with a hearing impairment that would interfere with their ability to listen to recorded music were excluded.

Data Collection and Instruments

Participants completed two questionnaires at baseline, the Participant Demographic and Music Interest Questionnaire (developed by the authors) and the CFS. Burns, Sledge, Fuller, Daggy, and Monahan (2005) stressed the importance of assessing the needs and preferences of patients with cancer in regards to music prior to intervention. Identifying factors that affect intervention effectiveness promotes development of meaningful and effective music interventions. The CFS, a 20-item instrument, was used to assess the nurse's effectiveness in caring. At the end of the pilot study, participants were mailed the CFS and asked to complete two qualitative items that addressed their experiences with music listening.

Music Listening

At the time of recruitment, participants were given the choice of using a CD player or an MP3 player. Participants were educated on the use of the selected delivery modality and were given their choice of listening to their preferred music selections (Smolen, Topp, & Singer, 2002). Infection control measures were implemented to prevent transmission of any infectious organisms through headsets.

Nurse Focus

For this pilot project, the nurse's role was to initiate, cultivate, and sustain a caring–healing relationship by engaging the patient in the use of music listening as a healing modality. Nine female Caucasian nurses ranging in age from 20 years to greater than 50 years were recruited.

Data Collection and Instruments

Data were collected at baseline and completion of the project. Nurses completed a demographic questionnaire and the CFS-CPV. The CSF-CPV was used to assess the nurse's perception of the effectiveness of the care he or she provides. Using the CFS to assess patients and the CFS-CPV to assess nurses, the investigator can determine if the nurse's report of effectiveness in caring coincides with an increase or decrease in the patient's perception of effectiveness in caring (J. W. Nelson, personal communication, July 7, 2008). Two focus groups were held following completion of the pilot project to allow nurses to share their insights and/or experiences during the pilot project. The focus group sessions were audio taped and transcribed verbatim without identifying information.

Interaction Procedure

Nurses were informed when a patient was enrolled in the project and asked to spend a minimum of 10 minutes per cycle engaging the patient in an interaction supporting "music" as the caring–healing modality. The Nurse and Patient Interaction Script was used as a guide for this interaction. The team and I provided ongoing feedback to staff nurses in supporting this skill development.

DATA ANALYSIS

Descriptive statistics were used to analyze demographic and music interest information on the patient participant and nurse participant sample. Due to the small sample size, data from the pre- and postsurvey using the CSF and CSF-CPV were also analyzed using descriptive statistics. Qualitative content analysis (Krueger, 1998) was used to assess data provided on the patients' postintervention qualitative questionnaires and from the nurse participant focus groups.

FINDINGS

Patient participants were predominantly female and over the age of 40. The majority of participants (n = 11) indicated having a prior background in music such as playing an instrument or singing in the choir. Their preferred choice of music was Country Western. Surprisingly, all but one patient participant chose to use the MP3 player. Nurse participants were female and were under the age of 50. All nurses reported a previous background in music such as playing an instrument or singing in the choir. Nurses indicated enjoying music across a wide range of genres (Table 15.1).

Data from the CFS indicated that patients perceived a high sense of effectiveness in caring by nurses both before and after the music-listening intervention. Data were collected from 14 participants preintervention and 10 participants postintervention. One of the participants passed away during the postintervention data-collection period and three participants did not return postsurveys. The mean patient participant prepilot score was 6.4 ± 0.4 (on a scale of 1–7) and the postpilot mean score was 6.5 ± 0.3. Data from the CFS-CPV indicated that nurses similarly perceived that they were effective in their caring for their patients. Data were collected from nine nurses pre- and postintervention. The mean pre- and postpilot nurse participant scores were 6.3 ± 0.3 and 6.5 ± 0.4, respectively, and not different from patient-participant ratings. Table 15.2 highlights the top three Caritas, that patients and nurses

TABLE 15.1 Baseline Demographics of Patient and Nurse Participants

	PARTICIPANTS	
DEMOGRAPHIC VARIABLES	PATIENT (N = 14)	NURSE (N = 9)
Sex		
Male	5	0
Female	9	9
Age		
20–29 years	1	1
30–39 years	0	2
40–49 years	5	4
≥ 50 years	8	2
Music importance in life*	7 ± 2	7 ± 2
Confidence using		
CD player*	8 ± 3	9 ± 2
MP3 player*	4 ± 4	5 ± 4

Note: *Mean ± SD on a scale of 1–10.

TABLE 15.2   Caritas Consistently Experienced and Delivered

SURVEY STAGE	PATIENT EXPERIENCED: CFS	NURSE DELIVERED: CFS-CPV
Pre-pilot		
	Caring with loving kindness	Caring with loving kindness
	Caring processes for decision making	Caring processing for decision making
	Acceptance of feelings	Instilling faith and hope
Post-pilot		
	Caring with loving kindness	Caring with loving kindness
	Caring processes for decision making	Caring processes for decision making
	Development of helping, trusting relationships	Being open to miracles

"strongly agreed" were delivered. Care delivered with loving kindness and the use of caring processes in decision making were two Caritas that both patients and nurses rated highly. Patient and nurse participants were less likely to *strongly agree* with the statements about the delivery of spiritual care. This was reflected by a majority of statements focused on spiritual care as in which they were *neutral*, or they said they *slightly agree* or *agree*. There was a similar pattern of lower ratings by patient and nurse participants on items addressing individual spiritual beliefs and practices and the creation of a healing environment. In addition, patient participants did not view their nurses as being open to miracles.

Data from the patient-participants' post-intervention surveys indicated that the personal benefits of music listening were creating a sense of relaxation and supporting personal autonomy through a "choice" of music. One patient participant wrote: "I did enjoy it [music]! Hoping not to have any [chemotherapy] but would enjoy having the option each time." Another patient participant replied, "[Music] helps to curb anxiety instead of using medication."

Similarly, the qualitative data generated in the focus groups indicated that nurses (*n* = 12) perceived the personal benefits of listening to music for patients and themselves. Nurses reported that listening to music created a sense of calmness both personally and environmentally. One nurse participant stated, "I've heard the nurses say, it's so nice to hear [music]. It's so relaxing. It's so much better when we hear music on the unit. It's not as chaotic and it's [music] healing for us too when it's a busy productive day. It's great to have that release through music as well," Listening to music opened the "doors" to new meaning for nurses and their patients. One nurse stated, "I think for some patients we are seeing a side of them that we didn't necessarily see before." Music became a part of the nurses' day-to-day activities when they practiced. They began to play CDs during their shift while they finished charting and preparing the unit for the next day. The team observed nurses sharing music stories and memories with each other.

Nurses acknowledged that the delivery of spiritual care was the most challenging aspect of providing holistic care when the results of the CSF and CSF-PV were shared with them in the focus groups. Nurse participants reported feelings of comfort and competence in discussions of end-of-life issues but admitted they were uncomfortable with initiating and engaging in interactions addressing spirituality. Concerns expressed by nurses were: a lack of education about religious beliefs, absence of skills to perform spiritual assessments, and time demands. Nurses attending the focus group expressed a commitment to engage in the delivery of spiritual care with their patients. One nurse suggested, "If you ask a patient . . . what brings you peace or where do you find joy?—those are spiritual things . . . helping them to identify their spirituality . . . [Nurses] learning new ways to phrase things with patients will be helpful for us helping them spiritually." Creating a "caring moment" by exploring a patient's interest in spiritual music was identified as a strategy they would use in the future.

DISCUSSION

The literature corroborates the project's findings of patient satisfaction (Weber et al., 1997) and self-expression (Daykin et al., 2007; O'Callaghan, 2001) when listening to music as a caring–healing modality within the context of the nurse–patient interaction. The music-listening intervention supported patient autonomy through patients' ability to select the music they preferred in an environment with few choices (Burns et al., 2005). Music listening as a caring–healing modality also contributed to nurses' well-being and improved their work environment. Many of the nurses were surprised by the "unexpected" benefit of self-expression with music listening. When both the nurse and the patient can engage in self-expression as part of an interaction during a caring moment, they are able to connect on a deeper level, thus promoting a caring–healing experience.

Data from the CFS and CFS-CPV indicated the need to address spiritual beliefs and practices in nurse–patient interactions. Patients and nurses both believed that the spirituality dimension of care was lacking from their interactions. Focus groups engaged nurses in open, respectful dialogue while reflecting on their role in providing spiritual care. These reflective activities supported integration of Watson's human caring theory's 10 Caritas Processes into their daily practice (Watson & Foster, 2003).

Instruments that measure caring–healing behaviors within the context of a nurse–patient interaction are limited. Use of the CFS and the CFS-CPV in the practice settings provides insights into nurse–patient interactions from both perspectives. Results of our project indicate that integration of the human-caring theory and use of the CSF and CSF-CPV instruments can influence nursing's day-to-day practice as well as guide future research. As nursing establishes its own voice, credibility, professional autonomy, and accountability for our sacred work in caring, healing, and health, our commitment to our profession, to society, and to humanity will ensue.

MERGING MY JOURNEY WITH OTHERS: NURSING IMPLICATIONS

Nursing in the 21st century is deficient in using nursing theories to guide practice. Nursing practice is largely driven by other disciplines, which has had a negative impact on nurses and the profession of nursing. As nurses have fallen short of directing their own discipline, job satisfaction, pride and passion for the profession, and lack of autonomy and credibility also have suffered. The importance of using nursing theory in practice is essential for nursing's survival. The interaction of nursing theory with practice transforms and guides efficient and effective nursing care through direct nursing goals (Meleis, 2007). Theory in practice also promotes nursing satisfaction because nursing knowledge, encompassing core beliefs and values, is guiding nursing's actions. Nursing theory provides a common language among practitioners, theorists, researchers, and educators (Meleis, 2007). According to Watson (2008), a profession that does not have its own language will not exist. Therefore, it is important for nurses to name, declare, articulate, and act upon the phenomena of nursing and caring for the profession to continue its holistic, sacred work and promise to humanity.

Several nursing implications can be drawn from nurse–patient interactions using music listening as a caring–healing modality. As nurses, we need to acknowledge and support our patients' individual, spiritual belief systems in order to foster caring–healing interactions. Music listening as a caring–healing modality in an outpatient chemotherapy setting can bring personal benefits to patients (e.g., relaxation and sense of autonomy) and can bring "unexpected" personal benefits to nurses (e.g., creating a sense of calmness and finding meaning). By using music listening in the context of the nurse–patient interaction, patients and nurses are able to self-discover their own healing practices, promoting health and well-being. Incorporating caring–healing modalities within the nurse–patient relationship upholds holistic practices that focus on the "wholeness" of the individual, including need for spiritual care, and strengthens our profession of nursing.

Through this journey of doctoral work and education, I found the way-markers back to my core profession, "Nursing." As a team, we became "open" to the way-markers guiding our path. Our team rediscovered the "gifts and blessings" that nursing provides for others and ourselves. Together, Ana and I discovered that our journey has just begun in exploring the complementary role of PhD- and DNP-prepared nurses working in a clinical setting. The DNP degree is an exciting option for nurses choosing to obtain a terminal degree in practice. This new doctorate-of-practice role is just beginning to emerge in clinical nursing and organizational systems. As time progresses, the number of DNP professionals will increase and their contributions to the profession of nursing and health care will be present. In the meantime, the journey needs to move forward, starting with academia and systems collaborating to bring this role to the forefront. Without recognition, the significance of such a role will never be valued. As nurses choose to advance their education and lead an evidence-based practice, we strongly advocate the importance of being open for way-markers along their journeys to enhance healing environments through a collaborative practice.

REFERENCES

Burns, D. S., Sledge, R. B., Fuller, L. A., Daggy, J. K., & Monahan, P. O. (2005). Cancer patients' interest and preferences for music therapy. *Journal of Music Therapy, 42*(3), 185–199.

Daykin, N., McClean, S., & Bunt, L. (2007). Creativity, identity and healing: Participants' accounts of music therapy in cancer care. *An Interdisciplinary Journal for the Social Study of Health, Illness and Medicine, 11*(3), 349–370.

Edwardson, R. E. (2011). Imagining the DNP role. In M. E. Zaccagnini & K. W. White (Eds.), *The doctor of nursing practice essentials: A new model for advanced practice nursing.* Sudbury, MA: Jones & Bartlett.

Evans, D. (2002). The effectiveness of music as an intervention for hospital patients: A systematic review. *Journal of Advanced Nursing, 37*(1), 8–18.

Ferrer, A. J. (2007). The effect of live music on decreasing anxiety in patients undergoing chemotherapy treatment. *Journal of Music Therapy, 44*(3), 242–255.

Krueger, R. A. (1998). Analyzing and reporting focus group results. In M. Flemming & D. E. Axelsen (Eds.), *The focus group kit* (pp. 79–95). Thousand Oaks, CA: Sage.

Meleis, A. (2007). *Theoretical nursing, development and progress* (4th ed.). Philadelphia, PA: Lippincott Williams & Wilkins.

O'Callaghan, C. (2001). Bringing music to life: A study of music therapy and palliative care experiences in a cancer hospital. *Journal of Palliative Care, 17*(3), 155–160.

O'Callaghan, C., Sexton, M., & Wheeler, G. (2007). Music therapy as a non-pharmacological anxiolytic for pediatric radiotherapy patients. *Australasian Radiology, 51,*159–162.

Pothoulaki, M., MacDonald, R., & Flowers, P. (2005). Music interventions in oncology settings: A systematic literature review. *British Journal of Music Therapy, 19*(2), 75–83.

Quinn, J. F., Smith, M., Ritenbaugh, C., Swanson, K., & Watson, M. J. (2003). Research guidelines for assessing the impact of the healing relationship in clinical nursing. *Alternative Therapies in Health & Medicine, 9* (Suppl. 3), A65–A79.

Richards, T., Johnson, J., Sparks, A., & Emerson, H. (2007). The effect of music therapy on patients' perception and manifestation of pain, anxiety, and patient satisfaction. *MEDSURG Nursing, 16*(1), 7–15.

Smolen, D., Topp, R., & Singer, L. (2002). The effect of self-selected music during colonoscopy anxiety, heart rate, and blood pressure. *Applied Nursing Research, 16*(2), 126–136.

Watson, J. (1999). *Postmodern nursing and beyond.* Philadelphia, PA: Churchill Livingstone.

Watson, J. (2001). Post-hospital nursing: Shortage, shifts, and scripts. *Nursing Administration Quarterly, 25*(3), 77–82.

Watson, J. (2002). Intentionality and caring–healing consciousness: A practice of transpersonal nursing. *Holistic Nursing Practice, 16*(4), 12–19.

Watson, J. (2006). Walking pilgrimage as caritas action in the world. *Journal of Holistic Nursing, 24*(4), 289–296.

Watson, J. (2008). *Nursing: The philosophy and science of caring* (Rev. ed.). Boulder, CO: University Press of Colorado.

Watson, J., & Foster, R. (2003). The Attending Nurse Caring Model: Integrating theory, evidence and advanced caring-healing therapeutics for transforming professional practice. *Journal of Clinical Nursing, 12,* 360–365.

Weber, S., Nuessler, V., & Wilmanns, W. (1997). A pilot study on the influence of receptive music listening on cancer patients during chemotherapy. *International Journal of Arts Medicine, 5*(2), 27–35.

16

CaritasHeartMath™ in the Emergency Department Setting: The Impact of Self-Care on Practitioners

Diane Raines, Peggy McCartt, and Pamela Turner

"What if we could give our staff a tool that they could use to manage stress in the moment in the Emergency Department?"

*T*his was the question we asked after hearing Jean Watson, founder of the Watson Caring Science Institute (WCSI), and Robert Browning, director of Development with HeartMath, speak at one of Dr. Watson's Caritas consortiums. They propose that organizations that use Dr. Watson's theory of human caring as a foundation for nursing practice consider the impact HeartMath might have when combined with both caring theory and science. HeartMath, a nonprofit research and education institute, has been working in heart science and stress reduction for almost 20 years. Founded by Doc Childre, HeartMath was developed as a way to teach people how to reduce stress and improve health and performance. HeartMath uses practical techniques derived from scientific research on the psychophysiology of stress, emotions, and the interactions between the heart and brain which enhance the heart–brain communication and coherence within individuals and organizations. The techniques help to calm the heart and the rest of the body while increasing mental acuteness and overall performance by bringing more balance to the autonomic nervous system.

HeartMath techniques seemed congruent with our caring-science work and offered the possibility of an additional tool that nurses could use in self-care—a key precept of caring theory. We believed the combination of HeartMath and caring science in return would help our employees learn to better manage their stress, which could: reduce sick time; increase employee morale; lead to more coherent communication and optimal mental clarity and creativity; and greater patient satisfaction.

HISTORY

Baptist Health is a faith-based, mission-driven, not-for-profit hospital system in northeast Florida. Serving the community for over 55 years, Baptist has over 8,000 employees in five hospitals, the region's largest home health agency, and over 100 primary care and specialty providers located in traditional physicians' offices and urgent care settings. Baptist's mission and values have guided the system and its nurses to provide excellent care with compassion and respect. Baptist Health is currently the largest Magnet health system in Florida. In addition, for 15 years the community has named Baptist Health nurses as "the best" in the National Research Corporation's Health Market Guide Survey.

Overtime, Baptist Health has developed a relational culture that emphasizes the importance of each individual in creating the best possible environment for patients, families, and staff. In orientation the chief operating officer tells new employees, "We believe our health system is distinguished by caring people dedicated to the service of others. It is the caring behaviors demonstrated by each one of us that distinguishes Baptist Health."

With that history as a backdrop, Baptist nurses selected Dr. Jean Watson's (2005) *theory of human caring* as our unifying nursing theory in 2004 when we began our Magnet journey. A team of nurse educators, leaders, and staff endorsed her theory because it most aligned with our prevailing culture of caring and was applicable to all areas of practice. We later developed a philosophy and model of caring to help guide clinical practice.

Nursing Philosophy

Baptist Health's philosophy is: The foundation for nursing excellence is *caring relationships.* Nurses at Baptist Health achieve excellence in practice through a collaborative approach where knowledge, compassion, caring, respect and acceptance are valued and modeled.

"Nurses work with all disciplines as colleagues committed to the common goal of safe, scientifically based quality patient and family care achieved in an atmosphere of caring and respect."

Model of Caring Relationships

With the theory of human caring as a guide, Baptist nurses created nursing model of care describing six tenets of nursing practice—education, research, evidence-based clinical practice, quality and performance improvement, stewardship, and patient/family/community partnerships (Figure 16.1). Over the past 7 years we have engaged with caring theory and science in a number of ways. We have participated in Dr. Watson's Caritas consortium, where we learned from others who

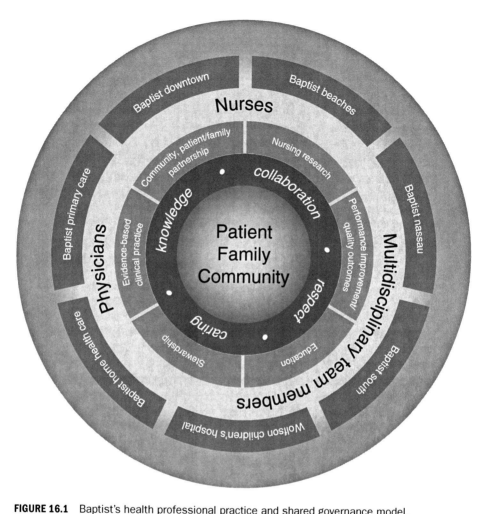

FIGURE 16.1 Baptist's health professional practice and shared governance model. (Baptist Health, 2010)

manifest the theory of human caring. Dr. Watson has taught our leaders and staff, challenging them to bring the Caritas Processes to life both personally and professionally. We have trained seven nurses as Caritas coaches through the WCSI. Their influence from this ongoing training is intended to broaden our exposure to caring science and help us find ways to make the science real. Their work includes creating a Caritas garden by staff, writing a book of caregiver stories that inspire others, changing the environment of a busy surgical service to one of caring and engagement, and creating a healing-arts pilot. In addition, all of our staff participates in the Spirit of CareGiving™, a 2-day retreat where staff members focus on their possibilities and the choices they make in life and where self-care is emphasized regardless of role.

In addition to our engagement with caring science, we emphasize professional development in evidence-based practice (EBP) and nursing research. We have eight EBP mentors trained at Arizona State University, two of whom are PhD nurse researchers. This team has successfully led our staff to develop EBP projects and submit nursing research projects to Baptist's institutional research committee (IRC) to expand the knowledge of our practitioners and advance their nursing practice. "Show me the evidence" is more than a play on a famous movie tag line—it is increasingly the way our nurses think when presented with ideas and information. Thus, the combination of caring science and EBP positioned us well to consider a project that would allow us to research the impact of a scientifically based skill set that enhances self-care.

PREPARATION

Researchers, Caritas coaches, and nurse leaders came together to discuss the feasibility of piloting CaritasHeartMath at Baptist Health. This would be part of a national pilot conducted by the Watson Caring Science Institute and HeartMath. The pilot was designed to integrate and systematically implement, demonstrate, and assess the impact of blending caring science with science of the heart. Specific tools and techniques developed by HeartMath would be taught and reinforced in the context of the theory of human caring and a caring-science environment. HeartMath techniques enable practitioners to control their responses in stressful situations by applying heart-centered breathing techniques coupled with the intentional generation of heartfelt positive emotions to bring their heart rhythms into a balanced state. This *emotional shift* is a key element of the technique's effectiveness. Positive emotions appear to excite the system at its natural resonant frequency and thus enable coherence to emerge and to be maintained naturally without conscious mental focus on one's breathing rhythm. This is because input generated by the heart's rhythmic activity is actually one of the main factors that affect our breathing rate and patterns. When the heart's rhythm shifts into coherence as a result of a positive emotional shift, our breathing rhythm automatically synchronizes with the heart, thereby reinforcing and stabilizing the shift to systemwide coherence (Institute of Heartmath, 2010).

The pilot oversight group felt that the emergency department (ED) staff could most benefit from immediate stress reduction. Staff within the ED is exposed to the pressures of time, criticality, and incredible emotional turmoil on a daily basis. Turnover in our EDs was higher than in many other units, and staff exhibited overt signs of stress including frequent callouts, leaves of absence, and so on. We determined to focus on one primary area for ease of implementation and selected the largest ED at Baptist Health's flagship hospital. This ED is a tertiary care facility is in an urban setting in northeast Florida. There are 57 adult ED beds; 47 are acute care and 10 are fast track or nonacute care beds and sees 70,000 patients a year. It is a Level 2 trauma center and a Baker Act receiving facility for behavioral health patients. The facility is stroke certified and accredited by the Society of Chest Pain Centers. There are 135 staff; 95 are registered nurses (10% of whom have a national certification in emergency nursing) and 45 are unlicensed staff including assistive-care personnel, patient-care advocates, transporters, and others. We elected to invite all staff, not just nurses, to participate. In addition, we opened up participation to educators, other ED directors within the system, and local academic faculty who also embrace Dr. Watson's theories in their curriculum and who educate nurse practitioners in emergency medicine.

FUNDING

In order to participate, we needed to secure funding for the education and staff time for those participating. Costs included 12 hours of classroom training, food, and supplies. We were extraordinarily blessed to have a donor through the Homeyer Institute for Nursing Research and Education at Baptist, a privately funded institute established to enhance nurse competency in our health system. The Homeyer funding allowed us to participate in the pilot without taxing the ED budget.

STUDY BACKGROUND

The PhD RN researchers served as the principal investigators (PIs) for the pilot study. The initial proposal described the study as blending caring science with leading-edge research on the relationship between the heart and the brain and how this relationship affects physical and emotional health and human performance. The proposal described the specific education sessions, the techniques related to heart-centered breathing, and the intentional generation of heartfelt positive emotions that would be taught and reinforced, and the validated assessments that would be used to assess participants' pre- and post-experiences. The CaritasHeartMath pilot project was described as an effort to provide education and techniques for staff to integrate self-care and caring concepts with the ability to use strategies to manage stressful situations in the present. An additional purpose of the study was to determine how the staff's response to training could positively affect the overall patient-care experience. Ultimately, the purpose was to equip our caregivers in a highly stressful environment with tools and techniques that allowed them to manage their stress and reinforce the importance of self-care in order to care for others. IRC approval was obtained for the pilot to begin in the fall of 2009. The CaritasHeartMath training model is designed to touch and transform the hearts, minds, and hands of the practitioners. The pilot project integrates the philosophy/theory/science of human caring/Caritas nursing (http://www.watsoncaringscience.org) with science of the heart. Compassionate Caritas heart-centered science methods, techniques, and modalities draw upon the latest HeartMath and caring-science research, which deepens the humanity of the practitioner. The program is designed to extend and sustain the Caritas practices and caring-science model in the piloted area and, ultimately, throughout the system. HeartMath skills and techniques would provide a mechanism for the personal transformation of the practitioners and their human-caring practices.

HeartMath's transforming stress program elements offer participating staff new tools and strategies for managing stress and increasing consistent caring practices in the face of their daily challenges. It provides tools to help individuals recognize stress and lack of clarity as it is happening. This process occurs through grounding specific theory-guided practices: "pausing," "centering," "breathing," radiating love and compassion from the heart center, helping to sustain Caritas ways of being/becoming. This scientifically based practice allows one to shift consciousness and intentionality *in the moment*. These tools are based on more than 15 years of research by the nonprofit Institute of HeartMath. The CaritasHeartMath program offers a unique, theoretical, philosophical, ethical, and scientific framework for transforming professional practices. It contributes to the foundation for creating authentic caring-science institutions and restoring human caring–healing for practitioners and patients alike.

As a national pilot site, we would participate in preparing nurses and other selected staff in a series of advanced training programs in Watson's Caritas nursing integrated with techniques developed by WCSI and HeartMath. The participating staff would develop depth of personal and professional knowledge, skills, and techniques to practice intentional conscious, heart-centered, Caritas-loving approaches for self and others. The program would nurture authentic, compassionate, caring–healing relationships, developing communities of caring, thus transforming the culture of health care systems beyond medical-technical foci alone.

SIGNIFICANCE AND PRACTICE IMPLICATIONS

Numerous studies (Beck, 2000; Boughn, 2001; Boughn & Lentini, 1999; Kelly, Shoemaker, & Steele, 1996; Kersten et al., 1991; Pillitteri, 1994; Stevens & Walker, 1993; Williams, Wertenberger, & Gushuliak, 1997) have established an iterative theme of "caring for others" as the major motivating factor for both men and women choosing health care as a career. Yet, health care workers are continually confronted with having to practice based on a task-oriented, highly technological, biomedical model as opposed to a model of human caring that influenced them to the profession in the first place. This challenge is compounded by the current shortage of health care providers and a fast-paced health care environment. It is reported that providers who are not able to practice within a caring context are characterized as hardened, oblivious, robot-like, frightened, and worn down (Swanson, 1999). Conversely, providers are much more satisfied, fulfilled, purposeful, and knowledge seeking when caring is present in their nursing practice (Watson, 2002).

Purpose

The overarching purpose of the project is to provide staff the knowledge and the skills to nurture authentic, compassionate, caring–healing relationships with themselves, their coworkers, and the patients they care for in the ED. The intent is that this authentic, caring perspective of delivering care will transcend to the day-to-day milieu of the ED, transforming it to a sustainable environment of care and compassion, which ultimately benefits the patients and families. Ultimately, future patients may benefit if the program demonstrates that nurses' caring behaviors were enhanced, thereby improving the quality of patient care and the patients' overall experience in the ED.

PARTICIPANTS

After obtaining permission from the IRC at Baptist Health, information sessions about the study were conducted at staff meetings by the nurse researchers and chief nursing officer who explained the purpose of the study. Because one of the schools of nursing in the community provides an educational, advanced, registered-nurse-practitioner tract in emergency nursing, their faculty were included in the informational sessions because they rotate through the ED and provide student and staff support when present. After the informational sessions were held, the nurse researchers provided e-mail and phone-contact information via postings on staff lounge boards so those interested in participating could contact one of them. The nurse researchers had no direct-line supervision over any staff who chose to participate, thereby protecting their anonymity. The management team was instructed not to encourage staff's enrollment in the project to avoid any implications of coercion. Any questions related to the project prior to implementation were addressed by the PIs. The PIs obtained informed consent and provided the staff with the dates when the training would take place.

Employees who knew in advance that they would be leaving the ED within the projected time frame of the study were excluded. The funded number of staff participants went up to 120, to include ED clinical leaders, interdisciplinary staff, Caritas coaches, and select Jacksonville University faculty. Prior to implementation of the project, staff in the ED were required to complete the National Institutes of Health (NIH) Protection of Human Subjects education module.

A participant was included in the study upon completion of the NIH education module and the Consent for Participation in a Clinical Research Study. Once enrolled in the study, the participants then attended the 12-hour CaritasHeartMath education program. There were no anticipated discomforts or risks related to participating in the project.

In the 3 weeks between the classes and pre- and post-testing, Caritas coaches and the PIs rounded in the ED to give brief reviews on the heart-centered breathing techniques, reinforce caring theory, and so on. Approximately eight sessions were held for staff on both shifts. Beginning in February 2010, at the request of the assistant nurse managers from the ED, the Caritas coaches began meeting with them on a monthly basis for coaching and caring-science work. The leadership group felt that they wanted to reinforce the HeartMath techniques with the staff and wanted coaching on how to better care for their staff. The focus on the coaches moved from individual staff participants to ED leadership.

STUDY DESIGN

The study is a pre-test, post-test design using a convenience sample. Instruments are as follows:

1. Personal and Organizational Quality Assessment (POQA-R) (Appendix 16.1) Program effectiveness was assessed through analysis of pre- and post-training measurements using an instrument created by the Institute of HeartMath. The instrument, titled Personal and Organizational Quality Assessment (POQA-R), is a validated assessment tool designed to provide an overview of personal and job-related constructs. This 80-item survey measures physical stress symptoms, psychological health, resilience, emotional competencies, organizational climate, and work performance. Examples of these constructs are:

- Personal: fatigue, anger management, distress, and vitality
- Physical stress symptoms: inadequate sleep, body aches, rapid heartbeats
- Job-related: satisfaction, productivity, clarity, communication, and social support

Participants completed the POQA-R prior to participating in the CaritasHeartMath education program and immediately after participating in the education program. The instrument was administered by the project development director of HeartMath.

2. Caritas Patient Assessment Score (CPAS) (Appendix 16.2)
A questionnaire, titled the Caritas Patient Assessment Score (CPAS), is given to patients treated in the ED to complete at the time of discharge. The CPAS is a four-item instrument designed to measure patients' assessments of caring processes and willingness to recommend the hospital. The scale was adapted from the 20-item Caring Factor Survey (Nelson, 2008), which has satisfactory reliability and validity. The CPAS contains four items reflecting four Caritas Processes measured on a 5-point scale (*never* to *always*), a single item assessing the patient's willingness to recommend the hospital, and a single open-ended item asking if there are any caring or uncaring moments the patient would like to share. Exclusion criteria consist of patients who are not able to speak English; are younger than 18 years; have been admitted; and those presenting with a behavioral health issue, traumatic injury, and/or assault. The CPAS was distributed to patients in the ED pre- and post-staff participation in the CaritasHeartMath education program to determine the program's effect on the patients' perceptions of care and compassion they received in the ED. Questionnaires were distributed by the ED staff and will be collected for up to 2 years. There are no patient personal identifiers on the CPAS questionnaire that could link responses back to individual patients. Box-type receptacles were strategically placed in the ED for the patients to deposit their completed questionnaires to further protect the anonymity of patients' responses.

3. Baptist Downtown ED Patient Satisfaction Survey
In addition, patient responses from the Baptist Downtown ED's Patient Satisfaction Survey, provided through NRC Picker, were reviewed both retrospectively prior to the staff's participation in the CaritasHeartMath education program, and prospectively after participation in the education program to determine the effect of the program on the patients' perceived patient-care experience in the ED. At the time, the Baptist Downtown ED Patient-Satisfaction Survey consists of 64 items intended to evaluate how satisfied a patient is with the services received in the ED. The survey is mailed by NRC Picker to a randomly selected group of patients who have been treated in the ED. Patients are provided a stamped envelope to mail the completed survey to NRC Picker for processing.

DATA ANALYSES

The data were analyzed using descriptive and inferential statistics jointly by the PIs, WCSI, and HeartMath.

POQA-R SCORES

Demographics

Demographics revealed that the majority of participants work full time with greater than 2 years with the organization. Fifty-two matched pairs completed education and evaluations. Results were divided into two categories: Personal Quality and Organizational Quality.

Personal Quality

The Personal Quality results demonstrated improvement in all categories of personal stress. Of the 10 grouped constructs, seven achieved highly significant results ($p<.001$). These were in gratitude, calmness, fatigue, anxiety, anger management, resentfulness, and stress related to symptoms.

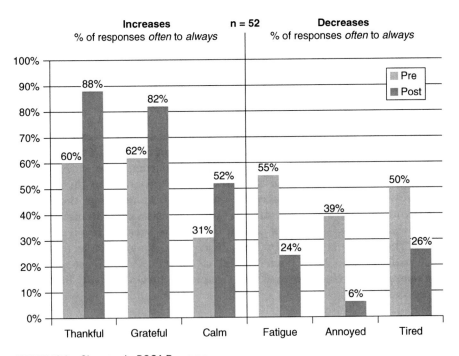

FIGURE 16.2   Changes in POQA-R scores.

TABLE 16.1   Specific Items From POQA-R

PERSONAL QUALITY	PRE	POST	CHANGE
I feel thankful.	60	88	+47%
I feel grateful.	62	82	+32%
I feel calm.	31	52	+68%
I feel peaceful.	31	55	+77%
This is an organization where people feel a sense of appreciation for one another.	33	56	+70%
I feel worried.	46	25	−46%
I feel there is never enough time.	60	37	−48%
I feel like leaving the organization.	8	2	−75%

Of the 10 grouped constructs, two achieved significance at $p < .05$: positive outlook and motivation (Figure 16.2).

Table 16.1 illustrates examples of specific items from the POQA-R that reflect the caring theory where participants reported feeling the construct "*Often/Always.*"

Organizational Quality

The Organizational Quality Assessment results revealed few statistically significant changes. Most attributes started at average and all but one saw improvement. The highest statistical change was in intention to quit.

Caritas Patient Assessment Scores

Patient perceptions of caring were collected at three time points: before staff education, in the interval between the two caring education sessions, and following staff education. The CPAS (Modified) scale contains four items with five possible response options ranging from *never* (1) to *always* (5). Possible scale scores range from 4 to 20. The scale exhibited satisfactory, internal-consistency reliability (Cronbach's alpha of .92).

There were 653 surveys that were completed and used for analysis. In general, the majority of patients perceived caring practices to be provided always during their ED visits. A one-way analysis of variance was performed to evaluate differences before, during, and after staff education.

TABLE 16.2   Change in CPAS Scores

CPAS-MODIFIED SCORE	N	MEAN	SD
Before education	183	19.01	2.322
Between education sessions	334	18.90	2.553
Following education	136	19.10	2.054

No statistical differences were found among the three data-collection periods. Table 16.2 presents the number of patients, the mean, and the standard deviation of scores for the three data-collection points.

The vast majority (665, or 99%) of the 671 patients who answered the question would recommend the ED to someone they love.

NRC Picker Patient-Satisfaction Scores

We compared the trends in nurse-sensitive items to determine if there were any changes in results over the course of this pilot project. The resulting line graph is noted in Figure 16.3.

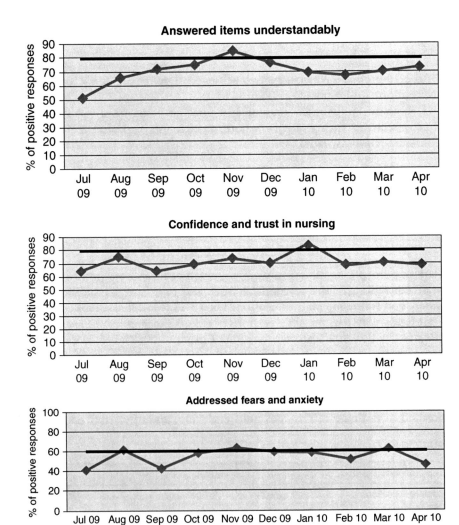

FIGURE 16.3   Nurse-sensitive items, pattern over time. (National Research Corporation, 2010)

There was an upward, positive trend in the November–January time frame of the pilot in the three areas that address nurse caring.

NEXT STEPS

The ED is a complex environment where multiple strategies are being deployed to enhance staff and patient satisfaction. The preliminary results of this pilot study demonstrated that education and training regarding caring-science and HeartMath techniques for ED staff improved their personal outlook related to stress and depression behaviors. We also observed positive patient-satisfaction and perception results that tracked staff results. Although there may have been intervening variables that also affected the scores, there were none as focused and intentional as the CaritasHeartMath training during this period.

The request by the ED leadership to pull back from staff support and focus on their skill set came as a surprise but came in response to dialogue with them about how to enhance and sustain the results with the staff. Although all the leaders were part of the initial training and experience, it was clear that they felt the need to enhance their skill set before they were expected to be models for the staff. This is a lesson learned for us. If we had the opportunity to do this again, we would explore ways to educate the leadership first and make sure they had solid footing before moving to the staff.

In the process of focusing on the leaders, we have had minimal direct focus with the staff. We have seen their use of the techniques decline by their own report, and leaders' observations decline. We also have experienced a decline in the patient-satisfaction scores. The participants completed the second round of assessment in the summer of 2010 with the POQA-R instrument, and we would anticipate a decline in those results as well.

It is clear that CaritasHeartMath is a behavioral technique that requires not just intellectual knowing but behavioral reinforcement. Because the preliminary results were so powerful in this group, we have been able to obtain funding to train two staff members to be HeartMath instructors, meaning we will have competent staff on site to educate and reinforce training in the future.

In conjunction with this effort, we continue to build more of a Caritas environment in the ED through our leadership coaching and dialogues, creating a Caritas sacred space for staff and using art in the environment. We believe that in order to translate caring science into practice, one must use multiple techniques over time.

REFERENCES

Baptist Health, Jacksonville, Florida. (n.d.). *Nursing.* Retrieved October 20, 2010, from http://www.e-baptisthealth.com/

Beck, C. T. (2000). The experience of choosing nursing as a career. *Journal of Nursing Research, 39*(7), 320–322.

Boughn, S. (2001). Why women and men choose nursing. *Nursing Health Care Perspective, 22*(1), 14–19.

Boughn, S. & Lentini, A. (1999). Why do women choose nursing? *Journal of Nursing Education, 38*(4), 156–161.

Institute of HeartMath. (n.d.). *www.heartmath.org.* Retrieved August 15, 2010, from http://www.heartmath.org/mission/vision

Kelly, N. R., Shoemaker, M., & Steele, T. (1996). The experience of being a male student nurse. *Journal of Nursing Education, 35*(4), 170–174.

Kersten, J., Bakewell, K., & Meyer, D. (1991). Motivating factors in a student's choice of nursing as a career. *Journal of Nursing Education, 30*(1), 30–33.

National Research Corporation. (n.d.). *www.nationalresearch.com.* Retrieved August 15, 2010, from http://hcmg.nationalresearch.com/Default.aspx?DN=7, 1,Documents

Pillitteri, A. (1994). A contrast in images: Nursing and nonnursing college students. *Journal of Nursing Education, 33*(3), 132–133.

Stevens, K. A., & Walker, E. A. (1993). Choosing a career: Why not nursing for more high school seniors? *Journal of Nursing Education, 32*(1), 13–17.

Swanson, K. M. (1999). What's known about caring in nursing science: A literary meta-analysis. In A. S. Hinshaw, S. Feetham, & J. Shaver (Eds.), *Handbook of clinical nursing research* (pp. 31–60). Thousand Oaks, CA: Sage Publishing.

Williams, B., Weternberger, D. H., & Gushuliak, T. (1997). Why students choose nursing. *Journal of Nursing Education, 36*(7), 346–348.

Watson, J. (2005). *Caring science as sacred science.* Philadelphia, PA: F. A. Davis.

APPENDIX 16.1

𝒫𝒪𝒬𝒜-ℛ **Personal and Organizational Quality Assessment-Revised**

This survey is voluntary and confidential.
Only summary, anonymous data will be provided to your organization.

INSTRUCTIONS: Please fill in the boxes below with the requested dates and ID number. For the remaining items, FILL IN THE NUMBER of the response that describes you.

TODAY'S DATE
Month Day   Year

UNIQUE ID NUMBER

Please enter the last four digits of your social security number or a 4-digit number you can easily remember. This number is used for tracking responses over time. No attempt to identify you can or will be made. If you feel uncomfortable providing this information, you may leave it blank.

1. What is your GENDER?

① Male   ② Female

2. What is your MARITAL STATUS? (fill in one only)

① Single   ③ Partnered   ⑤ Divorced

② Married   ④ Separated   ⑥ Widowed

3. Roughly how old are you?

① Under 21   ③ 31-40   ⑤ 51-60   ⑦ Over 70

② 21-30   ④ 41-50   ⑥ 61-70

4. What is your approximate salary range?

① Under $20,000   ⑦ $70,000 - 79,999

② $20,000 - 29,999   ⑧ $80,000 - 89,999

③ $30,000 - 39,999   ⑨ $90,000 - 99,999

④ $40,000 - 49,999   ⑩ $100,000 - 149,999

⑤ $50,000 - 59,999   ⑪ $150,000 or more

⑥ $60,000 - 69,999

5. What is your highest level of EDUCATION? (fill in one only)

① Elementary   ⑥ Bachelor's Degree

② Junior/Middle School   ⑦ Some Graduate

③ High School   ⑧ Master's Degree

④ Technical School   ⑨ Doctorate Degree

⑤ Some College/Associate's Degree

6. Which of the following best describes your EMPLOYMENT STATUS? (fill in one only)

① Student   ⑤ Executive

② Laborer   ⑦ Engineer/Technical

③ Skilled or Clerical   ⑧ Retired

④ Management   ⑨ Unemployed

⑤ Professional   ⑩ Other

7. How many HOURS PER WEEK do you usually work?

① Less than 25 hours   ④ 41-50 hours

② 26-35 hours   ⑤ 51-59 hours

③ 36-40 hours   ⑥ 60 or more hours

8. How long have you been with this COMPANY or ORGANIZATION?

① 0 - 6 MONTHS   ⑤ 5 YEARS - 10 YEARS

② 6 MONTHS - 1 YEAR   ⑥ 10 YEARS - 20 YEARS

③ 1 YEAR - 2 YEARS   ⑦ 20 YEARS OR MORE

④ 2 YEARS - 5 YEARS

9. How long have you been in your CURRENT JOB or POSITION?

① 0 - 6 MONTHS   ④ 2 YEARS - 5 YEARS

② 6 MONTHS - 1 YEAR   ⑤ 5 YEARS - 10 YEARS

③ 1 YEAR - 2 YEARS   ⑥ 10 YEARS OR MORE

Please turn to the next page

PLEASE DO NOT WRITE IN THIS AREA

42794

(continued)

Reprinted from the Institute of HeartMath with permission.

$\mathcal{POQA}\text{-}\mathcal{R}$ Personal and Organizational Quality Assessment-Revised

INSTRUCTIONS:
Following is a list of words that describe feelings people sometimes have. Please FILL IN THE NUMBER which reflects how frequently you have felt the following during the LAST MONTH.

	NOT AT ALL	ONCE IN A WHILE	SOMETIMES	FAIRLY OFTEN	OFTEN	VERY OFTEN	ALWAYS
1. Resentful	①	②	③	④	⑤	⑥	⑦
2. Fatigued	①	②	③	④	⑤	⑥	⑦
3. Annoyed	①	②	③	④	⑤	⑥	⑦
4. Sad	①	②	③	④	⑤	⑥	⑦
5. Body aches (Joint Pain, Backaches, etc.)	①	②	③	④	⑤	⑥	⑦
6. Headaches	①	②	③	④	⑤	⑥	⑦
7. Rapid Heartbeats	①	②	③	④	⑤	⑥	⑦
8. Depressed	①	②	③	④	⑤	⑥	⑦
9. Exhausted	①	②	③	④	⑤	⑥	⑦
10. Blue	①	②	③	④	⑤	⑥	⑦
11. Appreciative	①	②	③	④	⑤	⑥	⑦
12. Relaxed	①	②	③	④	⑤	⑥	⑦
13. Anxious	①	②	③	④	⑤	⑥	⑦
14. Tired	①	②	③	④	⑤	⑥	⑦
15. My sleep is inadequate	①	②	③	④	⑤	⑥	⑦
16. Thankful	①	②	③	④	⑤	⑥	⑦
17. Indigestion, heartburn or stomach upset	①	②	③	④	⑤	⑥	⑦
18. Calm	①	②	③	④	⑤	⑥	⑦
19. Cynical	①	②	③	④	⑤	⑥	⑦
20. Muscle Tension	①	②	③	④	⑤	⑥	⑦
21. Grateful	①	②	③	④	⑤	⑥	⑦
22. Worried	①	②	③	④	⑤	⑥	⑦
23. Unhappy	①	②	③	④	⑤	⑥	⑦
24. Uneasy	①	②	③	④	⑤	⑥	⑦
25. Angry	①	②	③	④	⑤	⑥	⑦
26. Peaceful	①	②	③	④	⑤	⑥	⑦

27. Over the last month my health has been:

Excellent	Good	Average	Fair	Poor
①	②	③	④	⑤

28. Fill in the bubble on the line below that indicates how stressed you have been in the past month:

Most Calm I've Ever Been ○—○—○—○—○—○—○—○—○—○—○—○ Most Stressed I've Ever Been

(continued)

Following is a list of statements that describe the way people sometimes feel or think about themselves. Please FILL IN THE NUMBER which reflects how frequently you have felt or thought the following during the LAST MONTH.

Scale: NOT AT ALL / ONCE IN A WHILE / SOMETIMES / FAIRLY OFTEN / OFTEN / VERY OFTEN / ALWAYS

#	Statement	1	2	3	4	5	6	7
29.	My life is deeply fulfilling	①	②	③	④	⑤	⑥	⑦
30.	Dynamic	①	②	③	④	⑤	⑥	⑦
31.	I get upset easily	①	②	③	④	⑤	⑥	⑦
32.	I find it difficult to calm down after I've been upset	①	②	③	④	⑤	⑥	⑦
33.	I feel loved by my spouse/partner	①	②	③	④	⑤	⑥	⑦
34.	I feel optimistic about the future	①	②	③	④	⑤	⑥	⑦
35.	I wake up and look forward to each day	①	②	③	④	⑤	⑥	⑦
36.	Motivated	①	②	③	④	⑤	⑥	⑦
37.	I am pleased with my life	①	②	③	④	⑤	⑥	⑦
38.	I sometimes have urges to break, throw or smash things	①	②	③	④	⑤	⑥	⑦
39.	I sometimes have a short fuse	①	②	③	④	⑤	⑥	⑦
40.	Enthusiastic	①	②	③	④	⑤	⑥	⑦

We are asking about your feelings and experiences over the LAST MONTH. Please FILL IN THE NUMBER which reflects how much you AGREE or DISAGREE with the following statements as they apply to you, your job and place of employment during the LAST MONTH.

Scale: STRONGLY DISAGREE / DISAGREE / SLIGHTLY DISAGREE / NEUTRAL / SLIGHTLY AGREE / AGREE / STRONGLY AGREE

#	Statement	1	2	3	4	5	6	7
41.	I constantly work at full capacity	①	②	③	④	⑤	⑥	⑦
42.	We listen carefully to each other at work	①	②	③	④	⑤	⑥	⑦
43.	People's roles and responsibilities are made clear	①	②	③	④	⑤	⑥	⑦
44.	I strive as hard as I can to be successful in my work	①	②	③	④	⑤	⑥	⑦
45.	There is tension between management and staff	①	②	③	④	⑤	⑥	⑦
46.	My work is usually interesting and stimulating	①	②	③	④	⑤	⑥	⑦
47.	Other people know me by the long hours I keep	①	②	③	④	⑤	⑥	⑦
48.	I feel good about what I do at work	①	②	③	④	⑤	⑥	⑦
49.	The quality of communication at work is excellent	①	②	③	④	⑤	⑥	⑦
50.	The goals of my organization are clear to me	①	②	③	④	⑤	⑥	⑦
51.	I accomplish all my objectives at work	①	②	③	④	⑤	⑥	⑦
52.	I feel there is never enough time	①	②	③	④	⑤	⑥	⑦
53.	I feel good about the future of the organization	①	②	③	④	⑤	⑥	⑦
54.	My efforts make a big difference in my organization	①	②	③	④	⑤	⑥	⑦
55.	I am proud of the company I work for	①	②	③	④	⑤	⑥	⑦

(continued)

We are asking about your feelings and experiences over the LAST MONTH. Please FILL IN THE NUMBER which reflects how much you AGREE or DISAGREE with the following statements as they apply to you, your job and place of employment during the LAST MONTH.	STRONGLY DISAGREE	DISAGREE	SLIGHTLY DISAGREE	NEUTRAL	SLIGHTLY AGREE	AGREE	STRONGLY AGREE
56. I really like the way I'm treated by my supervisor	①	②	③	④	⑤	⑥	⑦
57. I feel pressed for time	①	②	③	④	⑤	⑥	⑦
58. I understand our business strategy	①	②	③	④	⑤	⑥	⑦
59. My work produces excellent results	①	②	③	④	⑤	⑥	⑦
60. I always approach my work with whole-hearted effort	①	②	③	④	⑤	⑥	⑦
61. The pace of life is too fast and I can't keep up	①	②	③	④	⑤	⑥	⑦
62. I feel a strong sense of rapport with my supervisor	①	②	③	④	⑤	⑥	⑦
63. I am creative and innovative	①	②	③	④	⑤	⑥	⑦
64. I feel conflict between work and personal priorities	①	②	③	④	⑤	⑥	⑦
65. I see a connection between the work I do and the company's strategic objectives	①	②	③	④	⑤	⑥	⑦
66. I feel very supported by my supervisor	①	②	③	④	⑤	⑥	⑦
67. It takes a lot of effort to sustain my performance level	①	②	③	④	⑤	⑥	⑦
68. I feel very useful in my job	①	②	③	④	⑤	⑥	⑦
69. I always know how my supervisor wants me to utilize my time	①	②	③	④	⑤	⑥	⑦
70. I am able to speak out without fear of the consequences	①	②	③	④	⑤	⑥	⑦
71. I feel like leaving this organization	①	②	③	④	⑤	⑥	⑦
72. My work is very challenging	①	②	③	④	⑤	⑥	⑦
73. We have great confidence about being successful in the future	①	②	③	④	⑤	⑥	⑦
74. I feel like quitting my job	①	②	③	④	⑤	⑥	⑦
75. People respectfully express different points of view during meetings	①	②	③	④	⑤	⑥	⑦
76. People where I work feel free to express their opinions	①	②	③	④	⑤	⑥	⑦
77. My work is often recognized and appreciated by my superiors	①	②	③	④	⑤	⑥	⑦
78. When people talk about the current state of our organization, most of the stories are about good news (e.g. innovations, achievements, new and better practices, etc.)	①	②	③	④	⑤	⑥	⑦
79. My job gives me a sense of accomplishment	①	②	③	④	⑤	⑥	⑦
80. I am always highly productive	①	②	③	④	⑤	⑥	⑦
81. I work with people who don't get along with each other	①	②	③	④	⑤	⑥	⑦
82. This is an organization where people feel a sense of appreciation for one another	①	②	③	④	⑤	⑥	⑦
83. My job requires me to use all of my abilities	①	②	③	④	⑤	⑥	⑦
84. I'm aware of power struggles between co-workers that damage morale	①	②	③	④	⑤	⑥	⑦
85. Doing my tasks well substantially contributes to my organization	①	②	③	④	⑤	⑥	⑦

Thank You Very Much For Your Participation!

APPENDIX 16.2

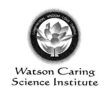

Watson Caring
Science Institute

Caritas Patient Assessment Score©

DIRECTIONS: When answering the questions, please consider the overall CARE you have received during this hospital stay. Please check the one best answer.

During this hospital stay:	Never	Rarely	Occasionally	Frequently	Always
My caregivers consistently provide care to me with loving kindness.					
My caregivers respond to me as a whole person, helping to take care of all my needs and concerns.					
My caregivers have a helping and trusting relationship with me.					
My caregivers have created a healing environment that recognizes the wholeness of my body, mind, and spirit.					

Would you recommend our hospital to someone you love?

Yes ☐   No ☐

We invite and honor your willingness to share any notable caring or uncaring moments you may have experienced during your hospital stay?

Thank you for sharing and completing our survey!

Caritas Patient Assessment Score© (CPAS©), Copyright by Watson Caring Science Institute. Visit: www.watsoncaringscience.org.

Adapted from: Nelson, J.W., Watson, J., & InovaHealth. (2009). Caring Factors Survey (CFS). In J. Watson (Ed.), Assessing and Measuring Caring in Nursing and Health Sciences. (2nd Edition, pp. 253-258). New York: Springer.

Modified for Jacksonville Baptist.

SECTION IV

International Measurement of Caritas: Exemplars From the Field

17

First Measurement of Caritas in Italy

Giuliana Masera

*R*eception of patients/clients in the health care environment can be defined as a quality indicator of the personalization and humanization of health care services. It is the opportunity for the first caring moment and is essential in setting the tone for the care that will occur from admission to discharge. This study examined the perception of caring in an elder care center in the province of Piacenza, Italy, which is located in the northwestern portion of the country. It was the first study to undertake an empirical approach to translate, test, and describe the results from the Caring Factor Survey (CFS) designed for use in Italy.

The moment dedicated to a user's reception takes on a decisive value both for the importance of the moment itself and for the complexity of the relational and empathetic relationship even before the nurse establishes a clinical relationship with the person. The patient's perception of caring the moment he or she is received in the facility cannot be understated, nor can it be turned into a simple bureaucratic practice. It requires the person who is receiving the patient to consider and anticipate the patient's every need, including physical, spiritual, and emotional/mental.

On this subject, several health units have elaborated projects relative to reception (see Project of the Veneto Region Health Unit n. 19, 1998/1999). The attention given to the dimension of the relational quality within the limits of "improving the provision of the services of all the operative Units, with particular attention to: reception, comfort, bookings and waiting-times," aims at increasing the quality of sociomedical services and at consolidating the positive image of an administrational organization. Objectives of this kind envision nurses maintaining a constant relationship with patients from the moment of their reception to the moment of their discharge.

If reception becomes a quality indicator, the instruments through which to measure it become important, and the CFS developed by Nelson, Watson, and Inova Health (2008) constitutes a valid instrument. The CFS is being used increasingly in the United States as an important instrument for assessing the standard of satisfaction in holistic terms of the users and of the care given them by the staff within the facilities. This evaluation scale has application for public and private facilities that include both acute and chronic care. Legler, Sramek, Conklin and Diamond review in Chapter 4 how it has been shown to be useful for patients and their family members. This is especially useful in situations where patients cannot speak for themselves, such as in dementia or acute illness. Leger et al. reveal in Chapter 4 how the family has been shown to be a satisfactory proxy for the care being given to the patient.

PROCEDURES

The CFS had to be translated from English to Italian in preparation for its administration to residents of the Prospero Verani Nursing Home. The author of this study translated the survey and presented the translated version to the managers, nurses, and health care supervisors of the nursing home for content validation. Each statement was considered by the group and agreed upon at a meeting that took place on October 20, 2007. The discussion took place until there was 100% agreement among the group that the wording of the items in Italian was consistent with that in English.

The CFS was then administered on October 22–24, 2007, to 16 guests of a nursing home, Healthcare Residence Prospero Verani, in Fiorenzuola d'Arda in the province of Piacenza, Italy.

PRESENTATION OF THE RESULTS

The overall Cronbach's alpha was .86 and would not have increased even if an item had been deleted. This indicated that it was a relatable tool to measure caring in Italy. Results of the descriptive statistics revealed variance for each of the 10 concepts of caring, with some scores as low as 2.5 (promotion of expression) to as high as 7.0 for all 10 items in the CFS. The highest mean score was for perception of caring being given with loving kindness (mean score 6.91). The lowest mean score was for allowing expression of feeling, both positive and negative (mean score 5.31). Each of the 10 concepts of caring, plus the total CFS score, was above the midpoint of 4.0 on a 1–7 scale, indicating that, in general, there was agreement that all caring concepts were operational. The total CFS score, that is, all caring concepts combined, was 5.98 (Table 17.1).

DISCUSSION

Loving kindness was perceived by patients because it had the highest-ranking score. It received a score of 6.9 on a 1–7 Likert-type scale.

Development of trusting relationships was ranked second, and it is believed that it was facilitated through direct relationship building

Table 17.1 Descriptive Statistics of 16 Respondents

	N	MINIMUM	MAXIMUM	MEAN	STD DEVIATION
Loving kindness	16	6.00	7.00	6.9063	.27195
Trusting relationship	16	4.50	7.00	6.3438	.81074
Faith and hope	16	4.00	7.00	6.1563	1.01191
Healing environment	16	3.00	7.00	6.1250	1.08781
Teach and learn	16	3.50	7.00	6.0313	1.24457
CFS total	16	4.70	6.85	5.9750	.64135
Problem solving	16	4.50	7.00	5.9375	.98107
Holistic care	16	4.00	7.00	5.8438	.99530
Spiritual support	16	2.50	7.00	5.6563	1.26120
Allow miracles	16	4.00	7.00	5.4375	.87321
Promote expression	16	2.50	7.00	5.3125	1.23659
Valid N (listwise)	16				

between care providers and patients and also among the guests of the facility. For example, care providers put people with the same cognitive level at the same dining table or in the same bedroom in order to stimulate communication between the guests.

One of the patients who responded to the survey had provided a comment stating that the environment was indeed beautiful; this comment is consistent with the fourth-highest score. However, it should be noted that the patient who commented on the beautiful environment also stated that no matter how beautiful the environment was, it was not enough to heal him or her, which reveals that caring is multifaceted.

Items 6 and 8 related to patients' feelings as to whether they were taught in an individual way to maximize their learning. It is posited that those who reported a neutral answer—there were some who gave it a score as low as 3.5—may have reported this because they consider themselves self-sufficient and, hence, do not need teaching. Those who reported high scores for teaching may have been responding to the work of the physiotherapists, who made extended efforts to ensure that the patients understood their mobilization. In addition, nurses constantly checked that the patients understood the importance of following the prescribed treatment to maximize their health.

Creative problem solving was in the lower half of the caring concepts. The high scores reported by patients for creative problem solving as a process of caring may be in part due to the respect shown to them for their personal religious beliefs.

Holistic care—attention to body, mind, and spirit—was ranked among the lowest of the caring factors. Those who selected *neutral* and *slightly disagree* justified their answers by saying that they find it difficult to externalize feelings and worries to caregivers, which makes it hard for caregivers to tend to each aspect of a person. The answers were generally positive with guests reporting that they were always consoled and sustained by the staff in moments of difficulty and depression, although there was room for improvement.

Spiritual support was third to last, with the lowest score of 2.5 being reported. This response alludes to the underlined possibility that, as patients, their beliefs were respected but not encouraged and supported by caregivers.

Miracles received a neutral answer by a majority of the guests because they never talked about miracles with the staff; or because, having had chronic diseases for several years, they did not believe in miracles; or because they were afraid that the health care team would make fun of them ("They'll think I'm mad!").

For those who did report a positive answer regarding belief in miracles, the reason may have been that guests' recovery was always encouraged and that there always was a feeling of hope regarding the future. Guests' relatives also were given a great deal of attention by the health care team.

It was interesting that staff promoting expression of feelings was ranked last by patients. Those who selected *neutral* and *slightly disagree* may have done so because they are reserved by nature and, therefore, do not feel the need to show their feelings, or because seeing how busy the staff were with their work, they were afraid "to waste their time." Patients who reported they *strongly agree* and *agree* to the expression of emotion confirmed the open-mindedness of the staff in allowing guests to speak openly about their feelings.

CONCLUSION

From the answers emerging from the CFS, originated by Nelson, Watson, and Inova Health (2008), to this study in Piacenza, Italy, it appears that there are rank-order perceptions of the caring factors within Watson's theory of Caritas. It may be deduced that reception; kindness; good manners; encouragement to react; support, not only physical but also moral and spiritual; and, above all, abstention from judgment—therefore, *tolerance, respect, responsibility, and hospitality*—are necessary elements for the care and satisfaction of people's individual needs. Within this theoretical framework, these concepts of Caritas are important to make guests feel that they are in a warm and loving embrace.

According to Emmanuel Lévinas (1980), a philosopher and Jewish theologian, we experience *responsibility* not as something rational and predictable, but, on the contrary, as something unpredictable that just *happens* to us without our conscious will or consent being engaged. Among the many examples of this idea that Lévinas provides, that of *the face* is crucial. The face, he says, "*is* by itself and not by reference to a system." By this he means that no amount of detail about the way someone looks can ever capture what it *is* to be that person; there is always something left over from such calculations, and what is left over is precisely and simply *him or her—his or her uniqueness.*

Jacques Derrida (1996), a French philosopher, introduced the concept of *hospitality*: Genuine hospitality before any number of unknown others is not, strictly speaking, a possible scenario. If we contemplate giving up everything that we seek to possess and call our own, then most of us can empathize with just how difficult enacting any absolute hospitality would be. Despite this, however, Derrida insists that the whole idea of hospitality depends on such an altruistic concept and is inconceivable without it. In fact, he argues that it is this internal tension that keeps the concept alive.

Derrida (2000) claims that "we thus enter from the inside: the master of the house is at home, but nonetheless he comes to enter his home through the guest who comes from outside" (p. 125). Lévinas (1969) asserts that hospitality is "the concrete and initial fact of human recollection and separation" (p. 172).

According to Florence Nightingale (1859), nursing was a spiritual practice, and spirituality was considered intrinsic to human nature and a potent resource for healing. She was clear about nursing being a calling, and she articulated nursing's healing role, that of being and working in harmony with nature. In this heritage, nursing, and its focus on caring and healing in harmony with nature and environmental conditions, was a form of values-guided, artful practice attending to basic human essentials, grace and beauty. In awakening to the humanity of nursing, according to Jean Watson (1979), nurses are invited, if not required, to repattern their own field of being (Heidegger, 1971) in the direction of an expanded caring–healing consciousness by becoming more clear about nursing's heritage and values-based practices. These tasks are carried out from a deep philosophical tradition that calls upon us to cultivate a caring consciousness and an ethic of caring as foundational for our practice. It is vital that this ethic of caring is present at the reception of the guests. This study illustrates the beginning of understanding the ethic of caring more deeply in relationship to love, humanness, and healing in Italy.

REFERENCES

Derrida, J. (1996). *Sull'ospitalità* [Of Hospitality]. Milano: Baldini e Castoldi.
Derrida, J. (2000). *Of hospitality* (R. Bawlby, Trans.). Stanford, CA: Stanford University Press.

Heidegger, M. (1962). *Being and time* (J. Macquairre & E. Robinson, Trans.). London: SCM Press.

Heidegger, M. (1971). *Essere e tempo* [Being and time]. Milano: Longanesi & C.

Lévinas, E. (1969). *Totality and infinity* (A. Lingis, Trans.). Pittsburgh, PA: Duquesne University Press.

Lévinas, E. (1980). *Totalità e infinito. Saggio sull'esteriorità* [Totality and infinity]. Milano, Italy: Jaca Book.

Nelson, J., Watson, J., & Inova Health. (2008). Development of the Caring Factor Survey© (CFS), an instrument to measure patient's perception of caring. In J. Watson (Ed.), *Assessing and measuring caring in nursing and health science* (2nd ed.). New York, NY: Springer.

Nightingale, F. (1859/1992). *Notes on nursing: What it is and what it is not.* Philadelphia, PA: Lippincott.

Project of the Veneto Region Health Unit n. 19. (1998/1999). Retrieved June 22, 2011, from http://archive.forumpa.it/forumpa2000/regionando/veneto/asl19adria/progettoaccoglienza.pdf

Watson, J. (1979). *Nursing: The philosophy and science of caring.* Boston, MA: Little, Brown.

18

Utilization of the Clinical Caritas Process in a Selected Tertiary Hospital in the Philippines

Patricia Clarisse V. Reyes, Diana Marie Avecilla-Millare, Mae Shela S. Cruz, Princess M. Ramos, Elena O. Rubis, John Carlo G. Villamero, and Margaret May A. Ga

Caring is the essence of nursing and the most central and unifying focus for nursing practice (McEwen & Willis, 2002). It is the most valuable attribute nursing has to offer to humanity (Fitzpatrick & Whall, 2005). Patricia Benner describes caring as the essence of excellent nursing practice (Benner, Tanner, & Chesla, 1992). Caring means that persons, events, projects, and things matter to people (Potter & Perry, 2007).

Just because caring is a complex human phenomenon, it does not mean we should not try to capture as much of it as possible. By having instruments to address caring, there are more possibilities for developing knowledge of caring and learning more about how patients, nurses, and systems may benefit. At best, these measurements serve as quality indicators of caring and point back toward the deeper aspects behind the measurements. In doing so, clarification of assumptions can be made as well as reconciliation between ontological and epistemological assumptions within the various theoretical/conceptual systems of caring. Finally, the results may lead to a better fit among research traditions, design methods, and the processes used for creative emergence: the use of extant as well as new forms of caring inquiry (Watson, 2002).

According to Professor Jean Watson, caring for patients is premised on 10 caring processes collectively known as the Clinical Caritas Process. It is these 10 processes that make up the construct of caring.

The Clinical Caritas Process is an emerging model of transpersonal caring that moves from carative to caritas. *Caritas* is a Latin word that means "to cherish, to appreciate, to give special attention, if not loving, attention to"; it connotes something very fine that is indeed precious. Caritas conveys love and allows love and caring to come together for a new form of deep transpersonal caring. This relationship between love and caring connotes inner healing for self and others, extending to nature and the larger universe, unfolding and evolving within a cosmology that is both metaphysical and transcendent with the coevolving human in the universe (Watson, 2007).

The interpersonal process in a caring environment involves human beings interacting with each other with dignity and respect. However, as health care needs become complex, technology is incorporated into the caring environment. With technology becoming part of the caring environment, care complexity escalates. As care becomes complex, it is vital that nurses' and patients' perceived values of caring behaviors become congruent (Sombillo, 2006).

The study describes the extent of use of the Clinical Caritas Process by staff nurses as perceived by patients according to the following core components of the Caritas Processes: (1) loving kindness; (2) instilling faith and hope; (3) spiritual beliefs and practices; (4) helping, trusting relationship; (5) promotion of expression of feelings; (6) decision making; (7) teaching and learning; (8) healing environment; (9) holistic care; and (10) miracles.

The study focused on adult medical-surgical patients confined in the tertiary hospital. From the list of patients confined in the medical-surgical floors of the hospital, 51 met the criteria of the study. The study also describes the use of the Clinical Caritas Process by staff nurses as perceived by patients belonging to different categories of patient acuity. Categories include the following: (1) minimal care patients; (2) moderate care patients; (3) total care patients; and (4) critical care patients. Finally, the study also described the difference between the extent of use of the Clinical Caritas Process by staff nurses as perceived by patients between and across all patient categories.

MATERIALS AND METHODS

The instrument used was the Caring Factor Survey (CFS), a survey questionnaire developed in the United States to provide support in measuring care as perceived by patients (Nelson, Watson, & Inova Health, 2008). Twenty items were created by the authors of the tool, two questions for each Caritas Process, and all items were validated by other experts in Caritas Processes. The CFS uses a 1–7 Likert scale with higher scores indicating a greater sense of caring from the patients' perspectives as indicated in the following: 1, *strongly disagree*; 2, *disagree*; 3, *slightly disagree*; 4, *neutral*; 5, *agree*; 6, *slightly agree*; and 7, *strongly agree*.

The CFS was administered to a total of 51 patients in an acute care setting in the Philippines: 15 of the patients were from the minimal care category, 17 from the moderate or partial care category, 13 from the total care category, and 6 from the critical care category.

Data obtained from the questionnaires were tabulated and treated statistically. For the purpose of conveying extent of Caritas use, the mean scores for each of the respondents were qualitatively interpreted as follows:

6.14 to 7.00—Very Great Extent (that Caritas Process was used by the nurse)
5.28 to 6.13—Great Extent
4.41 to 5.27—Above Average Extent
3.54 to 4.40—Average Extent
2.67 to 3.53—Below Average Extent
1.81 to 2.66—Low Extent
0.94 to 1.80—Very Low Extent

RESULTS

Cronbach's alpha for the CFS was .98. No item, if deleted, would have resulted in an increased alpha.

Descriptive statistics revealed a range of 1–7 for one or more of the Caritas Processes. All mean scores were above the midpoint of 4.0, which indicates that there was a general perception of Caritas for each concept (Table 18.1).

TABLE 18.1 Descriptive Statistics Aggregate Data

	DESCRIPTIVE STATISTICS				
	N	MINIMUM	MAXIMUM	MEAN	STD DEVIATION
Holistic care	51	2.00	7.00	6.1765	1.00411
Promote expression of feelings	51	2.00	7.00	6.0686	1.07712
Practice loving kindness	51	1.50	7.00	6.0588	1.29864
Helping and trusting relationship	51	1.50	7.00	6.0490	1.14129
Instill faith and hope	51	1.50	7.00	6.0098	1.14669
CFS total score	51	1.60	7.00	5.9745	1.02637
Healing environment	51	1.00	7.00	5.9412	1.12981
Teaching and learning	51	1.50	7.00	5.9118	1.11223
Problem solving	51	2.00	7.00	5.8824	1.26723
Spiritual beliefs and practices	51	2.00	7.00	5.8627	1.03479
Allow miracles	51	1.00	7.00	5.7843	1.21349
Valid N (listwise)	51				

Comparison of the mean scores by care level, minimum to critical care, using a one-way ANOVA, revealed no significant differences using an alpha of .05. Patterns of the bar graph, comparing levels of care, revealed the critical care level as the highest level of care but had the lowest scores. These patterns are noted in Figure 18.1.

Upon further examination of the mean scores to understand the extent of use of the Caritas Process, it was understood that generally the Clinical Caritas Process was used by staff nurses to a great extent (recall mean range for great extent was 5.28 to 6.13) in the tertiary hospital. All of the 10 core components of the Caritas Processes were used to a great extent; holistic care ranked first. Allowing miracles was last in rank.

The Clinical Caritas Process was used by staff nurses to a great extent as perceived by all patients, regardless of category. Use of the Clinical Caritas Process was perceived highest by the total care patients and lowest by critical care patients, as discussed previously.

There is no difference in the extent of use of the Clinical Caritas Process by staff nurses as perceived by patients between and across all categories. However, it should be noted that this was a small sample and thus underpowered, which is a limitation of this study. To adequately examine the differences of these four categories of care, there would need to be 180 for an effect size of 0.25, power of 0.80 while using an alpha of .05.

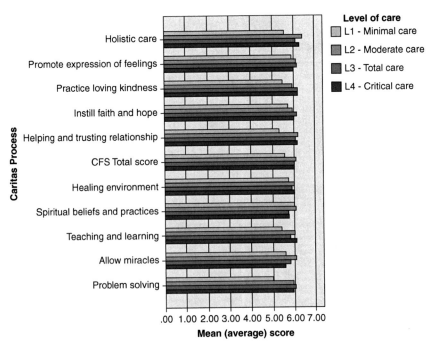

FIGURE 18.1   Mean scores for all levels of care.

CONCLUSION

Patients, regardless of their care requirements, whether minimal, moderate, total, or critical, perceived the staff nurses to be using the Clinical Caritas Process. A larger sample size is needed to validate this further.

RECOMMENDATIONS

Based on the findings and conclusion of the study, the following recommendations were offered:

1. The CFS should be used as a screening tool for probationary nurses.
2. Spirituality sensitivity trainings in the form of retreats, seminars, workshops, programs, and Bible studies should be provided to the staff nurses.
3. The Clinical Caritas Process should be included in the primary health care subjects.
4. The concept of spirituality should be given more focus in the personal, moral, and social development subjects so as to enhance the spirituality of nursing students.
5. Second-year students should pass spirituality-assessment tests to become eligible for the Bachelor of Science in Nursing program.
6. More studies on the Clinical Caritas Process should be conducted so as to support and strengthen the theory.

These recommendations are in various stages of implementation at the Makati Medical Center School of Nursing. Additional studies with larger sample sizes will help establish an understanding of the effect the recommendations may have had on perception of Caritas within each level of care.

REFERENCES

Benner, P., Tanner, C., & Chesla, C. (1992). From beginner to expert: Gaining a differentiated clinical world in critical care nursing. *Advances in Nursing Science, 14*(3), 13–28.

Fitzpatrick, J., & Whall, A. (2005). *Conceptual models of nursing: Analysis and application* (4th ed.). Upper Saddle River, NJ: Pearson Prentice Hall.

McEwen, M., & Wills, E. (2002). *Theoretical basis for nursing.* Philadelphia, PA: Lippincott Williams & Wilkins.

Nelson, J., Watson, J., & Inova Health. (2008). Development of the Caring Factor Survey© (CFS), an instrument to measure patient's perception of caring. In J. Watson (Ed.), *Assessing and measuring caring in nursing and health science* (2nd ed.). New York, NY: Springer.

Potter, P. A., & Perry, A. G. (2007). *Fundamentals of nursing* (6th ed.). St. Louis, MO: Mosby Elsevier.

Sombillo, R. (2006). Comparison of nurses' and patients' perceptions of caring behaviors. *Philippine Journal of Nursing.* 76(1)

Watson, J. (2002). *Assessing and measuring caring in nursing and health science.* New York, NY: Springer.

19

Reflection as a Process to Understand Caring Behaviors During Implementation of Relationship-Based Care in a Community Health Service in England

Allison Tinker, Janina M. Sweetenham, and John Nelson

*T*his chapter explores the use of reflection as a technique for supporting the introduction of relationship-based care (RBC; Koloroutis, 2004) into four pilot teams working in a community health service in England. The effective implementation of RBC requires health professionals to engage closely with their emotions as well as their intellect, and so guided reflection was explored to establish whether it could serve as an effective learning method in embedding the principles of RBC in community practice.

The implementation of RBC was aided by the use of three questionnaires designed and psychometrically tested by John Nelson, president of Healthcare Environment. These are: the Self-Care Questionnaire and the Compassionate Care Questionnaire (Care Provider Version), which are both based on Watson's theory of caring, and the Healthcare Environment Survey (HES). Of the 34 staff members, 32 (94%) responded to at least one of the three surveys sent. When the majority of the staff responds like this, it gives the opportunity to use the data for decision making because it reflects the perceptions of almost every staff member. The joint reflection and interpretation of the data by management and staff allow for the identification of action aimed at refining the environment and infrastructure of RBC.

A WORLD PILOT

RBC is a model for transforming practice in which relationships between the patient, family, and caregivers lie at the heart of care delivery. It argues that safe, quality care is achievable only when therapeutic, growth-promoting relationships exist between all parties. Implementing RBC brings congruence to an organization and offers a platform for valuing the good things that already exist, and for creating consensus on the things that need further development.

Outcomes of a successful implementation of RBC include: individual and team commitment; effective resource awareness and use; organization-wide alignment with its corporate vision, mission, and values; and, most important, excellent clinical outcomes, patient/family satisfaction, and staff satisfaction.

The National Health Service (NHS) in the United Kingdom is divided broadly into acute hospital-located facilities and community-based services. In the light of contemporary government initiatives, senior staff within Rotherham Community Health Services (RCHS) decided to implement RBC, in conjunction with Choice Dynamic International,[1] a company licensed by Creative Health Care Management[2] to deliver RBC in the UK. Because RBC has not previously been implemented in a service that is entirely community focused, this would also serve as a world pilot.

The NHS is held in high regard at the national and international levels. From its inception in 1944 by Bevan, with his vision for health care "from the cradle to the grave," to the current day, it has gone through a plethora of reforms, restructuring, and redesigning. However, the heart of the NHS continues to pump to the same beat, to provide quality care, free at the point of delivery. In the current political and economic climate, this is proving to be a monumental task.

The recent government White Paper, "Equity and Excellence: Liberating the NHS" (Department of Health [DOH], 2010) outlines the challenges ahead:

- A 45% management cost reduction over the next 4 years
- The devolution of primary care trust commissioning to a centralized governing body
- The move to general practitioners commissioning consortia
- Reduction in hospital admissions and length of stay
- A proactive, case-management approach to manage patients with long-term conditions; shared decision making will be the norm: *"no decision about me without me"*
- Increased use of assistive technology
- A new consumer champion, Health Watch England, located in the Care Quality Commission
- Patient safety is above all else

Simply put, the government is talking about the transformation of front-line services to meet the targets by making cost-efficiency savings,

[1]Choice Dynamic International, *drsue@choice-dynamic-int.com*
[2]Creative Health Care Management, Inc., Minneapolis, http://www.chcm.com

increasing productivity, and ensuring that quality care is maintained within the financial envelope agreed upon by provider and commissioner, as outlined in service specifications. Previous change effort in the NHS has focused on: moving organizational boundaries; deploying resources differently; and introducing new jobs, tools, targets, and techniques (Plesk, Bibby, & Garretts, 2004). However, modifying structures alone is insufficient and will not achieve the transformation required in complex health care organizations.

In early 2010, RCHS found itself at a transitional stage, soon to merge with Rotherham Foundation Trust, whereby the acute and community services would be integrated with the subsequent need to transform services. If underlying patterns in the system remain unchanged and unchallenged—that is, decision making, power bases, and intergroup communication—the transformation that is so badly required may indeed fail, resulting in a repeated pattern of reorganization, restructuring, and redesigning.

Within this political context, senior staff in RCHS saw RBC as a way of keeping the focus of care on the patient and family. RBC is an ideal model for supporting clinicians through the process of change; it challenges preconceived ideas on caring and healing environments and reignites clinicians' passion for the service they provide.

The implementation of RBC into a community setting has generated a number of challenges, not the least of which is because the examples offered in the literature refer to acute hospital environments. The language and cultures are different: this is due not just to the diversity between American English and English spoken in the UK, but also because of the significant differences between the community context and environment and those found in an acute hospital. Furthermore, the nature of teams and patient assignment/allocation are not the same. Community professionals usually work in isolation in patients' own homes; they do not have colleagues, equipment, and facilities at their fingertips. Their challenges are consequently unique to this environment and the lead professional coordinating and/or delivering care may not be a nurse: he or she may be from a different professional background such as physiotherapy or occupational therapy.

For health professionals working in the community environment, the supporting structures found in institutional health care settings are not physically present. Consequently, community practitioners must make the clinical judgment in isolation, based on their own knowledge, skill, ability, experience, and intuition. They do not have the chance to easily "check it out" with a colleague.

RBC proposes a transformational change in the "ways and means" of health care, beginning with a revisiting of the service's philosophy. Organizations, by their very nature, may be large and unwieldy, and they alone do not govern the culture of health care—it is the people within that organization who create its future. Every individual employee has a part to play in implementing new initiatives such as RBC. External consultants can work with the health board's strategic leaders to suggest ways to enhance and develop services, but the responsibility for true success lies with each member of staff changing the way he or she thinks about health care, about his or her practice, and about the way he or she relates to patients and their families.

The concepts of the Self-Care Questionnaire and the Compassionate Care Questionnaire are both based on Watson's concept of caring within her theory of Caritas. Essentially, Watson asserts that if one cares for self and others using her 10 concepts, the recipient of care will feel authentic compassion, even love, and thus initiate an internal cascade of healing from decreased cortisol, increased oxytocin, increased IgA, and increased DHEA, which is referred to as the engagement hormone and the opposite of cortisol. In addition, feeling compassion and love will facilitate the person who is feeling cared for to access his or her frontal lobes to make better decisions. Care begins with caring for self, which ensures the capacity to care for patients as well as to model such behavior for their development.

In Rotherham, it was suggested that one technique that could support the required changes in practice, attitudes, and thought processes was that of "reflection" and its application to practice. It was proposed that all professional groups used reflection as a learning tool and that the existence of an organization-wide policy addressing this concept meant that it could be used within the multidisciplinary teams involved in the pilot study. Furthermore, the organization already had a policy relating to clinical supervision in which structured, guided reflection was expected to occur to facilitate professional development.

Much of the literature addressing the importance of reflection incorporates aspects of "self-care" similar to elements of Watson's theory of Caritas: practicing compassion (for self and others), promoting expression of all feelings, creative problem solving, teaching creatively to ensure learning, creating an environment conducive to healing/growth, and allowing the extraordinary to happen. These ideas are all addressed in the three questionnaires used to gather baseline data. Importantly, research using these questionnaires in the United States has shown there is a moderately strong relationship between self-care and compassion fatigue and burnout. In other words, employees who do not care for themselves are at highest risk of disengaging with the patient and of eventual burnout over the job. This has implications such as lower productivity, increased sick calls, and reports from patients of poor caring attitudes of health providers.

"Reflective practice" can also be seen to represent an important concept called "participative action research" in which the researcher presents data gathered from questionnaires. These data are then interpreted and applied by the professional practitioner, supported by the analysis of the researcher. It is important that frontline users interpret the data and work with leaders/managers to change systems and processes appropriately. Statisticians can then use the staff interpretation to add to the model of research to make sure that the proper variables are being measured, thus enhancing validity and reliability and reducing the likelihood of error. This process, based on sociotechnical systems theory (Trist & Bamforth, 1951), states that an organization will be effective only if the employees are informing the process. It is well known that staff's participative competence is the essence of empowerment and success within decentralized organizations.

Within the Rotherham study, reflective practice would therefore be addressed as a technique to facilitate the implementation of RBC as well as an approach to support the participative action research process underpinning its implementation.

THE IMPORTANCE OF REFLECTION

Reflection is more than a concept; it is a method of learning, a philosophical process that adds value to the individual's personal and professional life (Reid, 1993). There are, however, many definitions of reflection, but common characteristics suggest that reflection is an active process that involves analysis of self, others, and the context using existing knowledge as a reference point. It involves new learning, and it links theory and practice in a real and dynamic way. Furthermore, if reflection is related to work and formally structured, practice and action become the catalyst for the application or generation of knowledge. This reverses the traditional view of theory and practice as being philosophically and practically disengaged. Bridging the perceived theory/practice gap is one of the major reasons for the widespread adoption of reflection into professional education.

Reflection was proposed by Schön (1998) as a way of exploring and understanding what professional do. Schön was concerned about the limitations of basing such an understanding on the dominant rational/technical models of thinking. He argued for adopting a more existentially focused approach that could enable the individual to create a framework to carry learning forward into new situations. Usher (1997) identified technical-rationality as "the dominant paradigm which has failed to resolve the dilemma of rigour versus relevance confronting professionals" (p. 143).

Schön focused on "reflection-in-action" and "reflection-on-action" to explore the understanding of "artful doing." Reflection-in-action suggests thinking on one's feet. It addresses the exploration of experience and emotion and links them to "theories-in-use" (Argyris & Schön, 1974). Thus, new understanding is achieved that then informs future practice. As a result of this learning, professionals then test out their theories.

As a result of reflective processes, the individual's repertoire of experience is extended so that novel situations are seen as both different and familiar. The individual uses the prior experience as a precedent and then applies it in a unique way to the new context.

The literature is littered with benefits associated with structured reflection (Argyris & Schön, 1974; Boud, Keogh, & Walker, 1985; Boyd & Fales, 1983; Burns & Bulman, 2000; Ghaye, 2005; Jarvis, 1992; Johns, 2002; Mezirow, 1981; Schön, 1998; Schutz, 2007). These include:

- Attitude change arising from the resolution of cognitive dissonance generated during reflection
- Development of self-awareness and personal empowerment
- Enhancement of critical-thinking processes that illuminate knowledge
- The increased ability to articulate the nature/meaning of practice and the professional role
- A greater awareness of the dynamic interaction between theory and practice
- Enhanced understanding of interpersonal/intrapersonal and political and social issues

Many of these issues are also addressed through the questionnaire items. For example: professional patient care includes staff perception of continuity of care with the patient, collaboration with other team members, care planning, and creating a relationship with the patient. Professional growth refers to what the staff feel they are learning professionally. Autonomy refers to the staff's perception of being able to use their knowledge and skills to do the job they know they are supposed to do.

Undergraduate programs for nursing and allied health professionals in the UK agree that reflection and reflective practice are essential if their students are to become safe, competent practitioners. Such individuals place the patient at the center of care; they are willing to question their own practice and are open and honest enough to encourage their colleagues to critique shared experiences. Reflective practice enables the professionals to improve their clinically focused skills and to extend their awareness and understanding of the true meaning of joining their chosen professional body. It is only through interactive, reality-based discussions about care that a code of conduct becomes alive. Furthermore, such supervised reflection (usually as part of clinical supervision) enables responsibility, authority, and accountability to be explored using such techniques as appreciative inquiry (Cooperrider & Whitney, 1999), resulting in the individual's recognition of authentic experiential learning.

As undergraduates, nurses and allied health professionals are taught a variety of reflective practice models and the ways to apply them, and they are encouraged to record their learning in portfolios, log books, and reflective journals.

Despite this common recognition of the importance of reflection, the reality is that the theory is not always applied in subsequent practice. Most health professionals believe themselves to be reflective; however, when prompted further, the offered descriptions often relate to "mental percolation" in which an experience is described and conclusions drawn. In the absence of a structured process of reflection, a critical scenario may be run and rerun through the mind, underscoring the emotional fallout rather than producing an objective, analytical experience resulting in professional learning and development.

REFLECTIVE PRACTICE IN A COMMUNITY ENVIRONMENT

We know that reflective practice has the potential to bridge the gap between theory and practice, but clinical practice is full of complex situations with competing goals and conflicting perspectives—the "swampy lowlands" of practice (Schön, 1983). We would also suggest that community-based practice offers further layers of murkiness to the swamp. Understanding and delivering care in this context requires a whole new focus. Culturally specific knowledge must embrace how to deal with an infected wound in an unhygienic house, or how to approach a relative whom you suspect of harming a patient, or ensuring that the care for a terminally ill patient is maintained and uninterrupted in the presence of a feuding family.

Community professionals, such as the district nurse or domiciliary physiotherapist, may be dealing with such issues every day. The need for rapid decision making in clinical practice does not allow for careful consideration and debate, resulting in a type of performance anxiety where there is no room for being wrong. Self-evaluation in this context is clearly not appropriate, but the knowledge acquired experientially is undoubtedly valuable and is indeed valued by learners above classroom learning.

The challenge for those involved in the continuing education of health professionals is to encourage them to critically reflect on the complex issues faced in the community environment. However, once in practice in the community setting, it is the skills of the practice teacher that are essential in helping students to genuinely understand the difference between "knowing-in-action" and "reflection-in-action" (Schön, 1983).

To divorce knowledge from its historical, social, and political context and the personal, social, and professional interests influencing it is unrealistic and goes against the principle of personalized, patient-centered care advocated within RBC. The opportunity to interpret practice or critique the context of practice is as important as the opportunity to be self-reflective and critical.

It is imperative, therefore, that the clinician has a safe environment in which to explore such issues, beginning with personal attitudes and resultant emotions arising from challenging circumstances. As Schutz (2007) states, emotions are so closely related to values that in order to truly reflect on our practice, we need to recognize individual values and assess events against that framework. Structured reflection enables this reevaluation of perspective arising from the mental indigestion of stressful practice. For those professionals who may not have a positive attitude toward reflection and clinical supervision, this cognitive discomfort may never be relieved, resulting in emotional overload and burnout.

During the initial discussions about implementing RBC in Rotherham, we recognized the value of reflection and decided to consider how it could support effective interprofessional working.

INTERPROFESSIONAL WORKING

Over the last decade there has been a move to interprofessional learning on all undergraduate health and social programs with the drive to "work together" and agree to "joined up working—indeed, to simply modernize working patterns (DOH, 2000).

The need for closer working and greater collaboration, coordination, and communication between the different professional groups has been highlighted in the UK by a number of major inquiries into varying aspects of health and social care, especially relating to child protection, mental health, and vulnerable adults. The importance of professionals recognizing and valuing their colleagues' competence and abilities cannot be underestimated. Fundamentally there is a need to challenge traditional boundaries and professional tribalism (Carlisle, Cooper, & Watkins, 2004; Smith & Roberts, 2005). The focus for different professional groups working in multidisciplinary teams should be the patient. The unifying force must be an agreed vision of collective values and beliefs that are aimed at serving the "best interest of the patient."

Professional development programs need to give opportunities for multidisciplinary teams to have the chance to reflect together on their interprofessional relationships. Such an approach will help collaborative effort, so crucial in today's health environment (Ross, King, & Firth, 2005).

As Ghaye (2005) suggests, this requires the development of a level of emotional intelligence/literacy that enables staff to respect and trust each other. He identifies two key attributes in this: the acknowledgment of the same values and the recognition/articulation of team goals. Covey's (2006) "speed of trust" demands the presence of integrity in character and recognition of clinical competency. Fundamental to reflective practice is a feeling of trust and the specific demonstration of trusting behaviors that affect the pattern of relationships within and beyond teams, resulting in a team's ability to think and act differently.

The HES data collected in Rotherham found statistically significant differences between the four pilot teams in the following areas: professional growth, teamwork, job satisfaction, autonomy, pride in the organization, distributive justice, workload, and the total HES score. Because trust is based on commonly held understanding and values, these findings would bear greater investigation.

"Mutual trust is a virtuous circle of anticipation and action whose initiation always requires a leap of faith beyond the available evidence" (Schön & Rein, 1994).

Certainly this has been reflected in RCHS. Despite the findings from the data, the perceived experience of professionals suggests that the development of multidisciplinary teams has caused a cultural shift in which allegiance to uniprofessional practice has given way to multiprofessional practice. As the teams striving to implement RBC explored and agreed on beliefs, values, and goals, a transformational change occurred. Is it possible that, in the few weeks between the initial data being collected and the completion of the first RBC workshops, a profound shift has occurred that would nullify the significant difference identified in the data immediately above?

Professional identity and functions remain the same, but integration and collaboration on care interventions are patient focused. Furthermore, interdependent practice is actively chosen and adopted. The teams have learned to overcome organizational structures, limitations, and traditional, professional boundaries to achieve successful integration.

The RBC program and the associated reflective workshops create a safe environment to debate, discuss, explore, and critique individual beliefs and values underpinning the care they give to patients. The art of care delivery is also celebrated. This exploration of patient-focused philosophy has also served to emphasize the value and importance of relationships between team members.

Together with a range of knowledge-enabling processes, the demonstration and display of attitudes and behaviors reflecting care for each other has created the solid foundation of an effective, reflective team. The key to sustaining this transformation lies in the relationship between clinical supervision and reflection, because learning through exploration, critical analysis of practice, and self-evaluation is essential in the ongoing evolution of person-centered care.

CLINICAL SUPERVISION

Clinical supervision in the UK has followed a number of models over the last 20 years. It has been set up as a one-to-one interaction between the practitioner and another specifically designated professional; sometimes the "other person" has been the individual's line manager or the manager of a similar service from a different organization. Some places have used group supervision where entire teams come together or a group of staff at the same organizational level have shared their experiences. Different professional groups have approached the idea of clinical supervision in a variety of ways. All policies relating to clinical supervision identify specific roles to be used within the process, but these roles have different names and functions and there may be no clear, coherent approach.

Historically, RCHS recognized that there was discord and ambiguity between nursing and allied health professionals relating to clinical supervision and the associated roles of mentor, preceptor, and supervisor. Similarity of language did not reflect similarity of construct.

Consequently, a working party was established with representatives from the nursing and therapy professions that produced a set of agreed-upon standards for practice. The resultant policy was ratified across the organization and published as the Policy for Clinical Supervision (NHS Rotherham Community Health Services, 2008b). The purpose of the document is clear: "To enable clinicians to reflect on practice to recognise their strengths and weaknesses to support the development of practice knowledge and skills thereby achieving and maintaining local and national standards."

The policy clarifies the roles, functions, and responsibilities of the supervisor and supervisee; it identifies the process and training, modes of delivery, and how to record the learning. Despite the detail of the policy, which incorporates semistructured documents for logging learning, there is no mention of using reflective models to guide the supervisee's thinking and the supervisor's structure. It may be that an assumption is made that professionals will adopt a relevant model for this purpose, but perhaps it needs to be made explicit. Johns's (2002) view is that reflection needs to be guided because practitioners need help to see beyond themselves and require the support and challenge to confront and resolve contradiction in daily practice. Successful implementation of clinical supervision needs to go beyond a positive endorsement of the concept, toward an active and committed engagement with the process. The challenge facing practitioners is to find the time and energy to invest in their ongoing personal and professional growth and development.

It could be argued that the lasting benefits of reflection and reflective practice may be realized only if clinicians internalize the process and continue to work in a reflective manner throughout their careers. Such an approach also needs full endorsement by the employing organization. Effective clinical supervision must include interactive discussion whereby autonomous clinicians use reflective practice to explore the weight of responsibility, authority, and accountability that comes with professional practice. This is the arena where clinicians hold the mirror before them and truly account for the care that they give.

RESULTS USED WITHIN REFLECTIVE PRACTICE AT ROTHERHAM

Cronbach's alpha for all three measures used to evaluate that state of affairs of caring and the work environment performed well. For the Compassionate Care Questionnaire, Care Provider Version (CCQ-CPV), Cronbach's alpha was .89. Cronbach's alpha for the Self-Care Questionnaire was .89. Cronbach's alpha for the HES was .97. Established reliability provided confidence to discuss the results within the context of reflective practice.

Of 35 employees, 29 (85%) responded to the Self-Care Questionnaire; 32 responded to the CCQ-CPV, a 91.4% response rate; and 28 responded to the HES, an 82% response rate. An 80% response rate or greater was desired for reflective practice to ensure that the results represented the large majority of staff.

Results of the Self-Care Questionnaire reveal that staff members take time to develop helping and trusting relationships within their lives. This was the highest-ranked score. The lowest-ranked score was the response to treating themselves with loving kindness. It is noted that all scores are above the midpoint of 4.0, but loving kindness is barely above 4.0, which indicates that within the distribution of scores, almost half of the respondents do not feel loving kindness toward oneself. All 10 concepts of self-care, based on Watson's theory of caring, are noted in Figure 19.1.

For the CCQ-CPV, it is noted that all variables were above 5.0. The scores for the CCQ-CPV were dramatically higher when compared to the Self-Care Questionnaire. It was especially interesting to note that loving kindness was the top-ranked variable in the CCQ-CPV, with a mean score well over 6.0. It was interesting to contrast this to the Self-Care Questionnaire where nurses apply loving kindness to others but not self. The lowest-ranked variables related to allowing patients to believe in miracles. The rank order of caring behaviors enacted toward patients, as perceived by nurses, is noted in Figure 19.2.

When looking at the work environment scores, it is noted that satisfaction with the team manager was the highest and workload was the lowest. All variables except workload were above 4.0, indicating more satisfaction than dissatisfaction with the work environment, both socially

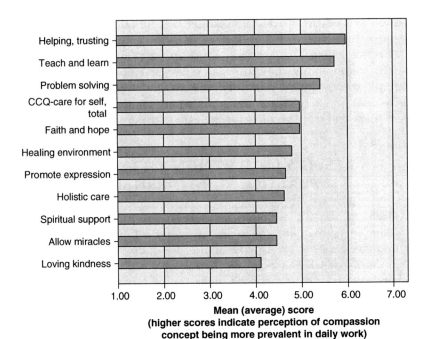

Mean (average) score
(higher scores indicate perception of compassion
concept being more prevalent in daily work)

FIGURE 19.1   Rank order of self-care scores.

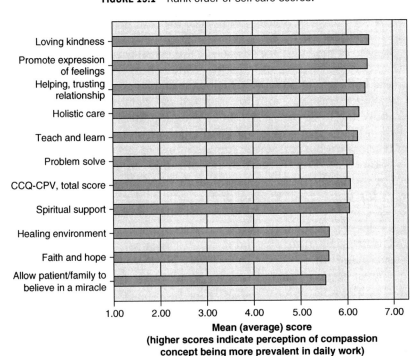

Mean (average) score
(higher scores indicate perception of compassion
concept being more prevalent in daily work)

FIGURE 19.2   Compassionate Care Questionnaire–Care Provider Version scores

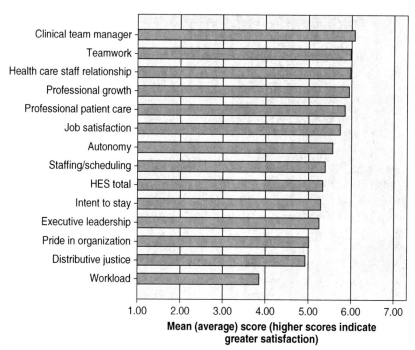

FIGURE 19.3   Rank order scores of the Healthcare Environment Survey (HES).

and technically. The rank order scores of the work environment are noted in Figure 19.3.

When examining how these measures and constructs related to each other, it was noted the total HES score relating to perceived competence in compassionate care. The correlation of .42 is considered a moderate correlation and was found to be statistically significant. This informs us that as the environment improves, our ability to provide compassionate care improves.

It was also identified that the environmental variable of pride in the organization had a statistically significant (alpha .05) correlation with self-care (Pearson's correlation: $r = .48$). It should be noted that pride in the organization is the employees' pride and engagement with the organization. It is about the employee going the second and third mile for the organization.

It was identified that professional growth has a moderate correlation with self-care and this finding was statistically significant, using an alpha of .05. It is likely that those who conduct self-care experience greater release of oxytocin and other hormones that give access to the frontal lobes, which are the critical-thinking portion of the brain. It would be interesting to know if those who do self-care also make better clinical judgments. It may also be that those who do self-care also take time to learn. Further discussion and scientific investigation are warranted.

PRACTICAL SUPPORT FOR REFLECTION

We recognize that some staff members within our pilot teams are very comfortable with the ideas, methods, and models available for reflection; but some are not. The support workers in the teams whose roles combine caring practice with administrative duties were not knowledgeable about the theoretical aspects of reflection but found it helpful to "talk through" specific experiences with their professional colleagues. If RBC is to be implemented effectively, everybody needs to be reflecting on their interactions with patients and their families. We proposed using a straightforward checklist that could be used to structure such talk-throughs, but that could also be explored in greater depth for deeper reflection. We offered this to the pilot teams with the understanding that if they already have a suitable model that works for them, they should continue to use it, but if they do not, they should try the LEARN framework. We will evaluate its use as we monitor the rollout of RBC.

LEARN: THE PROCESS OF REFLECTION

L	**Location**—Put yourself and the situation into context. ■ What were you thinking/feeling at the time? ■ What was the context of the event/situation?
E	**Exploration**—Consider your response. ■ What factors may have contributed to your response? ■ Were you pleased/dismayed/surprised about the way you responded?
A	**Assumptions**—Explore your mindset. ■ What assumptions did you make about the situation or people within it? ■ Did those assumptions help you or hinder you in dealing with the issue?
R	**Realization**—Recognize the way you now think/feel. ■ What have you learned as a result of going through this process? ■ How do you feel about what you have learned?
N	**New application**—How will you take your new awareness into the future? ■ In the future will you handle a similar situation in the same way or would you do it differently? Why/why not? ■ How can you prepare yourself to deal with a similar situation differently?

Created in 2000 by J. M. Sweetenham.

CONCLUSION

Through guided reflection alone, individual practitioners may not be able to solve all the challenges posed by such initiatives as RBC, but it offers the potential for teams to become part of something greater— reflective health organizations. Such organizations are curious and eager to learn; they consider how they are regarded by stakeholders, how they perform, and how they can improve (Ghaye, 2005). Within these organizations, reflection is seen as both a catalyst for learning and a response to it, just as reflective practice can be both proactive and reactive in nature.

The implementation of RBC across the first wave of teams in Rotherham is, at the date of this publication, still being rolled out. Lessons are being learned daily and the process may be compared to action research (Lewin, 1948), in which the approach is continually illuminating knowledge and understanding, which is then applied to subsequent action. Indeed, reflective practice is seen as representative of participative action research.

Clearly, we need more information and are further considering more detailed research to uncover issues of relevance relating to staff perceptions about reflection and clinical supervision. We also need to explore further the differences indicated in the baseline data and consider the correlation between those findings and the data from the grids. Furthermore, we need to consider how we may help staff to review and reflect on the meaning of data gathered during the process, and how best to facilitate them to directly affect the action-planning processes that arise from the interpretation of these data.

Our focus now is to extend this research and to test out the impact of guided reflection on the embedding of the principles of RBC in community practice.

ACKNOWLEDGMENT

The authors would like to thank Dr. Sue Smith, director of Choice Dynamic International, who holds the license to deliver RBC in the UK. Her leadership, encouragement, and support have been much appreciated.

REFERENCES

Argyris, C., & Schön, D. (1974). *Theory in practice: Increasing professional effectiveness*. San Francisco, CA: Jossey Bass.

Bevan, A. (1944). *White Paper: A National Health Service*. London: Department of Health.

Boud, D., Keogh, R., & Walker, R. (Eds.). (1985). *Reflection: Turning experience into practice*. London: Kagan Page.

Boyd, E. M., & Fales, A. W. (1983). Reflective learning: Key to learning from experience. *Journal of Humanistic Psychology, 23*(2), 99–117.

Burns, S., & Bulman, C. (2000). *Reflective practice in nursing* (2nd ed.). Oxford: Blackwell Science.

Carlisle, C., Cooper, H., & Watkins, C. (2004). "Do none of you talk to each other?": The challenges facing the implementation of interprofessional education. *Medical Teacher, 26*(6), 545–552.

Cooperrider, D., & Whitney, D. (1999). *Appreciative inquiry: Collaborating for change.* San Fransisco, CA: Berrett-Koehler.

Covey, S. M. R. (2006). *The speed of trust.* New York, NY: The Free Press.

Department of Health (DOH). (2000). *The NHS plan.* London: Author.

Department of Health (DOH). (2010). *Equity and excellence: Liberating the NHS.* London: Author.

Ghaye, T. (2005). *Developing the reflective healthcare team.* Oxford: Blackwell.

Jarvis, P. (1992). Reflective practice and nursing. *Nurse Education Today, 12,* 174–181.

Johns, C. (2002). *Guided reflection, advancing practice.* Oxford: Blackwell.

Koloroutis, M. (Ed.). (2004). *Relationship-based care: A model for transforming practice.* Minneapolis, MN: Creative Health Care Management.

Lewin, K. (1948). Time perspective and morale. In G. W. Lewin (Ed.), *Resolving social conflicts; Selected papers on group dynamics.* New York, NY: Harper & Row.

Mezirow, J. (1981). A critical theory of adult education and learning. *Adult Education, 32*(1), 3–24.

NHS Rotherham Community Health Services. (2008a). *Clinical preceptorship pack.* Retrieved from http://websrv.rotherhampct.nhs.uk/?FileID=13669

NHS Rotherham Community Health Services. (2008b). *Policy for clinical supervision.*

Plesk, P., Bibby, J., & Garretts, C. (2004). *Mapping behavioural patterns, summary booklet.* London: NHS Modernisation Agency.

Reid, B. (1993). But we're doing it already! Exploring a response to the concept of reflective practice in order to improve its facilitation. *Nurse Education Today, 13,* 305–309.

Ross, A., King, N., & Firth, J. (2005, January 31). Interprofessional relationships and collaborative working: Encouraging reflective practice. *Online Journal of Issues in Nursing, 10*(1). Retrieved from http://www.nursingworld.org/ojin/topic26/tpc26_3.htm

Schön, D. (1998). *The reflective practitioner: How people think in action.* Brookfield, VT: Ashgate.

Schön, D., & Rein, M. (1994). *Frame reflection: Towards the resolution of intractable policy controversies.* New York, NY: Basic Books.

Schutz, S. (2007, September). Reflection and reflective practice. *Community Practitioner, 80*(9), 26–29.

Smith, J., & Roberts, P. (2005). An investigation of occupational therapy and physiotherapy role in a community setting. *International Journal of Therapy and Rehabilitation, 12*(1), 21–29.

Trist, E. L., & Bamforth, K. W. (1951). Some social and psychological consequences of the longwall method of coal-getting. *Human Relations, 4*(8), 3–38.

Usher, R. (1997). *Adult education and the postmodern challenge.* London: Routledge.

20

A Chinese Cultural Perspective of Nursing Care in Macao, China

Michelle Ming Xia Zhu, Grace Ka In Lok,
Selwynne Wan Cheong, Sarah Sio Wa Lao,
and Joe Pak Leng Cheong

The Caring Factor Survey (CFS) was developed by John Nelson from Healthcare Environment, by Jean Watson from the Watson Caring Science Institute, and by Karen Drenkard and Gene Rigotti from Inova Health System (Nelson, 2008). The core of CFS is to assess the human attribute of Caritas. The original version of CFS bears 20 statements that are based on the caring factors emphasized in Watson's caring theory. However, the 10-item Traditional Chinese version of the Caring Factor Survey (CCFS) for measuring caring behaviors has not been developed.

As such, this study examined the reliability and validity of the 10-item Traditional Chinese version of the CFS in measuring the caring behaviors of nurses in hospitals. Moreover, the Caritas Processes (Watson, 2005), as perceived by patients and caregivers in Macao, are also assessed in this study.

In order to proceed with the study, however, translation of the English questionnaire into Chinese was done and content validity was verified. The patients and caregivers, selected by convenient sampling, and data were collected by using the new CCFS.

A total of 261 patients and patients' caregivers participated in this study with a response rate of 98%. Cronbach's alpha of the CCFS was 0.87 and the Content Validity Index (CVI) was 0.86. The mean score of the CCFS[1] was 52.80 ± 8.64, with approximately half of the participants (54.2%) rated higher than the mean scores. Participants in the gynecological and obstetrical ward rated higher scores (54.56 ± 9.97) than those in other wards.

In general, the overall response of the participants reflected that the caring behaviors of the nurses among the hospitals in Macao are satisfactory.

---

[1] The CCFS summed the scores of all items instead of the average of all items like other CFS studies in this book and as is the norm for CFS use.

The 10-item CCFS has shown good validity and reliability for measuring caring behaviors in Chinese settings.

BACKGROUND

Caring is a complex process because it occurs between nurses and patients. Nurse–patient interactions encompass a wide range of attitudes and behaviors in the humanistic, relational, and clinical domains of nursing practice and constitute the main vehicles for promoting quality care in nursing (Maltby, Drury, & Fischer-Rasmussen, 1995). Nonetheless, caring itself is an abstract concept that is difficult to explain, assess, or measure. Whereas caring can be understood as an attitude, a behavior, or just a word, it is commonly expressed in various ways. In response, Dr. Jean Watson's theory of transpersonal caring has become familiar to nurses and nursing worldwide. Her philosophies of caring and Carative Factors are presented as a measurable process within the clinical environment. A major challenge in this field of caring science, as Dr. Watson refers to it, is that caring as an inherent and personal experience for oneself is expressed differently in varied cultures (Watson, 2005). In this regard, caring-measurement instruments, such as the Caring Behavior Inventory (CBI) (Wolf, 1986) and Caring Nurse–Patient Interactions Scale (CNPI-Scale) (Cossette et al., 2005), developed in the West, may not be appropriate for Eastern cultural settings. For its part, nursing in China is often seen as a concept borrowed, or adapted, from the West. Indeed, definitions in Chinese nursing textbooks are translated from Western literature. To date, there have been only a few studies for developing measurement tools for investigating the concept of caring in care recipients; for instance, for patients from Chinese cultural backgrounds.

This study thus examined the reliability and validity of the 10-item Traditional Chinese version of the CFS, whose English version was originally developed by Nelson, Watson, Drenkard, and Rigotti in 2006 (Drenkard et al., 2005). In addition, the study also established the perception of caring among the Chinese study participants.

LITERATURE REVIEW

Concept of Caring

As previously stated, caring, while at the root of nursing, is also difficult to define conceptually. Jean Watson, one of the most noted nursing theorists in the world, has developed a humanistic philosophy and a theory about caring. For Watson, caring is the core element of nursing and caring in nursing is more than an aptitude or avocation but a science (Ryan, 2005). Watson's human caring theory attempts to define nursing as an emerging discipline and distinct health profession. Moreover, she makes explicit nursing values, knowledge, and practices of human caring that tend toward subjective, inner-healing processes and the life world of the experiencing person, requiring unique caring–healing arts and a framework called "Carative Factors" that complement conventional medicine, but stand in contrast to "curative factors."

More precisely, caring is the process of Caritas that is manifested in practice in many forms, and within this process both nurse and patient possess the potential to benefit and grow (Jesse, 2010). As emphasized by Watson, the main concepts of the Carative Factors include the following (Jesse, 2010):

- transpersonal healing
- transpersonal caring relationship
- caring moment
- caring occasion
- caring healing modalities
- caring consciousness
- caring consciousness energy
- phenomenal file/unitary consciousness

In summary, the perception of caring and the caring perception should exist once the connection between nurse and patient bonds.

Nonetheless, results obtained from caring from nursing behaviors do seem to be subjective and difficult to ascertain. In addition, nurses working in different clinical areas perceive caring differently. For example, surgical nurses might perceive caring in more technical and professional terms than nurses working in medical wards. However, it is not known if this observation is the result of differences among nurses before entering their respective clinical areas or if exposure to these clinical areas influences perceptions of caring. In fact, many studies have focused on identifying organizational and structural factors in health care delivery that relate to patient outcomes (e.g., Meurer et al., 2002).

Caring Perception in Chinese Culture

The profession of nursing was first established in the West in the late 19th century. To the Chinese, nursing was regarded as a new and Western concept. In the previous decades, Chinese patients recognized that the physical nursing care provided in acute hospitals was more important than psychological care (Davis, Hershberger, Ghan, & Lin, 1990; Holroyd, Cheung, Cheung, Luk, & Wong, 1998). This may reflect the fact that Chinese nurses concentrated on those practical and accessible behaviors—such as "looking after," "nurturing," or "treating" patients—but they lacked psychological and spiritual caring capabilities (Pang et al., 2004). In the modern era, the nurse's role should be transformed so as to help people to adapt to dynamic states influenced by their natural and human environment. As such, caring has been referred to as the essence of nursing. It is what helps nurses perform more humanely, enhancing their capacities to bond within the nurse–patient relationship (Wolf et al., 1998).

Caring, as an essential element of professional nursing, includes human nature, moral imperatives, trust and respect, nurturing of emotional expressions, interpersonal activities, and orientations toward healing behaviors (Lin & Chiou, 2003). In Chinese culture, religion (Confucianism and Mohism) influences people's perception of caring. In effect, people should be interdependent, bonded, and concerned with and for each other. Thus, the concept of "love others as oneself" is increasingly being taught within primary education. In this context, caring behaviors are not discussed in terms of intentionality, because these behaviors occur, or should occur, naturally.

Although Chinese nurses and patients usually do not mention "caring" too much in their daily practice, it is regarded as a personal accomplishment (Pan, 2008). Much of Chinese literature has focused on investigating the perceptions of caring behaviors rather than the essence of caring. Patients often are asked about how professional, polite, or skillful the nurses are as well as what type of support those nurses provide or could provide (Liu, Mok, & Wong, 2006). Similarly, Ma (2004) indicated that Taiwanese patients in intensive care units (ICUs) perceived "assistance in human needs" as one of the most important of caring behaviors. Assistance may include the ability of observation, professional knowledge and skills, time for treatment and medication, and so on.

From Watson's perspective, caring is demonstrated through nurse–patient interactions. Intimate interpersonal relationships through self-discipline, patience, kindness, and cooperation, rather than self-expression, are taken by the Chinese as an appropriate, expected, moral manner. When caring research shifted its focus to the meaning of caring in nursing, perspectives in caring research opened up for exploration.

In this regard, Chinese researchers conducted specific studies to investigate Chinese inpatients' perceptions of caring during hospitalization. Study outcomes indicated 10 core elements in caring: being kind and attentive, being friendly, paying close attention to patients, respecting patients, providing immediate response when needed, giving comprehensive care when needed, giving accurate treatment, providing health education, easing patients' suffering, and providing help at any time (Huang, Liu, & Yang, 2009). In places integrated with rich Oriental and Western cultures, such as, Hong Kong and Taiwan, the literature further noted three specifically Chinese cultural-caring components: expressive behaviors in patient understanding and respecting, providing holistic patient care through the illness, and serving as a patient advocate (Lin, 2004; Yam & Rossiter, 2000).

Caring Perception of Macao Patients

The Chinese (now the largest population in Macao) have strong roots in traditional Confucianism and Mohism. Thus, most Macao patients share a similar culture with people in Hong Kong, Taiwan, and China.

Because nursing is a Western science, developing the education of nursing has fallen behind in the East, especially in Macao. The first systematic program for nursing education was started 86 years ago, with Bachelor of Nursing Science programs launched just 10 years ago in the two nursing schools in Macao. Nevertheless, there was no course that specifically introduced the philosophy of nursing caring to nursing students. Rather, students were taught the concept of caring through nursing-related subjects. Furthermore, research studies in nursing domains have focused mostly on investigating patient (e.g., Lok et al., 2005) and health care satisfaction. Concurrent to the patient-satisfaction study just noted, comparatively poor attention was paid to patients' perceptions of caring in the East. In effect, the perspective of nursing care from a Macao patient seems to have been neglected. As a result, the evidence provided for improving the quality of nursing care in Macao is very limited.

Caring Factor Survey's 10-Item Chinese-Version Study

Watson believes that using her 10 "Carative Factors" allows nurses to go beyond an objective assessment of the patient toward a deep, personal caring relationship (which occurs when nurse and patient come together in a transpersonal moment) (Watson, 2005). At that moment, when the spirit of nurse and patient is present, transcendence, harmony, and healing will appear (Jesse, 2010). Theoretically, this kind of moment should be generated naturally. Nevertheless, because caring is a subjective sensation for human beings, it remains difficult to standardize for different nurses and patients within the practice setting.

The original 20-item CFS that was developed in 2006 was reduced to 10 items in 2008 (DiNapoli, Nelson, Turkel, & Watson, 2010). This scale was used to examine the human attribute of Caritas, or a connection between caring and universal love. It also measures and indicates nurses' use of physical, mental, and spiritual caring behaviors, as reported by the patients for whom they provide care. Persky, Nelson, Watson, and Bent (Watson, 2008) had originally reported on the reduction of the 20-item CFS as a more convenient way to measure caring.

In this study, a 10-item version was translated into Chinese and examined for reliability and validity. The caring experiences of the patients and the caregivers, which include the duration of hospitalization, frequency of admission, and frequency of interaction with nurses, were the demographic variables included in this study.

METHODOLOGY

Conceptual Framework

The philosophy of Watson's caring theory and the literature indicated that caring experiences and demographic variables were the basic influential factors proposed for measuring patients' perceptions of caring. Figure 20.1 shows the conceptual framework of this study.

Research Aims and Objectives

This study was aimed to assess the reliability and validity of the 10-item Traditional Chinese version of CFS. In addition, the perception of caring in nursing was explored from the inpatients who received nursing care service under a Chinese context. The results of the study recommended nursing care improvements and nursing education amelioration in Macao. The objectives were to

1. examine the reliability and validity of the 10-item Traditional Chinese version CFS;
2. assess the perception of caring in nursing from patients and their caregivers;
3. explore the differences of caring perception among various wards;
4. analyze the relationship between caring experience and perception of care.

Research Design

This was a quantitative and cross-sectional research study. The 10-item Traditional Chinese version of CFS was the instrument used to examine the patients' perceptions of caring.

Research Instrument

The 10-item CFS was translated and modified into a Chinese version and called the Chinese Caring Factor Survey (CCFS). The CFS was first translated from English into Chinese with some modifications by a bilingual team

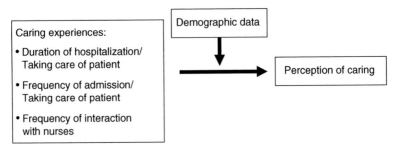

FIGURE 20.1 Conceptual framework of this study.

of experienced nursing educators, academic staff, and clinical nurses. Then, backward translation was done by two bilingual linguistic academic staff. The CFS used a Likert-type scale ranging from 1 to 7; lower scores (1–3) indicated levels of disagreement, whereas 7 indicated the highest level of agreement. A rating of 4 indicated neutrality. All statements were phrased in positive language. The higher the score reported by the patients meant that the patients viewed the more caring nurses as those who honored their individual wholeness and unity of mind–body–spirit (Nelson, 2008). In addition, background data including demographic data, admission information, and hospitalization experience were considered in the CCFS.

Procedures

After ethical approval was obtained, the CCFS questionnaire was rated by trained investigators who assessed the internal consistency and reliability in the setting. The content validity of the CCFS was evaluated by an expert panel composed of two nursing college presidents, one head nurse, one assistant professor specializing in statistics, and one nursing educator who teaches nursing ethics. Patients or patients' family members/caregivers were also invited to participate and respond to each statement.

Samples

This study was carried out at an acute regional hospital in Macao that shared more than half of the total number of hospital admissions. According to the census data, the average number of daily new admissions of the two main hospitals of Macao is nearly 60 people and the number of beds in the target hospital is over 500 (Statistics and Census Service of Macao SAR Government, 2008). All participants were recruited for the study by convenience sampling between April 10 and April 30, 2010. The participants consisted of inpatients who were admitted for at least 2 days and inpatients' family members who stayed with the patients for at least 2 hours per day. Other inclusion criteria were participants had to be more than 18 years old, medically stable, able to communicate fluently in Chinese, and had no hearing impairment. Individual with psychiatric illness and cognitive impairment were excluded.

RESULTS

Demographic Data

A total of 261 patients and patients' caregivers were included in this study. The response rate was 98%. Participants included patients (75.8%), family members (20.7%), and caregivers (3.5%). The majority of the participants were Chinese (93.2%) and 94% were able to communicate in Cantonese. The age of the participants ranged from 18 to 98 years old, with most of them (31.7%) between 39 and 58 years of age; the mean age was 56.22 ± 19.0 years. Most of them (63.6%) were female, married (78.9%), and had been educated in primary school or below (45.2%). Most of the participants (48.8%) were admitted in the internal medicine departments, 64.4% of the patient participants were admitted in the hospital for less than 7 days, and 62.9% of the patients' family members or caregivers were taking care of the patients for less than 7 days. Demographic data of the participants are summarized in Table 20.1.

Patients had high scores (stronger perception of caring) with females rating higher than males. Participants between 59 and 78 years of age rated caring higher than the other age groups. Single participants scored higher than married participants. Those with lower education got higher scores. Patients who were admitted for 4–7 days and family members/caregivers who took care of the patients for 4–7 days obviously rated higher than other periods. Participants in gynecology and obstetrics rated higher scores (54.56 ± 9.97) than those in other departments.

Caring Factor Survey

The sample mean score of the CFS in this study is 52.80 ± 8.64 with approximately half of the participants (54.2%) scoring above the mean scores (Table 20.2). The item with the highest score was "My nurses have established a helping and trusting relationship with me during my time here" (5.78 ± 1.07). The item with the lowest score was "My nurses have responded to me as a whole person, helping to take care of all my needs and concerns" (4.80 ± 1.58).

Validity of the CCFS

The CVI was used to determine the appropriateness of the items. Five experts evaluated on each item of the CCFS on relevance, clarity, and simplicity. They were requested to rate among 1 (*not relevant*), 2 (*somewhat relevant*), 3 (*quite relevant*), and 4 (*highly relevant*). A CVI was computed by adding items that were rated as *quite relevant* (3) or *highly relevant* (4) and the total was divided by the total number of the experts. The item CVI ranged from 0.80 to 0.95, and the total CVI was 0.86 in the final version, indicating adequate content validity (Polit & Hungler, 1999).

Reliability Testing

Reliability is a major criterion of an instrument in order to assess the quantitative data adequately and accurately. The overall scale internal consistency with the Cronbach's alpha = .87 indicates high reliability of the 10-item Traditional Chinese version CFS.

TABLE 20.1 Summary of Demographic Data and CFS Mean Score ($n = 261$)

VARIABLE		FREQUENCY (%)	MEAN	SD
Participants' identity	Patients	75.8%	53.22	8.82
	Family members or caregivers	24.2%	51.73	7.79
Gender	Male	36.7%	52.44	8.07
	Female	63.3%	52.81	8.94
Age	18–38 years old	21.3%	51.96	8.26
	39–58 years old	31.7%	52.10	8.05
	59–78 years old	31.7%	54.73	9.39
	79–98 years old	15.3%	51.37	8.34
Marital status	Married	78.9%	52.71	8.53
	Single	21.1%	52.79	9.13
Nationality	Chinese	93.2%	52.90	8.77
	Portuguese	4.4%	53.09	5.07
	Others	2.4%	48.33	8.59
Common language use	Cantonese	94.0%	52.77	8.54
	Mandarin	5.2%	52.85	11.01
	Others	0.8%	56.00	7.07
Educational level	Primary school or below	45.2%	53.39	8.72
	High school	39.9%	52.47	8.78
	Diploma or above	14.9%	52.11	8.08
Department	Hospice and palliative care	3.9%	51.00	8.63
	Gynecology and obstetrics	10.4%	54.56	9.97
	Pediatrics	8.1%	53.55	7.78
	Internal medicine	48.8%	52.62	8.76
	Surgery	28.8%	52.53	8.30
Hospitalization days of patients	1–3 days	28.8%	51.29	9.68
	4–7 days	35.6%	54.38	6.90
	8–14 days	20.9%	53.83	10.74
	15–30 days	9.9%	54.32	7.97
	31 days or above	4.7%	46.89	10.65
Days of taking care of patients by family members or caregivers	1–3 days	25.9%	53.43	7.75
	4–7 days	37.0%	54.45	6.57
	8–14 days	14.8%	48.63	3.78
	15–30 days	16.7%	50.56	8.13
	31 days or above	5.6%	42.00	5.57

TABLE 20.2   Mean Score of CFS

INDIVIDUAL STATEMENT	n	MEAN	SD
1. My nurses have established a helping and trusting relationship with me during my time here.	252	5.78	1.07
2. Every day I am here, I see that the care is provided with loving kindness.	254	5.73	1.03
3. When my nurses teach me something new, they teach me in a way that I can understand.	253	5.43	1.23
4. My nurses have created a healing environment that recognizes the connection between my body, mind, and spirit.	251	5.42	1.23
5. The nurses honored my own faith, helped instill hope, and respected my belief system as part of my care.	253	5.29	1.19
6. I feel like I can talk openly and honestly about what I am thinking, because those who are caring for me embrace my feelings, no matter what my feelings are.	252	5.22	1.28
7. As a team, my nurses are good at creative problem solving to meet my individual needs and requests.	254	5.14	1.38
8. My nurses are accepting and supportive of my beliefs regarding a higher power, which allows for the possibility of me and my family to heal.	250	5.08	1.22
9. My nurses encouraged me to practice my own, individual, spiritual beliefs as part of my self-caring and healing.	252	4.91	1.36
10. My nurses have responded to me as a whole person, helping to take care of all my needs and concerns.	252	4.80	1.58

The corrected item-total correlation coefficients ranged from .52 (item 8) to .65 (item 5). The squared multiple correlation coefficients (R^2 values) indicated the proportion of variance in a given item that was shared with the other items, with higher values accounting for stronger consistency among the items (Polit & Hungler, 1999). The R^2 values in this study ranged from .35 (item 8) to .45 (item 5 and item 9). The coefficient alpha, if the item was deleted, ranged from .86 to .87. All of these correlations were found to be statistically significant at the .001 level. This finding explains that all of the items contributed to the overall high reliability; it was also apparent that none of the items seriously reduced the value of the coefficient alpha by being removed from the questionnaire (Polit & Hungler, 1999) (see Table 20.3).

The Internal Correlation of the CCFS

Spearman's rank-order correlation is a correlation coefficient that can indicate the extent of a relationship between variables measured on the ordinal scale (Polit & Hungler, 1999). Usually, if the coefficient is high, the strength

TABLE 20.3 Psychometrics for the CCFS (n = 261)

INDIVIDUAL STATEMENT	SMID	CITC	SMC	AID
1. Every day I am here, I see that the care is provided with loving kindness.	47.07	.63	.44	.86
2. As a team, my nurses are good at creative problem solving to meet my individual needs and requests.	47.66	.58	.41	.86
3. The nurses honored my own faith, helped instill hope, and respected my belief system as part of my care.	47.50	.629	.42	.86
4. When my nurses teach me something new, they teach me in a way that I can understand.	47.37	.58	.36	.86
5. My nurses encouraged me to practice my own, individual, spiritual beliefs as part of my self-caring and healing.	47.87	.65	.45	.86
6. My nurses have responded to me as a whole person, helping to take care of all my needs and concerns.	48.00	.58	.36	.86
7. My nurses have established a helping and trusting relationship with me during my time here.	47.02	.62	.44	.86
8. My nurses have created a healing environment that recognizes the connection between my body, mind, and spirit.	47.38	.51	.35	.87
9. I feel like I can talk openly and honestly about what I am thinking, because those who are caring for me embrace my feelings, no matter what my feelings are.	47.59	.62	.45	.86
10. My nurses are accepting and supportive of my beliefs regarding a higher power, which allows for the possibility of me and my family to heal.	47.71	.55	.39	.86

Notes: SMID, scale mean if item deleted; CITC, corrected item-total correlation; SMC, squared multiple correlation; AID, Cronbach's alpha if item deleted.

of correlation between the variables will be deemed great. In this study, Spearman's correlation analysis was conducted with the correlation coefficient of the CCFS, ranges from .25 to .59 ($P < .01$), which indicates that all of the items in the CCFS are showing a positive relationship. The detail of the Spearman's correlation coefficient is shown in Table 20.4.

DISCUSSION

The perception of nursing care in patients or their family members/caregivers is a crucial component in nursing, and there have been many instruments designed for measuring nursing care all over the world. Several of the scales identified that used Watson's theory included more than

TABLE 20.4 Item Correlation of the CCFS Chinese Version With Spearman's Rank-Order Correlation

	SPEARMAN'S RHO	ITEM 1	ITEM 2	ITEM 3	ITEM 4	ITEM 5	ITEM 6	ITEM 7	ITEM 8	ITEM 9	ITEM 10
Item 1	Correlation coefficient	1.000									
	Sig. (two-tailed)	.									
Item 2	Correlation coefficient	.52(**)									
	Sig. (two-tailed)	.000	.								
Item 3	Correlation coefficient	.53(**)	.47(**)								
	Sig. (two-tailed)	.000	.000	.							
Item 4	Correlation coefficient	.37(**)	.40(**)	.43(**)							
	Sig. (two-tailed)	.000	.000	.000	.						
Item 5	Correlation coefficient	.39(**)	.43(**)	.48(**)	.52(**)						
	Sig. (two-tailed)	.000	.000	.000	.000	.					
Item 6	Correlation coefficient	.45(**)	.39(**)	.42(**)	.42(**)	.46 (**)					
	Sig. (two-tailed)	.000	.000	.000	.000	.000	.				
Item 7	Correlation coefficient	.53(**)	.45(**)	.38(**)	.42(**)	.39(**)	.48(**)				
	Sig. (two-tailed)	.000	.000	.000	.000	.000	.000	.			
Item 8	Correlation coefficient	.46(**)	.43(**)	.32(**)	.33(**)	.30(**)	.41(**)	.59(**)			
	Sig. (two-tailed)	.000	.000	.000	.000	.000	.000	.000	.		
Item 9	Correlation coefficient	.37(**)	.38 (**)	.40(**)	.38(**)	.41()	.40(**)	.51(**)	.46(**)		
	Sig. (two-tailed)	.000	.000	.000	.000	.000	.000	.000	.000	.	
Item 10	Correlation coefficient	.36(**)	.25(**)	.39(**)	.39(**)	.42()	.42(**)	.33(**)	.27(**)	.53(**)	
	Sig. (two-tailed)	.000	.000	.000	.000	.000	.000	.000	.000	.000	.

Note: **Correlation is significant at the .01 level (two-tailed), $n = 261$.

22 items and most of them required more than 20 minutes to complete. The time-consuming and complicated scales may have lowered the respondent rate and affected the accuracy of the research. Thus, the development of a short, handy, and accurate scale for promoting clinical nursing quality is very important. In contrast, it took 10 minutes for patients or families to complete the CCFS.

This study showed that the CCFS has high internal-consistency reliability. The validity of the CCFS was indicated through content validation by stakeholders. As a result, the CCFS has proved to be an effective instrument for measuring the perception of caring from patients and family members or caregivers in hospitals under Chinese culture. The analysis provides support for the reliability of the CCFS because all of the items correlated in a significant level. However, several issues should be noted in relation to the correlation of items in the CCFS.

The CCFS will aid with the understanding of the meaning of caring for the Chinese population. The data in this study were collected by a few nursing students who were all trained to interpret the items of the CFS Chinese version with correct verbal expression. If the CFS Chinese version was interpreted by the patients or the family members themselves, the understanding of the meaning of caring may be affected, thus impacting the research results. This is because the concept of caring under Chinese culture is abstract and requires careful interpretation. Previous studies have found that the Chinese perceive caring as nurses giving quick responses to patient requests during their illness as well as implementing the treatments and medications on time (Holroyd et al., 1998; Ma, 2004). The Chinese tend to be concerned more about the physical wellness than the psychological, spiritual, and social aspects. Nurses in Macao are not keen to measure the perception of caring in patients; they pay more attention to patient satisfaction with the works that can be observed, such as the nurse's introduction of the environment to the patients (Lok et al., 2005). This phenomenon may be attributed to the passive or introverted feature of the Chinese, who are not familiar with expressing emotion and concern to others.

LIMITATIONS

This study was carried out to investigate the perception of caring from inpatients and their family members or caregivers at one hospital in Macao. The findings of this study may have been influenced by the organizational culture and may not represent all the points of view of the Chinese. In addition, this is the first study of its kind in Macao and thus it is impossible to compare it to other facilities' perceptions of caring. Despite these limitations, we think that it is the most appropriate approach for this study. The findings can provide Chinese patients' perspectives on caring and provide the guideline for nursing educators to improve the caring pedagogy in the nursing curriculum.

CONCLUSION

Constructing a measurement tool of perception of caring, which is based on Watson's caring theory, is a process of studying nursing care. The major concepts and definitions of Watson's 10 Carative Factors are indeed the philosophical foundation for nursing science. The results from this study show that nurses in Macao have been working hard to integrate concepts of caring in their daily nursing practice.

This study has been the first study of perception of caring in Macao, nevertheless the overall response from the participants reflects that the caring behavior of the nurses in this hospital within Macao is satisfactory. Moreover, the 10-item CCFS shows a good level of the validity and reliability in its measurement properties. This study can supply evidence for monitoring the clinical nursing quality and evolution of nursing education.

More studies should be conducted in exploring the essence of caring, the caring process, and caring outcomes in the health care setting of Chinese society. In addition, further studies can investigate the approach of integrating "caring" in the design of the nursing curriculum in Macao.

ACKNOWLEDGMENTS

First, we would like to express our deepest thanks to the five experts who helped and gave advices on the content validity of CCFS. Second, we need to give great thanks to Jimmy Cheong and Suzanne Lei, our colleagues who gave their invaluable time to translate and proofread the CCFS. Third, we are grateful to the data collectors, our students of Kiang Wu Nursing College of Macao, for their sparing no efforts conducting this project. In addition, we would like to thank the Research Committee of Kiang Wu Nursing College of Macao for the technical advice. Their support made this study possible.

REFERENCES

Cossette, S., Cara, C., Ricard, N., & Pepin, J. (2005). Assessing nurse–patient interactions from a caring perspective: Report of the development and preliminary psychometric testing of the Caring Nurse–Patient Interactions Scale. *International Journal of Nursing Studies, 42*(6), 673–686.

Davis, A. J., Hershberger, A., Ghan, L. C., & Lin, J. Y. (1990). The good nurse: Descriptions from the People's Republic of China. *Journal of Advanced Nursing, 15,* 829–834.

DiNapoli, P., Nelson, J., Turkel, M., & Watson, J. (2010). Measuring the Caritas processes: Caring factor survey. *International Journal for Human Caring, 14*(3), 15–20.

Drenkard, K., Nelson, J., Rigotti, G. & Watson, J. (2006). Caring factor survey. In J. Watson (Ed.), *Assessing and measuring caring in nursing and health sciences* (pp. 253–258). New York, NY: Springer Publishing Co.

Holroyd, E., Cheung, Y. K., Cheung, S. W., Luk, F. S., & Wong, W. W. (1998). A Chinese cultural perspective of nursing care behaviors in an acute setting. *Journal of Advanced Nursing, 28*(6), 1289–1294.

Huang, X. Z., Liu, Y. L., & Yang, C. (2009). *Nursing care: Application of Watson's caring theory in nursing* (1st ed.). Beijing, China: People's Military Medical Press.

Jesse, D. E. (2010). Jean Watson: Watson's philosophy and theory of transpersonal caring. In M. R. Alligood & A. M. Tomey (Eds.), *Nursing theorists and their work* (pp. 91–112). Maryland, MO: Mosby Elsevier.

Lin, P. F. (2004). Nursing care in Taiwan: A qualitative study. *The Journal of Health Science, 6*(1), 1–12.

Lin, Y. Y., & Chiou, C. P. (2003). Concept analysis of caring. *Journal of Nursing, 50*(6), 74–78.

Liu, J. E., Mok, E., & Wong, T. (2006). Caring in nursing: Investigating the meaning of caring from the perspective of cancer patients in Beijing, China. *Journal of Clinical Nursing, 15*(2), 188–196.

Lok, I. H., Fong, I. H., Kowk, W. S., Ao, C. I., Chan, L. W., Kuok, W. M., . . . Cheng, B. S. (2005). A patient-satisfaction survey in nursing care delivered by cardiac critical-care unit in a hospital in Macau. *Macau Journal of Nursing, 4*(1), 13–15.

Ma, S. C. (2004). A study of ICU patients' perceptions on nursing caring behavior. *Chang Gung Nursing, 15*(2), 156–164.

Maltby, H., Drury, J., & Fischer-Rasmussen, V. (1995). The roots of nursing: Teaching caring based on Watson. *Nurse Education Today, 15,* 44–46.

Meurer, S., Rubio, D., Counte, M., & Burroughs, T. (2002). Development of a healthcare quality improvement measurement tolls: Results of a content validity study. *Hospital Topics: Research and Perspectives on Healthcare, 80* (2), 7–13.

Nelson, J. (2008). Caring factor survey. In J. Watson (Ed.), *Assessing and measuring caring in nursing and health science* (pp. 253–260). New York, NY: Springer.

Pan, W. B. (2008). Caring factors. In J. C. Lee (Ed.), *Caring* (pp. 1101–1134). Taiwan, Taipei: Yeong Dah.

Pang, S. M. C., Wong, T. K. S., Zhang, Z. J., Chan, H. Y. L., Lam, C. W. Y., & Chan, K. L. (2004). Towards a Chinese definition of nursing. *Journal of Advanced Nursing, 46*(6), 657–670.

Polit, D. F., & Hungler, B. P. (1999). *Nursing research: Principles and methods* (6th ed.). Philadelphia, PA: Lippincott Company.

Ryan, L. A. (2005). The journey to integrate Watson's caring theory with clinical practice. *International Journal for Human Care, 9*(3), 26–30.

Statistics and Census Service of Macao SAR Government. (2008). Inpatients by medical specialty. In *Yearbook of Statistics 2008*(p. 142). Macao, China: Author.

Watson, J. (2005). *Caring science as sacred science.* Philadelphia, PA: F. A. Davis.

Watson, J. (2008). Caring factor survey. In J. Watson (Ed.), *Assessing and measuring caring in nursing and health science* (pp. 253–260). New York, NY: Springer Publishing Company.

Wolf, Z. (1986). The caring concept and nurse identified caring behaviours. *Topics in Clinical Nursing, 8*(2):84–93.

Wolf, Z. R., Colahan, M., Costello, A., Warwick, F., Ambrose, M. S., & Giardino, E. R. (1998). Relationship between nurse caring and patient satisfaction. *Medsurg Nursing, 7*(2), 99–105.

Yam, B. M. C., & Rossiter, J. C. (2000). Caring in nursing: Perceptions of Hong Kong nurses. *Journal of Clinical Nursing, 9*(2), 293–302.

SECTION V

International Comparison of Caritas

21

Comparison of Caritas in Health Care Facilities in Macao, China; Italy; the Philippines; and the United States as Perceived by Patients

John Nelson, Georgia Persky, Deanne Sramek, Guiliana Masera, Margaret May A. Ga, Michelle Ming Xia Zhu, Grace Ka In Lok, Iris Lawrence, and Alfonso Sollami

*T*his chapter combines all of the datasets from the previous 20 chapters that used the Caring Factor Survey (CFS) to measure patients' perceptions of Caritas (caring). Similarities as well as differences of countries are examined among 2,702 respondents, including data from Macao, China ($n = 261$), Italy ($n = 163$), the Philippines ($n = 51$), and the United States ($n = 2,227$). Five facilities were in Italy and seven were in the United States, which facilitated comparison of unit types in each respective country. Results revealed similarities across the globe alongside rank-order differences between countries and unit types. Data suggest that context is important when considering application of caring behaviors across the globe.

BACKGROUND

Research has shown that context is essential to consider within the application of caring concepts. The Canadian study by Cossette, Cara, Ricard, and Pepin (2005) examined caring from student nurses, perspectives. Cossette et al. (2005) found caring to be rated as less important by native-born students while concomitantly feeling more competent in caring when compared to nonnative students (Cossette et al., 2005). The authors assert that it may be because the native-born Canadian students have a more realistic understanding of caring within the Canadian culture (Cossette et al., 2005). The authors assert further that this finding indicates that ethnographic studies regarding caring should precede quantitative studies in caring so it is understood how caring is defined within the context of culture (Cossette et al., 2005). Another Canadian study using Watson's theory of caring elucidated the importance of negotiating cultural considerations when caring for patients who had immigrated to Canada from another country (Osborne, 1995).

One of the two studies from the United Kingdom found that patients' views of caring included both actions and attitudes of caring as essential if the patients were to feel cared for (McCance, 2003). These findings are consistent with Watson's theory of caring. Price (2006) argues that understanding the patients' idiosyncratic needs takes time and understanding, which may not become operational because of time constraints common to staff nurses.

A study in Iceland found that patients wanted nurses, most of all, to demonstrate clinical competence (Baldursdottir & Jonsdottir, 2002). Scottish patients reported it important to be heard, especially in the early formation of the nurse–patient relationship (Forchuk & Reynolds, 2001). It was important to the patient to voice perceptions even if the perceptions were negative (Forchuk & Reynolds, 2001). Allowing verbalization of both positive and negative perceptions is consistent with Watson's theory of caring (Watson, 1985). Patients from both Canada and Scotland identified the relationship with the nurse as important to their overall recovery (Watson, 1985).

Three studies were found that examined caring from a Chinese perspective (Arthur, Pang, & Wong, 2001; Holroyd, Cheung, Cheung, Luk, & Wong, 1998; Schofield, Tolson, Arthur, Davies, & Nolan, 2005). Arthur et al. (2001) used a quantitative approach to examine caring from the nurses' perspective and to evaluate the relationship of ability to care with level of technology. It was identified that the higher the level of technology the nurse worked within, the higher scores of ability in providing caring behaviors (Arthur et al., 2001). Holroyd et al. (1998) also used a quantitative method to examine perception of caring but as viewed by the patient in the Chinese culture (Holroyd et al., 1998). This study identified that within the Chinese culture, caring is viewed as contributory to perfect virtue (Holroyd et al., 1998). The Chinese culture expects interpersonal relationships to be kind, gracious, and sensitive (Holroyd et al., 1998). It is important that both people in the relationship respect one another to ensure no person in the interaction is disrespected or put to shame in any way (Holroyd et al., 1998). These expectations within Chinese relationships are consistent with the caring factors articulated by Watson (1985). Using the Care-Q, the researchers found that patients within the Chinese culture valued monitoring and follow-throughs and being accessible (Holroyd et al., 1998). Of the 59 items measured, clinical care that was reported to be least important to the patient included having the nurse sit with the patient, being asked what name the patient prefers to be called, and being touched (Holroyd et al., 1998). The lack of desire for individual care and attention was proposed to be due to the value in China of family and community in comparison to Western values of the individual (Holroyd et al., 1998; Schofield et al., 2005). In comparing this

Chinese study with Swedish and American studies that used the same research instruments, patients in all three countries desired close monitoring and follow-through, but the Chinese wanted care from physicians, not nurses (Holroyd et al., 1998). It was postulated that the Chinese view a stronger hierarchy between physicians and nurses as compared to Western health care; nurses monitor and report clinical status, but physicians provide care (Holroyd et al., 1998).

A study from Finland found that nurses reported physical care as the important aspect of caring, which is in contrast to what nurses often report as most important—the psychosocial aspects of the nurse–patient relationship (Greenhalgh, Vanhanen, & Kyngäs, 1998). Patients typically report the most important aspect of caring to be physical care (Greenhalgh et al., 1998).

Nurses' perceptions of caring in Ireland were found to be consistent with that of nurses in the United States, but the methods of executing the values of caring varied (Cammuso, 1994). Deady (2005) observed that nurses in the United States provided care based on interaction and mutuality between nurse and patient in contrast to more paternalistic care in Ireland (Deady, 2005). Deady's (2005) study revealed that psychiatric nurses in Ireland value understanding what is most important to their patients. Other studies suggest that intentionality between nurse and patient in establishing understanding of priorities in care may be what makes the nurse–patient relationship successful (Sherwood, 1997; Turkel & Ray, 2001).

A study from Scotland inquired about caring for families in accident and emergency departments from the nurse's perspective (Hallgrimsdottir, 2000). Ninety-six percent of the participants reported family care as a nurse's responsibility (Hallgrimsdottir, 2000). However, only 35% of the nurses reported evidence-based family care because most relied on the input of colleagues and personal friends on how to care for families (Hallgrimsdottir, 2000). Competence in family care is important to consider if a patient reports family care as a priority in caring. A multivariate analysis of nurses' perceptions of caring revealed two general domains as perceived by staff nurses and nursing students in Scotland: psychosocial caring and professional-technical caring (Lea, Watson, & Deary, 1998).

Watson et al. (2003) studied the priorities of caring activities in nurses from Spain and the United Kingdom (Watson et al., 2003). It was identified that nurses who provided care in the hospital setting had similar perceptions of caring, but the priorities of caring behaviors were different (Watson et al., 2003). It should be considered that such differences of priority of caring behaviors may exist within populations of patients from country to country as well.

Context should be considered within countries and different settings such as care for patients receiving electroconvulsive therapy (ECT) or patients with acute and/or chronic pain. Glynn revealed in Appendix H, page 419, that nurses performing ECT for patients were ranked highest by patients when asked about caring for all basic needs. It is reasonable to consider that, for a patient receiving ECT, the nurse must balance that care physically, emotionally, mentally, and spiritually. Herbst explains in Chapter 11 that patients in obstetrics who were experiencing pain were not receptive to a caring intervention that did not address their pain first before other caring behaviors.

Measuring patients' perceptions of caring in contrast to reporting perceived caring for patients by nurses is important because it has been identified that patients and nurses view and prioritize caring differently (Bassett, 2002; Chang, Lin, Chang, & Lin 2005; Drake, 1995; Hegedus, 1999; Kyle, 1995; Larsson, Widmark, Lampic, von Essen, & Sjoden, 1998; Proch, 1997; von Essen & Sjoden, 2003; Widmark-Petersson, von Essen, Sjoden, 2000). The CFS has been shown to be a valid and reliable instrument to use for measuring patients' perceptions of caring using Watson's theory of caring in multiple contexts across the globe including in Italy as described by Masera in Chapter 17, in the United States by Perksy, Felgen, Romano, and Nelson in Chapter 5, in Philippines as described by Reyes et al. in Chapter 18, and in China as described by Zhu, Lok, Cheong, Lao, and Cheong in Chapter 20.

METHODS

A secondary study was conducted of all the datasets from all chapters within this book that used the CFS for research.[1] An in-depth review of the background and methods can be found within each respective chapter, including the power analysis for each study. This chapter provides reference to each study, the number in each sample, and brings the analysis of comparisons deeper among the collective studies.

In 2006 there were 170 respondents who used the CFS, 266 in 2007, 419 in 2008, 678 in 2009, and in 2010 there were 969 patients or family members who responded to the CFS. Demographics that were examined included country, comparing patient and family response to caring, race, facility, and unit. Descriptive statistics (mean, minimum, maximum, and standard deviation) were used to understand rank order and variance for each concept of caring and the total score of caring, which was all 10 concepts combined. The general linear model (GLM) was used to examine the main and interaction effects of two concurrent demographics on perception of caring. Line graphs derived from the GLM procedure were used to more deeply understand patterns of demographics over time.

RESULTS

When comparing data from year to year, it was identified that 2006 had lower scores than 2007–2010 and the difference was statistically significant for all variables for all caring factors, except healing environment

---

[1] P. Glynn's data for patients receiving ECT were not included in the dataset. Her study can be found in Appendix H.

(alpha .05). On average, facilitation of a relationship with the patient and loving kindness were the two highest-ranked concepts of caring. The lowest-ranked concept, on average, across all 4 years was perception of spiritual support. These data are noted in Figure 21.1.

When comparing countries, it was found that Macao, China scored the lowest among the four countries measured and that the difference was statistically significant for all concepts of caring using an alpha of .05. Italy reported the highest score for caring for all concepts except holistic care and spiritual beliefs (Figure 21.2).

No statistically significant interaction (using an alpha of .05) was found for countries and time using the GLM. This was true for each

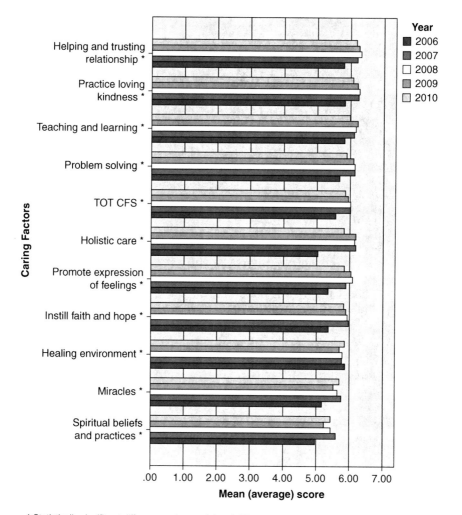

* Statistically significant difference using an alpha of .05.

FIGURE 21.1 Comparison of CFS scores, 2006–2010.

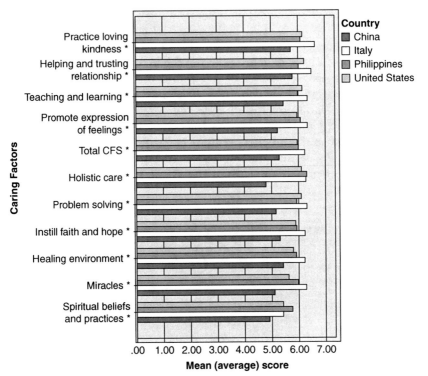

*Statistically significant using an alpha of .05.

FIGURE 21.2 Comparing caring factors among countries.

caring concept and the total CFS score. There was a main effect for a country for each concept and the total CFS score, which indicates that the difference between countries was sustained over time. Only Italy and the United States had data from several years that revealed a sustained difference between countries over time. The pattern for the main effect of the country that was generally true for each concept of caring and the total CFS score is noted in Figure 21.3.

A one-way ANOVA revealed statistically significant differences when comparing the 14 different facilities (using an alpha of .05). This was true for every concept of Caritas.

Different unit types were grouped together and compared. Fourteen different unit types from Italy and the United States were compared. There were 1,647 respondents to the CFS for the 14 unit types, including 163 from Italy and 1,514 from the United States (Table 21.1).

Eight of the 10 Caritas factors were found to differ between units and were statistically significant (using an alpha of .05). All but the caring concepts of problem solving and teach and learn were statistically significant. The total CFS score was also found to differ between units and was statistically significant (Figures 21.4 through 21.12).

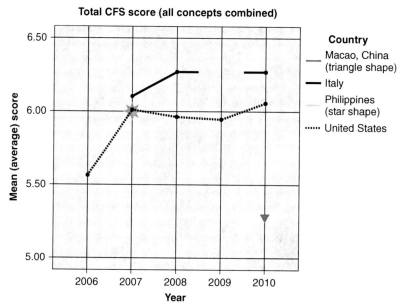

FIGURE 21.3 Main effect of country, total CFS score.

Table 21.1 Frequency of Respondents by Select Units

UNIT	AGGREGATE FREQUENCY	ITALY FREQUENCY	UNITED STATES FREQUENCY	PERCENT
Hospice	62	62	NA	3.8
Nursing home	16	16	NA	1.0
Cardiac surgery	20	20	NA	1.2
GI operative	50	50	NA	3.0
ICU	46	15	31	2.8
Neurology	143	NA	143	8.7
Psychiatric care	67	NA	67	4.1
Medical	441	NA	441	26.8
Labor and delivery	344	NA	344	20.9
Oncology	84	NA	84	5.1
Orthopedics	61	NA	61	3.7
Transplant	87	NA	87	5.3
Surgical	186	NA	186	11.3
Emergency dept.	40	NA	40	2.4
Total	1,647	163	1,514	100.0

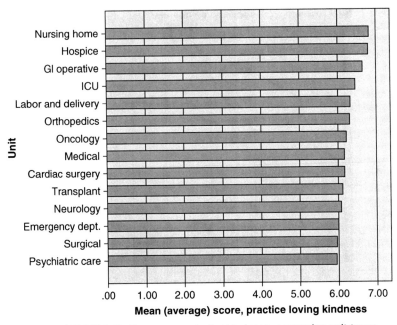

FIGURE 21.4 Caritas process, loving kindness, comparing unit types.

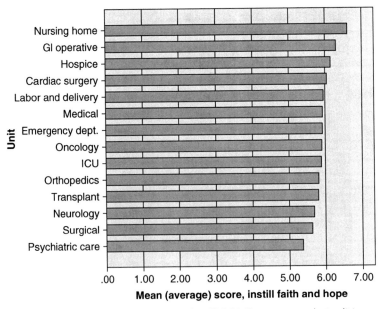

FIGURE 21.5 Caritas process, instill faith/hope, comparing unit types.

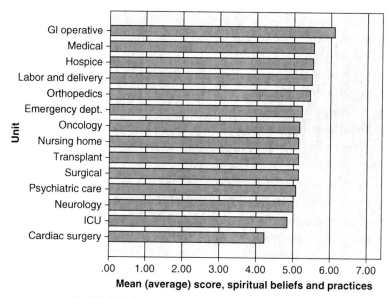

FIGURE 21.6 Caritas process, spiritual care, comparing units.

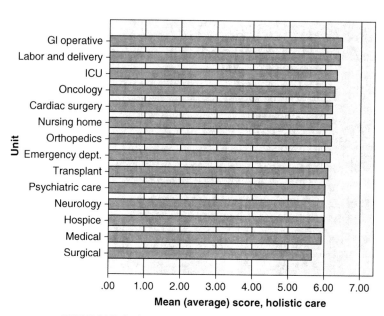

FIGURE 21.7 Caritas process, holistic care, comparing unit types.

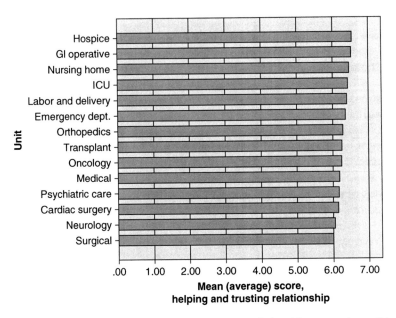

FIGURE 21.8 Caritas process helping/trusting relationship, comparing unit types.

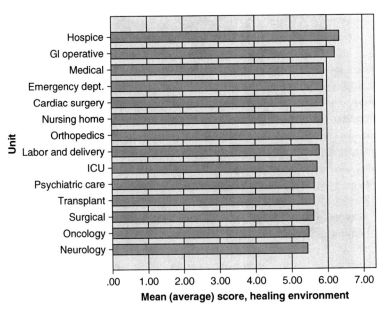

FIGURE 21.9 Caritas process healing environment, comparing unit type.

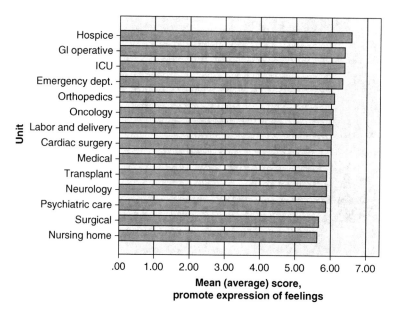

**Mean (average) score,
promote expression of feelings**

FIGURE 21.10 Caritas process promotes expression of feelings, comparing unit types.

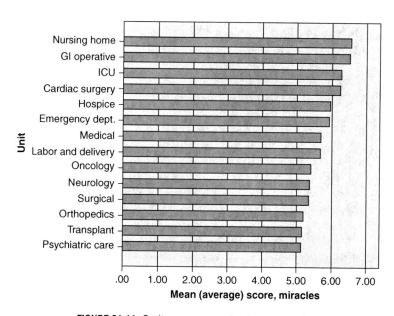

Mean (average) score, miracles

FIGURE 21.11 Caritas process miracles, comparing unit types.

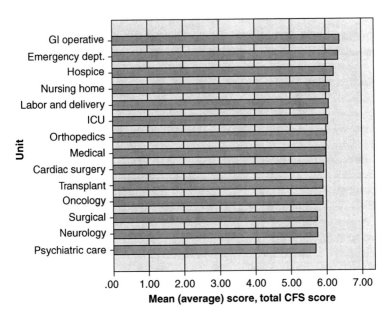

FIGURE 21.12 Total CFS score, comparing unit types.

Spiritual support was, on average, the lowest-scoring concept of caring as noted in Figure 21.6. The rank order of the 10 caring concepts was examined in each unit type. Results revealed that the concept for spiritual support was ranked last for the unit, except for the orthopedic unit where spiritual support was ranked ninth. In contrast, loving kindness was most frequently ranked number one, followed by facilitation of helping, trusting relationships (Table 21.2).

When comparing responses of the facilities that gathered data from the family as proxy, all concepts were compared and no differences were found for the total CFS score (using an alpha of .05). The only concept that was found to be statistically significant, when comparing patients ($n = 1,531$) and family members ($n = 215$), was the perception of being allowed to believe in miracles. It is noted that patients' scores (mean score, 5.58) were lower than those of patients' family members (mean score, 5.81) when asked about believing in miracles (Figure 21.13).

When comparing race, no differences were noted (using an alpha of .05). Race categories were used exclusively in the facilities in the United States and included Hispanic, White, non-Hispanic, Hispanic Black, non-Hispanic Black, Asian American Pacific Islander, Alaska Native American Indian, and Other.

Table 21.2 Rank Order of Each Caring Process, by Unit Type

UNIT	Q1 RANK LOVE KIND	Q2 RANK PROB SOLV	Q3 RANK INSTILL FAITH	Q4 RANK TEACH LEARN	Q5 RANK SPIRIT SUPP	Q6 RANK HOLISTIC CARE	Q7 RANK HELP/TRUST	Q8 RANK HEALING ENVIRONMENT	Q9 RANK PROMOTE EXPRESSION OF FEELINGS	Q10 RANK MIRACLES
Hospice	1	6	7	4	10	8	3	5	2	9
Nursing home	1	8	2	6	10	5	4	7	9	3
Cardiac surgery	6	1	7	3	10	4	5	9	8	2
GI operative	1	4	8	6	10	5	3	9	7	2
ICU	1	6	8	7	10	4	2	9	3	5
Neurology	1	3	7	5	10	4	2	8	6	9
Psychiatric care	4	5	8	3	10	2	1	7	6	9
Medical	3	4	5	2	10	8	1	7	6	9
Labor and delivery	4	5	7	3	10	1	2	8	6	9
Oncology	3	5	7	6	10	1	2	8	4	9
Orthopedics	1	3	8	5	9	4	2	7	6	10
Transplant	4	3	7	2	10	4	2	8	6	9
Surgical	3	4	7	1	10	5	1	8	6	9
Emergency dept.	6	5	8	3	10	4	2	8	5	9
All units combined	2	4	7	3	10	5	1	8	6	9

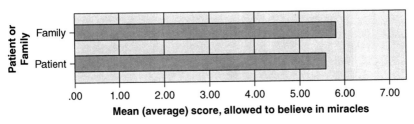

FIGURE 21.13 Patient and family responses, allowed to believe in miracles.

DISCUSSION

The lowest score in 2006 may have been due to that study being from a baseline study prior to implementation of any intentional caring intervention. Review of the respective studies revealed an increase in CFS scores after implementation of intentional caring which has been described in section I of Chapter 9 by Persky, Felgen, and Nelson, in section II of Chapter 9 by Rye, Sherman-Justice, and Fahrenwald, and Chapter 11 by Herbst.

Macao, China reporting the lowest score may be due to the concept of caring, especially so intentionally from nurses, which may be due to this being a cultural shift for China. Traditions of Confucianism and Mohism teach that people are naturally caring and, thus, intention of caring is a new and Western concept and described further in Chapter 20 by Zhu et al. Individual care traditionally is less preferred when contrasted to family or community care (Holroyd et al., 1998). In addition, there is a stronger hierarchy between physicians and nurses when compared to Western nations (Holroyd et al., 1998). Given these facts, the intentional and individual caring behaviors by nurses may take a while to integrate into the Chinese culture. In addition, individualizing care takes time and due to individualized caring concepts being new to care in China, it may be, as Price (2006) asserts, that current workload may constrain caring from becoming operational.

Findings from the 2006 to 2010 CFS data revealed loving kindness to be one of the top two caring concepts consistently around the globe and in most care-unit types. In contrast, spiritual support was ranked last. The low rank of spiritual care requires more careful consideration in light of spiritual care being an integral part of nursing care (Como, 2007). Patients want their personal belief systems to be part of their care (Nussbaum, 2003). In addition, the Joint Commission on Accreditation of Healthcare Organizations requires that spiritual assessment and spiritual care be offered to patients (Burkhart, Solari-Twadell & Haas, 2008; Joint Commission on Accreditation of Health Care Organizations, 2004).

Several potential outcomes for spiritual care exist, including increasing the likelihood that patients will adhere to their plan of care (Simoni, Frick, & Huang, 2006). Meador (2006) reported that more than two-thirds of participants assert that spiritual care should be part of their care.

Second, pursuit of supporting the patient spiritually may improve interdisciplinary care because it has been proposed by the American College of Critical Care Medicine for nurses and doctors to collaboratively integrate it into the patient's plan of care (Davidson et al., 2007). Third, it may assist with avoiding lawsuits/litigation (e.g., avoiding inadvertent blood transfusions for individuals whose belief system prohibits it). Litigation within health care trying to override those whose belief is not to be transfused due to spiritual beliefs generally fails (Gyamfi, Gyamfi & Berkowitz, 2003). Fourth, spiritual care has been shown to improve patient outcomes (Bowen, Baetz, & D'Arcy, 2006; Krebs, 2001; Tartaro, Luecken, & Gunn, 2005), including enhancement of coping with illness (Canada et al., 2006), alleviation of pain, decreased anxiety, decreased despair, and promotion of feelings of serenity (Renz, Mao, & Cerny, 2005).

It is the experience of the author of this chapter that spiritual care is not something all nurses are comfortable with. Providing competent spiritual care takes training. There are examples of formal spiritual training such as that cited by Koenig, George, and Titus (2004) at Duke University Medical Center, where they have developed a curriculum that incorporates spiritual care into their training of health professionals.

IMPLICATIONS

One of the greatest challenges in understanding the patients' needs for caring around the globe is the need for new models of analysis that go beyond the common use of mean scores. This chapter delineates how unique each country, facility, and unit is in relationship to perception and rank order of processes of caring. According to Watson (2005), caring is individual and dependent on the moment in time; there is no average caring moment. Thus it is imperative that nurses and health care professionals move beyond examination of the average score to understanding how to use other analytic methods such as fractals, nonlinear geometry, qualitative data, pattern analysis, and Parato mathematics. It is likely that these processes of analysis will be used in isolation at first, then to cross-validate findings in respective analyses. Finally, analysts, clinicians, academicians, engineers, architects, and other professionals can collaborate to generate new mathematical formulas that will integrate these or other methods of analysis. West (2007) cites that the use of fractal physiology by medicine over the last two decades has begun to revolutionize medical research. Such methods also can assist with understanding caring, to go beyond using the average to using the outlier and examination of the extremes of success. This will assist with understanding the context of caring. Each context is unique, thus understanding why and how caring works within each context will be the premise of success for each facility (Davenport & Harris, 2007).

It is asserted by the author of this chapter that there are patterns of love within each facility and on each unit that may be drawn geometrically using non-Euclidean geometrics. This is the concept of Phi, or the Fibonacci Code, that is evident in nature, art, and architecture (Hemenway, 2008). The challenge in delineating the pattern of love on each unit is creating an environment where the patient and staff are able to collaborate closely enough in an autonomous way that the caring needs and associated interventions are clearly understood and supported within architecture and systems that allow this caring to become operational. In addition, time itself introduces evolution of people, systems, and structure so the data are never exactly the same and described in more detail in Chapter 5 by Persky et al.

Understanding the patterns of love using multiple methods of analysis within an evolving environment will require innovation and mass collaboration. Innovative strategies such as mass collaboration have been shown to be extremely successful in Fortune 500 companies (Tapscott & Williams, 2008). One such group to tackle this is the Caring International Research Collaborative (CIRC), which is a research community of Sigma Theta Tau International (STTI), the honor society of nursing. The underlying premise of CIRC aligns with Thomas Kuhn's (1962) assertion that knowledge will grow exponentially once scientists share what they know. The group structure uses sharing groups, with each sharing group examining one construct. Examples of constructs are caring, workload, relationship-based care, self-care, architecture of caring concepts, and over a dozen other constructs that are examined within their respective sharing groups. Included within the sharing groups are nurses, academicians, engineers, architects, doctors, administrators, students, clinicians, ancillary staff from health care, consultants, and additional professionals who aid with understanding various facets of the caring moment. The aim of the entire CIRC group is to enhance the likelihood that a caring moment will occur with a patient, self, or coworker.

Most vital within this mass collaboration of CIRC, evolution of mathematics, and associated understanding is the involvement of staff and patients to interpret the data and assist with building models of research that are specified to their respective context. Mathematicians and regulators understand only the numbers but lack understanding of what the data are relating to or inferring within this respective context. Staff and patients should be the ones who are driving the data, not the mathematicians. If the staff and patients drove the data, the formulas would be more precise and thus produce less error and advance science.

Models that are generated by the staff, patients, and mathematicians can theoretically be interfaced and automated within electronic causal models that would recalculate with every new data point. Real-time calculations could theoretically produce outcome management systems that could proactively manage outcomes like patient falls and medication errors. Patients who understand this level of safety truly would feel cared for. Such electronic, staff-driven management of data could incorporate every concept of caring, including spiritual care, teaching needs that are patient specific, complex problem solving for patients, and every other caring process within Watson's theory of Caritas.

SUMMARY

Understanding caring within context is important for nurses to feel competent in the application of caring concepts (Cossette et al., 2005). What patients want may vary from Eastern to Western cultures (Holroyd et al., 1998; Schofield et al., 2005), and nurses need to understand this beyond the average score. Nurses and patients who are intentional in establishing mutual understanding of priorities of care may have the most success and satisfaction in the nurse–patient relationship (Sherwood, 1997; Turkel & Ray, 2001). Understanding what patients desire in care in each respective country, facility, and unit may facilitate not only satisfaction with care for the patient and staff, but also enhance compliance with the proposed and negotiated plan of care for healing, decrease morbidity and mortality, and decrease cost of care. Once caring interventions can be scientifically linked to improved outcomes, then it will be possible for nurses and health care facilities to be financially compensated for competence in Caritas.

ACKNOWLEDGMENTS

Acknowledgment goes to colleagues from the authors' class in Information Technology who assisted with literature review for spiritual care, including Mary Black, Kathrine Lund, Catherine Miller, and Christine Poe. Acknowledgment goes to graduate students from Italy who provided a copy of the data from their respective theses.

REFERENCES

Arthur, D., Pang, S., & Wong, T. (2001). The effect of technology on the caring attributes of an international sample of nurses. *International Journal of Nursing Studies, 38*(1), 37–43.

Baldursdottir, G., & Jonsdottir, H. (2002). The importance of nurse caring behaviors as perceived by patients receiving care at an emergency department. *Heart & Lung, 31*(1), 67–75.

Bassett, C. (2002). Nurses' perceptions of care and caring. *International Journal of Nursing Practice, 8,* 8–15

Bowen, R., Baetz, M., & D'Arcy, C. (2006). Self-rated importance of religion predicts one-year outcome of patients with panic disorder. *Depression and Anxiety, 23,* 266–273.

Burkhart, L., Solari-Twadell, P. A., & Haas, S. (2008). Addressing spiritual leadership: An organizational model. *The Journal of Nursing Administration, 38,* 33–39.

Cammuso, B. S. (1994). Caring and accountability in nursing practice in Ireland and the United States: Helping Irish nurses bridge the gap when they choose to practice in the United States. ED.D., Clark University.

Canada, L. L., Parker, P. A., deMoor J. S., Basen-Engqueist, K., Ramondetta, L. J., & Cohen, L. (2006). Active coping mediates the association between religion/spirituality and quality of life in ovarian cancer. *Gynecologic Oncology, 101,* 102–107.

Chang, Y., Lin, Y., Chang, H., & Lin, C. (2005). Cancer patient and staff ratings of caring behaviors: Relationship to level of pain intensity. *Cancer Nursing, 28*(5), 331–339.

Como, J. M. (2007). Spiritual practice: A literature review related to spiritual health and health outcomes. *Holistic Nursing Practice, 21,* 224.

Cossette, S., Cara, C., Richard, N., & Pepin, J. (2005). Assessing nurse–patient interactions from a caring perspective: Report of the development and preliminary psychometric testing of the caring nurse–patient interactions scale. *International Journal of Nursing Studies, 42*(6), 673–686.

Davenport, T. H., & Harris, J. G. (2007). *Competing on analytics.* Boston, MA: Harvard Business School Press.

Davidson, J. E., Powers, K., Hedayat, K. M., Tieszen, M., Kon, A. A., Shepard, E., et al. (2007). Clinical practice guidelines for support of the family in the patient-centered intensive care unit: American College of Critical Care Medicine Task Force 2004–2005. *Critical Care Medicine, 35,* 605–622

Deady, R. (2005). Psychiatric nursing in Ireland: A phenomenological study of the attitudes, values, and beliefs of Irish trained psychiatric nurses. *Archives of Psychiatric Nursing, 19*(5), 210–216

Drake, E. (1995). Discharge teaching needs of parents in the NICU. *Neonatal Network: The Journal of Neonatal Nursing, 14*(1), 49–53

Forchuk, C., & Reynolds, W. (2001). Clients' reflections on relationships with nurses: Comparisons from Canada and Scotland. *Journal of Psychiatric and Mental Health Nursing, 8*(1), 45–51

Greenhalgh, J., Vanhanen, L., & Kyngäs, H. (1998). Nurse caring behaviours. *Journal of Advanced Nursing, 27*(5), 927–932

Gyamfi, C., Gyamfi, M. M., & Berkowitz, R. L. (2003). Ethical and medicolegal considerations in obstetric care of Jehovah's Witnesses. *The American College of Obstetricians and Gynecologists, 102*(1), 173.

Hallgrimsdottir, E. M. (2000). Accident and emergency nurses' perceptions and experiences of caring for families. *Journal of Clinical Nursing, 9*(4), 611–619.

Hegedus, K. S. (1999). Providers' and consumers' perspectives of nurses' caring behaviours. *Journal of Advanced Nursing, 30*(5), 1090–1096.

Hemenway, P. (2008). *The secret code.* Logano, Switzerland: Springwood.

Holroyd, E., Cheung, Y., Cheung, S., Luk, F., & Wong, W. (1998). A Chinese cultural perspective of nursing care behaviours in an acute setting. *Journal of Advanced Nursing, 28*(6), 1289–1294.

Joint Commission on Accreditation of Health Care Organizations. (2004). *Spiritual assessment.* Retrieved February 21, 2008, from http://www.jointcommission.org/AccreditationPrograms/HomeCare/Standards/FAOs/Provision+of+Care/

Koenig, H. G., George, L. K., & Titus, P. (2004). Religion, spirituality, and health in medically ill hospitalized older patients. *Journal of the American Geriatrics Association 5*, 554–562.

Krebs, K. (2001). The spiritual aspect of caring—An integral part of health and healing. *Nursing Administration Quarterly, 25*, 55–60.

Kuhn, T. (1962). *The structure of scientific revolution.* Chicago, IL: Chicago Press.

Kyle, T. V. (1995). The concept of caring: A review of the literature. *Journal of Advanced Nursing, 21*(3), 506–514.

Larsson, G., Widmark, V., Lampic, C., von Essen, L., & Sjoden, P. (1998). Cancer patient and staff ratings of the importance of caring behaviours and their relations to patient anxiety and depression. *Journal of Advanced Nursing, 27*(4), 855–864.

Lea, A., Watson, R., Deary, I. J. (1998). Caring in nursing: A multivariate analysis. *Journal of Advanced Nursing, 28*(3), 662–671.

McCance, T. V. (2003). Caring in nursing practice: The development of a conceptual framework. *Research and Theory for Nursing Practice, 17*(2), 101–116

Meador, K. G. (2006). Spirituality and care at the end of life. *Southern Medical Journal, 99*, 1184.

Nussbaum, G. B. (2003). Spirituality in critical care. *Critical Care Nursing Quarterly, 26*, 214.

Osborne, M. E. (1995). Dimensions of understanding in cross-cultural nurse-client relationships: A qualitative nursing study. 207, University of Texas at Austin.

Price, B. (2006, August 23–29). Exploring person-centred care. *Nursing Standard, 20*(50), 49–56.

Proch, M. L. (1997). The development and validation of caring competencies for hospital staff nurses. 122, University of South Florida.

Renz, M., Mao, M. S., & Cerny, T. (2005). Spirituality, psychotherapy, and music in palliative cancer care: Research projects in psycho-oncology at an oncology center in Switzerland. *Support Care Cancer, 13*, 961–966.

Schofield, I., Tolson, D., Arthur, D., Davies, S., & Nolan, M. (2005). An exploration of the caring attributes and perceptions of work place change among gerontological nursing staff in England, Scotland and China (Hong Kong). *International Journal of Nursing Studies, 42*(2), 197–209

Sherwood, G. D. (1997). Meta-synthesis of qualitative analyses of caring: Defining a therapeutic model of nursing. *Advanced Practice Nursing Quarterly, 3*(1), 32–42.

Simoni, J. M., Frick, P. A., & Huang, B. (2006). A longitudinal evaluation of a social support model of medication adherence among HIV-positive men and women on antiretroviral therapy. *Health Psychology, 25*, 74–81.

Tapscott, D., & Williams, A. (2008). *Wikinomics, how mass collaboration changes everything.* New York, NY: Penguin.

Tartaro, J., Luecken, L. J., & Gunn, H. E. (2005). Exploring heart and soul: Effects of religiosity/spirituality and gender on blood pressure and cortisol stress responses (Electronic version). *Journal of Health Psychology, 10*, 753–765.

Turkel, M. C., & Ray, M. A. (2001). Research issues. Relational complexity: From grounded theory to instrument development and theoretical testing … synthesis of the research findings from a 5-year program of qualitative and quantitative studies. *Nursing Science Quarterly, 14*(4), 281–287.

von Essen, L., & Sjoden, P. (2003). The importance of nurse caring behaviors as perceived by Swedish hospital patients and nursing staff. *International Journal of Nursing Studies, 40*(5), 487–497.

Watson, J. (1985). *Nursing: Human science and human care.* Norwalk, CT: Appleton-Century-Crofts.

Watson, J. (2005). *Caring science as sacred science.* Philadelphia, PA: F. A. Davis.

Watson, R., Hoogbruin, A. L., Rumeu, C., Beunza, M., Barbarin, B., Macdonald, J., & McCready, T. (2003). Differences and similarities in the perception of caring between Spanish and UK nurses. *Journal of Clinical Nursing, 12*(1), 85–92.

West, B. (2007). *Where medicine went wrong, rediscovering the path to complexity.* Singapore: World Scientific.

Widmark-Petersson, V., von Essen, L., et al. (2000). Perceptions of caring among patients with cancer and their staff: Differences and disagreements. *Cancer Nursing, 23*(1), 32–39.

22

Nurses' Caring for Self: A Four-Country Descriptive Study (England, Israel, New Zealand, and the United States)

John Nelson, Michal Itzhaki, Mally Ehrenfeld, Allison Tinker, Mary Ann Hozak, and Sandy Johnson

*T*his chapter examines self-care as reported by 636 staff members who work in health care in four countries: England, Israel, New Zealand, and the United States. The Caring Factor Survey–Caring for Self (CFS-CS), premised on Watson's theory of Caritas, was the 10-item survey used to assess self-caring behaviors. Theoretically, if one cares for self using these 10 behaviors, Caritas for self will be perceived and, thus, integration/healing of body, mind, and spirit will occur. Results revealed differences among participating countries, facility, and unit type. Results also revealed that those with the highest self-care scores reported that their involvement with spirituality supported their belief that self-care is important.

Data in this chapter include those from previous chapters of this book, plus data from Israel and New Zealand (which is part of a larger project in self-care)—leaders of this project are identified in the acknowledgments at the end of this chapter. The largest sample, which came from the United States ($n = 528$), includes four different hospitals that used the CFS-CS. Studies these samples were derived from have been described in detail in Chapters 4 by Iris Lawrence et al. and 12 by Mary Ann Hozak and Maria Brennan. Samples 1 and 2 from Hozak and Brennan which is described in Chapter 12 had 347 and 80 respondents, respectively. Sample 3 from Johnson which is described in Appendix G had 87 respondents, and sample 4 from Lawrence and described in Chapter 4 had 14 respondents. The fourth sample, from England, has been described in Chapter 19 by Allison Tinker, Janina M. Sweetenham, and John Nelson. The fifth sample is from Israel ($n = 71$) and the sixth from New Zealand ($n = 8$). Similarities of countries as well as differences are examined among the 636 staff from health care who responded to this survey in 2010.

BACKGROUND

The Caritas Process of self-care is actually within Caritas Process 1, "Cultivating the Practice of Loving Kindness and Equanimity Toward Self and Others" (Watson, 2008). The CFS-CS was developed to measure caring of self, using all 10 concepts of Caritas. In more common language, this Caritas Process has been termed "loving kindness." Thus, loving kindness toward self is considered Caritas Process 1.

Other Caritas Processes follow in order. Caritas Process 2 is being sustaining and honoring one's own faith and hope. Caritas Process 3 is cultivation of one's own spiritual practices. Caritas Process 4 is taking time for relationships. Caritas Process 5 is being able to accept one's self, both the positive and negative. Caritas Process 6 is taking time to creatively solve problems within one's life. Caritas Process 7 is taking time for knowledge acquisition. Caritas Process 8 is creating a healing environment for oneself. Caritas Process 9 is tending to one's basic needs in life. Finally, Caritas Process 10 is allowing oneself to believe in the impossible; to believe in miracles.

METHODS

Methods for the four studies in the United States and the English study have been described in their respective chapters. The data from Israel and New Zealand are from a larger study that is looking at the relationship between self-care and compassion fatigue and burnout. Data from Israel were acquired by giving hard-copy surveys on self-care to 71 registered nurses who are learning at the Graduate Studies Program for Nurses (BA Program for Registered Nurses) at the School of Nursing, the School of Health Professions at Tel Aviv University. These nurses work at different hospitals and medical clinics at the center of Israel. Surveys were mailed to a survey management company so data could be entered and analyzed. There was a 100% response rate. New Zealand, in contrast, used an electronic survey to send to 200 nursing staffers and 8 were returned, a 4% response rate. Data from all six data sets were combined into a single data set using SPSS 19.0. Descriptive statistics and results from the ANOVA procedure are used to describe the similarities, rank order of self-care concepts, and differences between country and facility. An alpha level of .05 was selected to compare differences of mean scores between countries and facilities.

Two additional methods of analysis were used to understand the international data set of the CFS-CS more deeply. Pattern analysis of the bar graphs on unit/department comparisons were used when sample sizes were too small by unit, but an understanding of possible differences was desired. Finally, qualitative data were used to understand the high- and low-scoring CFS-CS scores. These concepts are consistent with Parato mathematics, using outliers to understand the extreme-success data points as well as the extreme-vulnerable scores in relation to self-care. Limitations of this process include lack of measuring possible, confounding variables. In addition, the small and unequal sample sizes within the four-country data set may lead to biases that must be considered within interpretation and possible follow-up studies.

RESULTS

Examination of the aggregate results revealed that respondents were most tentative to knowledge acquisition. Second was taking time for relationships, faith and hope, allowing miracles, tending to one's basic needs, taking time for problem solving, creating a healing environment, allowing one's self to look at both positive and negative personal qualities, spirituality, and treating oneself with loving kindness. All Caritas Processes were above the midpoint of 4.0 on the 1–7 Likert scale. These findings are graphically depicted in Figure 22.1.

Upon examination of the individual items in the CFS-CS, it is interesting to note that the items with the most nonresponders were those that related to spirituality and miracles (Table 22.1). Further examination of the mean scores revealed that each of the 10 Caritas Processes's scores

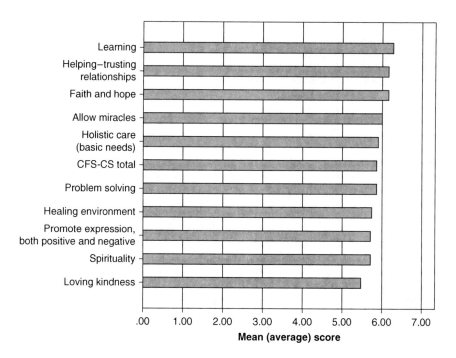

FIGURE 22.1   Aggregate scores, Caring Factor Survey–Caring for Self (CFS-CS).

TABLE 22.1 Descriptive Statistics, Caring Factor Survey–Caring for Self (CFS-CS)

CARITAS CONCEPT	n	MINIMUM	MAXIMUM	MEAN	STD DEVIATION
Loving kindness	635	1.00	7.00	5.4756	1.58282
Problem solving	635	1.00	7.00	5.8661	1.21610
Faith and hope	635	1.00	7.00	6.1465	1.20552
Learning	634	1.00	7.00	6.2776	1.05095
Spirituality	609	1.00	7.00	5.7192	1.44583
Healing environment	634	1.00	7.00	5.7445	1.39996
Relationships	634	1.00	7.00	6.1688	1.14020
Holistic care	633	1.00	7.00	5.9068	1.24620
Promote expression	634	1.00	7.00	5.7256	1.38615
Allow miracles	600	1.00	7.00	5.9750	1.32815
CFS-CS total	605	1.00	7.00	5.8864	1.01287

ranged from a low of 1.0 to a high of 7.0. Each process also had a standard deviation between 1.01 (learning) and 1.58 (loving kindness).

This size variance indicates that there are differences within the aggregate data, and demographics were examined further to identify where the differences may exist. The first demographic to be examined was differences between countries. An ANOVA procedure revealed that 8 of the 10 concepts of Caritas for self were statistically significant. The total CFS-CS score was also statistically significant using an alpha of .05. The only two items from the CFS-CS that were not statistically significant when comparing countries were the mean scores for relationships and loving kindness.

Upon examining patterns between countries, the sample from New Zealand had the lowest score for 7 of 10 Caritas Processes including relationships, learning, faith and hope, problem solving, loving kindness, holistic care (basic needs), and spirituality. The total CFS-CS score, which is all Caritas Processes combined, was also the lowest in New Zealand. The combined samples from the United States reported the highest mean scores for 9 of 10 Caritas Processes. The only process that did not have the highest score for the United States was faith and hope (Figure 22.2).

All countries but the United States had one facility only; thus the four facilities in the United States were examined to see if there were differences within the high scores reported in Figure 22.2. Using a one-way ANOVA, comparisons were made of the facility in California ($n = 71$ and described in Johnson, 2011), New Jersey sites 1 and 2 ($n = 347$ and 80, respectively, and described in Hozak & Brennen, 2011), and the facility in Florida ($n = 14$ and described in detail in Chapter 4 by Iris Lawrence et al.) Statistically significant differences were found for all but two of the CFS-CS items and the total CFS-CS score. This difference was found using

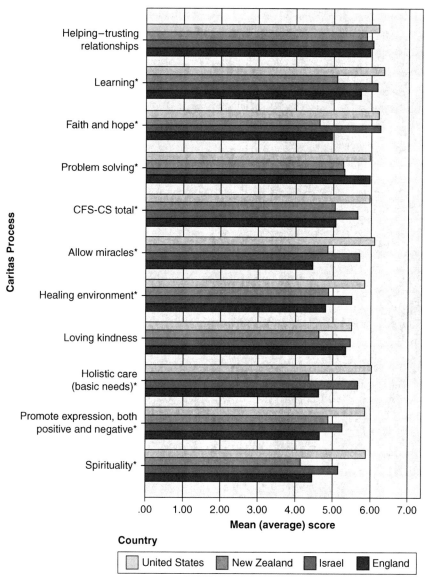

*Statistically significant difference using an alpha of .05.

FIGURE 22.2   CFS-CS mean scores, comparing countries.

an alpha of .05. The only two items in the CFS-CS that were not statistically significant were the reports of miracles and holistic care (Figure 22.3).

Examination of the patterns of the facilities in the United States revealed that the two facilities from New Jersey, which were from the same two-hospital system, scored the highest for 8 of 10 items in the CFS-CS. The only two items in the New Jersey facilities that were not the highest were perception of learning and miracles.

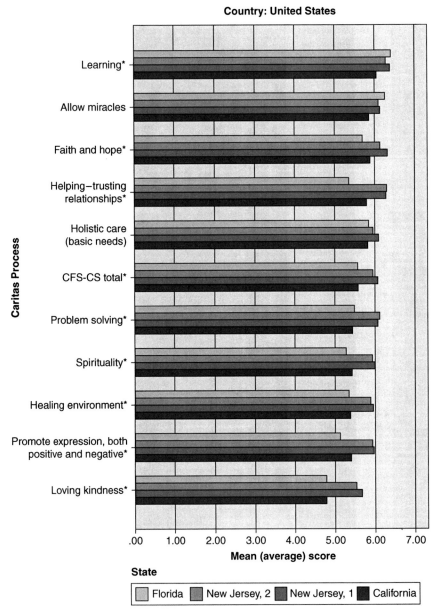

FIGURE 22.3 CFS-CS score by facility in the United States.

*Statistically significant difference using an alpha of .05.

It was further examined to see if there were differences between unit/department types. The units with at least five responders were graphed to compare differences. Numbers of respondents for each unit/department with five or more are noted in Table 22.2.

TABLE 22.2 Number of Respondents Per Unit/Department

UNIT	AGGREGATE	UNITED STATES	ISRAEL	ENGLAND	NEW ZEALAND
Home care/care management	66	34	3	29	–
Food/nutrition	58	58	–	–	–
Pediatrics	56	46	10	–	–
Environmental services/ housekeeping	46	46	–	–	–
Administration	45	45	–	–	–
Critical care	37	35	2	–	–
Operating room/theater	31	19	12	–	–
Emergency dept.	22	18	4	–	–
Education/training	21	17	4	–	–
Mental health	18	15	3	–	–
Obstetrics	16	13	3	–	–
Medical unit	13	3	10	–	–
Pharmacy	13	13	–	–	–
Telemetry	13	13	–	–	–
Radiology	12	12	–	–	–
Geriatrics	10	-	10	–	–
Patient access	9	9	–	–	–
Chronic hemodialysis	8	8	–	–	–
Endoscopy	7	7	–	–	–
Quality management	6	6	–	–	–
Patient relations	5	5	–	–	–
Recovery	5	5	–	–	–
Respiratory therapy	5	5	–	–	–
Surgical unit	5	5	–	–	–
Other	109	91	10	–	8
Total	636	528	71	29	8

The sample sizes were too small to evaluate for statistical significance when comparing differences between units using an alpha of .05. However, patterns with the bar graph of units reveal differences from unit to unit within the same facility. This pattern analysis was conducted for the United States and Israel, both of which had a variety of responding units. Only the total CFS-CS score was examined.

For the United States data, it is noted in Figure 22.4 that some units (e.g., operating room/theater) had a difference between facilities of more

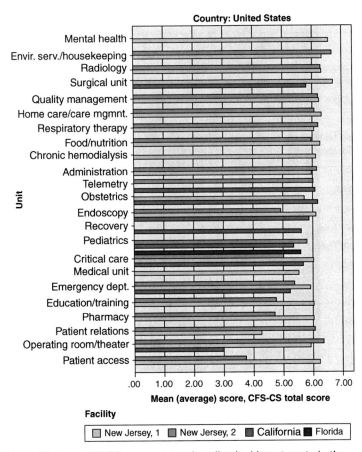

FIGURE 22.4   The total CFS-CS score, comparing all units/departments in the United States.

than 3.0, which on a 1–7 scale, with an adequate sample size, would be statistically significant using an alpha of .05. It is also noted that within the same system within New Jersey, departments (e.g., endoscopy) have a difference of greater than 1.0, which, based on the author's experience of doing statistics for over 10 years, would be statistically significant with an adequate sample size using an alpha of .05 with adequate power and effect size. The final comment regarding the United States data relates to the range of mean scores with several units' mean score being between 3 and 5; thus several within the distribution of each unit would be below 4.0. Scores below 4.0 indicate that the employees disagree that they are conducting self-care. This is discussed further in the chapter but identification of this element of the data is important.

Upon examination of the data from Israel, it is noted that all units/departments were above the midpoint of 4.0. Education/training, followed

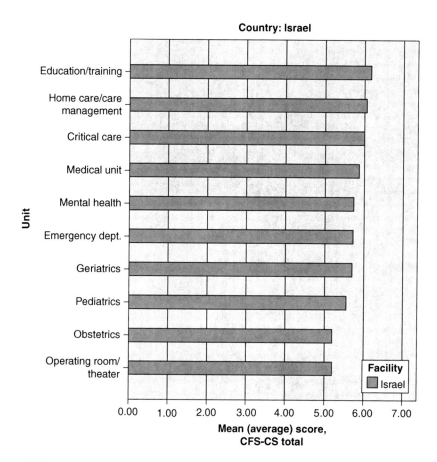

FIGURE 22.5 The total CFS-CS score, comparing all units/departments in Israel.

by home care, were the two highest-ranking units/departments for self-care. The operating room/theater was ranked last. Recall that the operating room/theater was also ranked lowest for the California hospital. The range from among the units was almost 1.0 (Figure 22.5).

Qualitative data were used to examine the thought processes of those who scored 6.5 or greater and those who scored 1.5 or less. The high scores are discussed first.

There were 195 who reported 6.5 or greater on a 1–7 scale, which represents 31% of the respondents. Among the 195 respondents who scored 6.5 or greater, 158 provided comments related to why they responded the way they did. The 158 comments were examined for themes and four were identified, including spirituality, view toward care for others as one cares for self, positive attitude, and family. The comments were themed, dummy coded, and bar graphed by frequency to understand prevalence of each theme of comments (Figure 22.6).

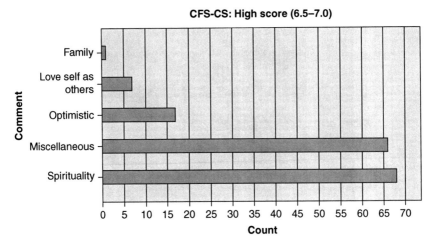

FIGURE 22.6 Comment themes for respondents with high CFS-CS scores (>6.5).

It is noted in Figure 22.6 that there were 68 comments that related to spirituality being the supporting reason they do self-care. Comments regarding spirituality included comments from all religions. It has been identified that religiosity and spirituality are not the same construct, but have overlap and both have positive benefits which are described in Chapter 1 by Nelson, DiNapoli, Turkel, and Watson. A few of the comments have been provided as quotes to illustrate views of how spirituality supports the behaviors of self-care. Each quote was taken from the response of a different individual:

I do believe in a higher power that guides me in caring for all of my needs and concerns and allows me to embrace who I am.

I believe in God and He has given me the ability to love and care for myself.

I am an individual who has a deep belief in God and Christ's teachings. Therefore I treat myself and others in a way that is pleasing to God.

Deep belief in loving kindness, middle ground, karma, tonglen to help others; gleaned from Buddhist teachings, readings and audio.

I attend bible study classes at my synagogue and have received training here that sensitizes me to my own spiritual needs.

Optimism was the second most common theme noted among the comments related to why the respondents responded as they did. Following are a couple of comments to illustrate this view:

Positive attitude and make the most and the best, given the situation.

Positive optimistic outlook on my life and the people affected by me.

Caring for self prior to caring for others was viewed as asserted by seven of the respondents. Two comments that illustrate this view are noted next:

> I need to care for myself so that I can give of myself to family, friends, coworkers and patients. I sometimes have to sacrifice some things in life to maintain rest and health. The big picture is that I can then be a better me.

> Believe I should take care of myself as I would someone else that I love.

Finally, for high-scoring individuals, the family was the fourth identified recurrent concept for promoting self-care. A couple of comments are noted next:

> My family support system is a big part of my life that allows me to maintain a positive outlook in life. Having a healthy marriage has also aided in answering these questions. I take the time to take care of myself first.

> Family upbringing.

Looking at the scores that were less than 1.5, there were only seven comments; thus, all scores that were less than 4.0 were examined because this is below the midpoint on a 1–7 Likert scale. There were 15 comments below 4.0 and all comments were themed or labeled. Miscellaneous comments included comments that were too brief to interpret for theming.

There were four who reported not doing self-care because there is no time. Other single reasons cited include feeling hopeless, feeling burned out, no belief in self, caring for others, being emotionally drained, and not being spiritual (Figure 22.7).

DISCUSSION

Acquiring knowledge was the highest-ranked score for the 10 caring processes, which is a valid high ranking for a knowledge-dependent profession like health care. In contrast, the lowest-scoring Caritas Processes were treating self with loving kindness and tending to one's spiritual life. This is most striking when considering the qualitative themes for those who scored high (6.5 or greater on a 1–7 Likert scale). According to those who scored high, the primary rationale for performing self-care was spirituality and caring for self before caring for others.

Differences were found between every demographic examined, including country, facility, and unit type. This is consistent with the concept of Caritas that it is not a generalizable concept (Watson, 2005). Thus, Caritas for self must be considered within the context of country,

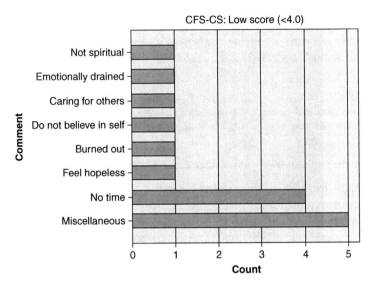

FIGURE 22.7 Comment themes for respondents with low CFS-CS scores (<4.0).

facility, and unit type. These findings are consistent with what was found in the international comparison for Caritas for patients—that concepts must be applied within context and described in detail in Chapter 21.

The use of quantitative data was most helpful by comparing demographics. Pattern analysis of the bar graphs assisted with understanding patterns when sample sizes were too small to detect differences and provided conversation for follow-up studies with larger sample sizes to evaluate if these differences can be replicated. Qualitative data were helpful in understanding the success factors for those who are most consistent with self-care, like spirituality and perspective to care for self first. This approach illustrates how different methods of analysis can be used in combination to facilitate conversations within context.

IMPLICATIONS

Results reveal that context must be considered within programs for self-care. This implies that methods to study an action plan for self-care must go beyond the use of Guassian mathematics, which relies on averages and variance. Comparisons of responses within the variance are helpful, as illustrated in this study, but other methods can be used to supplement understanding.

Outliers can be used for appreciative inquiry that pursues understanding what works well for the purpose of doing more of what works well. According to these data, exploration of spirituality of all faiths and beliefs should support the pursuit of self-care. Considering that spirituality is an aspect in which patients perceive that nurses do not interact within their jobs which is described in this chapter, it may be an aspect within health care that is not universally embraced. Further discussion and inquiry are warranted.

Another element of self-care that should be considered is the architecture of the facility itself. Does the architecture support the concepts of self-care becoming a reality? For example, the Caritas Process of relationships is facilitated by architecture that has cross sections and gathering spaces. Do units that have break rooms, spacious nursing stations, and hallways that crisscross, thus enabling individuals to interact, have higher scores for this concept of self-care? There is currently discussion, among researchers who authored this book, about examining the relationship of the concepts of Caritas and architecture. This same discussion of architecture could be applied to each of the 10 concepts of Caritas, spirituality, learning, and so on.

CONCLUSION

Self-care as it relates to caring for the patient is not understood at this point in the research trajectory. Prior to examining the relationship of self and patient care, more research within context needs to be conducted. In addition, the concept of how self-care, care for others, and the infrastructure relate needs to be examined within theoretical frameworks like that which is articulated by Dossey in the theory of integral nursing (2008). If we can understand self-care, Caritas as a healing intervention for patients and architecture of caring for self and others, we will likely be able to build structures and processes that facilitate Caritas as a central theme in health care.

ACKNOWLEDGMENTS

Acknowledgements to other researchers in the larger international study from the countries of Botswana, Ireland, Israel, New Zealand, Spain, and the United States. Individuals include M. Itzhaki, M. Ehrenfeld, B. Marshall, R. Vernon, D. Dignam, C. Rumeu, N.M. Seboni, N. Phaladze, M. Treacy, P. Larkin, G. Fealy, M. McNamara, and S. Johnson. A special thanks to Nancy Rollins Gantz and Kim Richards for providing the initial connection of these researchers.

REFERENCES

Dossey, B. M. (2008). Theory of integral nursing. *Advances in Nursing Science,* *31*(1), E52–E73.

Watson, J. (2005). *Caring science as sacred science.* Philadelphia, PA: F. A. Davis.

Watson, J. (Ed.). (2008). *Assessing and measuring caring in nursing and health* *science.* New York: Springer.

APPENDICES

Exemplars of Caritas From
Specific Populations

Appendix A

The Holistic Perspective of Nursing: The Caring Factor Survey in a Hospice in Italy

Sollomi Alfonso and Maria Cutrera

Over the centuries, the evolution of nursing has been continuous, including the succession of theories. The most current metaparadigm of nursing proposes the organizational structure of a conceptual/philosophical profession, and consists of four basic concepts: of person, environment, health, and nursing (Fawcett, 1984). From this metaparadigm, the nurse practitioner applies the plan to "care" for the person who has one or more needs and who cannot respond independently. At the core of this plan to care is the concept of caring, which Watson (2005) asserts requires specific skills that are specific to department and to patient. Therefore, application of caring within the profession of nursing requires a careful balance of science and humanism.

Today's health care environment mandates the nurse to accomplish many tasks within an ever-widening scope and responsibility of practice. This fact enhances the challenge to maintain balance of caring and science, especially in clinical areas like hospice where patients look for (and are entitled to) the human qualities of the nurse. Hospice patients look for someone to trust, a prepared companion to accompany him/her through a journey fraught with difficulty. Thus, it is the requirement of the hospice nurse to formulate principles capable of properly structuring the relationship of human care understood as a therapy as well as an attitude of interpersonal solidarity.

Lévinas (1991) interprets care as the fundamental moral principle, expressed with passion! Moreover, he opposes ethics of rights to an ethics of solidarity. The knowledge gained to "care" is special because it is intertwined with the intellectual appreciation of the value of the other. Care in this sense, especially within hospice, requires technical expertise and careful consideration of suffering. The awareness of suffering expresses a feeling of love toward the special characteristics of each individual, which assumes a common and shared responsibility for an ethic of aspiration and gratuity. According to Lévinas (1991), not all possess this skill to develop a good relationship as it requires training that affects the deep structures of personality. Well-skilled deliverers of care can themselves be a drug and yet be unaware of the total effect they may have (Levinas, 1991).

STUDY AIMS

In these structures, assistance more than ever must be considered in a "holistic" sense. From this consideration was born the purpose of a descriptive study, conducted in 2008, that aims to measure whether, in these structures in the provinces of Parma and Reggio Emilia, this caring philosophy is implemented and to know how the patients and/or family members perceive it—in fact, identifying an aspect of "quality" care provided. The purpose of this descriptive study assesses whether, within the philosophical structures in question in the provinces of Parma and Reggio Emilia, the philosophy of "Human Caring" is implemented and to what extent the patients and/or family members identifying the fact as an aspect of "quality" care provided.

THE SETTING: HOSPICE

The hospice is a residential structure designed to accommodate cancer patients in advanced stages of the disease or with symptoms of such severity that patients cannot be treated at home. The hospice, through the relief of symptoms, provides support systems to extend the life of the patient while providing support to the family.

Procedures

The administration of questionnaires took place from June 2008 to October 2008 in the following five hospice facilities:
1. Hospice "Casa Madonna dell'Uliveto"—Albinea (RE)
2. Hospice "La Valle del Sole"—BorgoTaro (PR)
3. Hospice di Fidenza (PR)
4. Hospice "Piccole Figlie" (PR)
5. Hospice di Langhirano (PR)

METHODS

Descriptive statistics were used to understand the mean, range, and standard deviation for each of the Caritas processes. Rank for each process was examined to understand which process may be more operational than others.

RESULTS

Results reveal all 10 Caritas Processes are above the midpoint of 4.0, indicating an overall perception that Caritas is in process within the hospice setting. However, the range and standard deviation reveal that every process is not uniformly perceived. Loving kindness was the highest-ranked process, while allowing to believe in miracles and being supported spiritually were the two lowest-ranked processes. The descriptive statistics are noted in more detail in Table A.1 and graphically depicted in Figure A.1.

DISCUSSION

Results revealed loving kindness, the central focus of the care philosophy, "Caring Human," is fully perceived as a characteristic element of assistance within the hospice setting. In contrast, spiritual support and allowing to believe in miracles were low. This underlines the "personal-intimate" aspect of Caritas.

The data collected and described here are a starting point for continuous improvement of the profession, specifically, in the delivery of caring behaviors. The relationship between health services and the user (patients, relatives, and visitors) is a complex, relational paradigm, within which it is possible to identify a set of specific processes and contexts of study. Recent policy changes have occurred in health services (crisis of the welfare state, administrative decentralization, corporatization, etc.)

TABLE A.1   Descriptive Statistics of All Caritas Processes in Hospice

CARITAS PROCESS	N	MINIMUM	MAXIMUM	MEAN	STD DEVIATION
Practice loving kindness	62	5.00	7.00	6.8065	.43753
Promote expression of feelings	62	3.00	7.00	6.5484	.80322
Helping and trusting relationship	62	2.00	7.00	6.5484	.95261
Teaching and learning	62	3.00	7.00	6.3710	1.04386
Healing environment	62	2.00	7.00	6.3548	1.08789
Problem solving	62	3.00	7.00	6.2742	1.01091
Total CFS	62	3.20	7.00	6.2694	.79457
Instill faith and hope	62	2.00	7.00	6.1935	1.18514
Holistic care	62	1.00	7.00	6.0645	1.30410
Miracles	62	3.00	7.00	5.9516	1.24700
Spiritual beliefs and practices	62	1.00	7.00	5.5806	1.54228

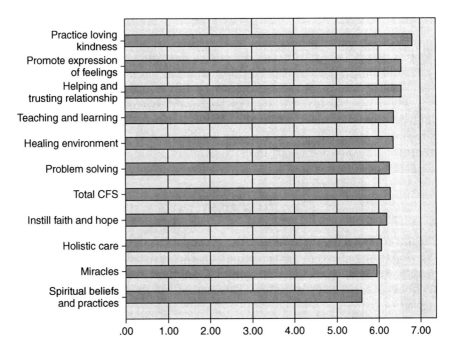

FIGURE A.1   Rank order of all Caritas Processes in the hospice (*n* = 62).

and have amended the trajectory of the nurse–patient interface. This requires a reexamination of how to deepen the understanding of caring within context, to ensure that reformulations of health care policy do not extricate the potential of healing and humanity of caring from the science of nursing. A possible next step for caring science in Italy may be the analysis of the ability of nurses, using the Caring Ability Inventory (CAI) test (Wolf, 2009), and/or the establishment of a multidisciplinary focus group in each local operating unit. The provision of health services, in fact, is increasingly tied to demand from the public and its opinion on satisfaction. In this sense, in our opinion, the rating scale used could have a double significance.

It is obvious that a decisive role is attributed to the person who receives the service; the patient and patient's family, in fact, become a central element around which strategies must be made compatible with the organizational environment, aimed at improving the perceived quality and, therefore, customer satisfaction.

REFERENCES

Fawcett, J. (1984). The metaparadigm of nursing: Current status and future refinements. *Image: The Journal of Nursing Scholarship, 16,* 84–87.

Lévinas, E. L'io e la totalità, in Entre nous. Essais sur le penser-à-l'autre, Grasset, Paris 1991; Italian translation: Tra noi. Saggi sul pensare all'altro, a cura di E. Baccarini, Jaca Book, Milano 1998, p. 47.

Watson, J. (2005). *Caring science as sacred science*. Philadelphia: F. A. Davis.

Wolf, Z. (2009). Caring behaviors inventory and new version of caring behaviors inventory for elders. In J. Watson (Ed.), *Assessing and measuring caring in nursing and health sciences* (2nd ed., pp. 253–260). New York: Springer Publishing.

Appendix B

Caring Behaviors of Community Health Nurses in a Barangay Health Center in Makati City, the Philippines

*Raffiel Jacinto, Kristal Capalungan, Katherine R. Gutierrez,
Sydrick D. G. Gutierrez, Iris Kate R. Llorca,
and Priscila L. Longanilla*

The researchers proposed this study after being exposed in the community to the caring behaviors of the community health nurses toward their clients. It was desired to more deeply understand nurse' ability to operationalize caring behaviors despite the perception that too many patients were coming in and out of the community's health center. Were the nurses able to concomitantly provide high-demand care and caring behaviors?

METHODS

Respondents for this study were the community health nurses and community residents. For the community health nurses, convenience sampling was utilized while purposive, non probability sampling was utilized for the community residents. The researchers utilized a researchers-made questionnaire to gather data regarding the caring behaviors of community health nurses. The respondents answered the items by checking the corresponding number to their answer using a Likert scale, with 5 being the highest ranking and 1 being the lowest. The data gathered were then tallied, analyzed, and interpreted to understand how nurses and patients reported the presence of five caring behaviors.

The five areas of interest and associated definitions were communication, competence, compassion, conscience, and commitment. A brief review of each area of interest is noted below.

1. *Communication* is the means to establish a helping–healing relationship (Potter, 2009). This is facilitated by attentive listening that involves absorbing both the content and the feeling the person is

conveying, without selectivity. Attentive listening conveys an attitude of caring and interest, thereby encouraging the client to talk (Kozier, 2004). According to Paulson (2009), caring nurses listened carefully to patients and responded to their individual, unique situations. Also, according to Kimble (2003), patients who feel cared for are more likely to communicate their needs more effectively, become active participants in their own care, and seek litigation less often.

2. *Competence* reflects caring in who consciously acquires and uses appropriate knowledge, skills, experience, and motivation and energy in assisting another person to grow fully (Roach, 2005).

3. *Compassion* is understood mainly in terms of empathy, the ability to enter into and, to some extent, share others' suffering (Tschudin, 2004).

4. *Conscience* is loyalty to oneself that should be respected in a person and in others as an innate right, and as a duty in responding to something greater than oneself. When conscience is allowed to be dulled or rationalized, it can result in behavior that may be less than admirable or excellent (Tschudin, 2004).

5. *Commitment* inspires us to be and do our best (Gordon, 2001).

Respondents, both nurses and patients, used the following guide for responding about perception of the presence of the five behaviors: 5 = always (10 out of 10 situations); 4 = often (7 out of 10 situations); 3 = sometimes (4 out of 10 situations); 2 = rarely (1 out of 10 situations); and 1 = never (0 out of 10 situations) (see Table B.1).

RESULTS

The extent of performance of caring behaviors of the community health nurses as perceived by themselves, according to the following components, shows that conscience is performed more often than the other components with a mean of 4.81. Compassion is ranked lowest as to the performance of caring behaviors with a mean of 4.43. The other components are as follows: competence mean was 4.73; communication was 4.58; and commitment

TABLE B.1 Qualitative Interpretation of Mean Scores

MEAN SCORE	QUALITATIVE INTERPRETATION
4.21–5.00	Very great extent
3.41–4.20	Great extent
2.61–3.40	Moderate extent
1.81–2.60	Minimal extent
1.00–1.80	No extent

TABLE B.2   Comparing Mean Scores of Community Health Nurses and Residents

RESPONDENTS	MEAN	COMPUTED T-VALUE	CRITICAL T-VALUE	DECISION
Community health nurse	4.62	4.83	1.96	Rejected
Residents	4.18			

mean was 4.56. Collectively, the grand mean of the caring behaviors as perceived by the community health nurses is 4.62.

The extent of performance of caring behaviors of the community health nurses as perceived by the community residents shows that conscience is still the most performed behavior as compared with the other components, with a mean of 4.39. Commitment was ranked lowest as to the performance of caring behaviors, with a grand mean of 3.89. The other components are as follows: competence had a mean of 4.35, communication was 4.16, and compassion had a mean of 4.11. The extent of performance of caring behaviors of community health nurses, as perceived by the community residents, was 4.18.

There is a large difference between the perceived performance of the caring behaviors of community health nurses themselves and community residents, with the effect size of 0.9 using Cohen's d.

In the hypothesis, the computed value of 4.84 is greater than the tabulated value of 1.96; thus the hypothesis was rejected, which means that there is a significant difference between the perceived performance of the caring behaviors of community health nurses themselves and community residents (see Table B.2).

CONCLUSION

The researchers therefore conclude that both community health nurses and community residents perceive the community health nurses, caring behavior differently.

RECOMMENDATIONS

Considering the aforementioned summary of findings and conclusion, the following was recommended:

To the *Nursing Educators:* Use the results of this study to put more emphasis on the utilization of the identified lowest components, specifically compassion and commitment of caring, when teaching the students.

To the *Community Health Nurse:* Utilize the results of this research to provide quality nursing care to the community residents by enhancing the caring behavior that is least utilized.

To the *Makati Health Department:* Use the results of the study to initiate programs like seminars and forums that are based on the least utilized components of caring behavior, particularly compassion and commitment, for continuous improvement of quality nursing care in the community health center. Examples could be:

- Nursing procedures update seminar
- Interpersonal relationship development programs
- Seminars for compassion and commitment in nursing
- Personal and professional development programs
- Customer service seminar

To the *future researchers:*
- Conduct a similar study that will include all the nurses in all the Barangay health centers in Makati and include a greater number of community residents as respondents.
- Conduct the same study that will include the sociodemographic profiles of both the community health nurses and the residents.
- Conduct the same study in different locations or on a larger scale and use the results of the study for a better understanding of the caring behaviors of community health nurses.

REFERENCE

Potter, P. A., & Perry, A. G. (2009). *Fundamentals of nursing* (7th ed.). St. Louis, MO: Mosby Elsevier.

Appendix C

Extent of Utilization of the Clinical Caritas Process as Perceived by Nurses in the Philippines

*Rea Anna B. Buenaventura, Gino Angelo S. Aloc,
Gernalyn M. Antonio, Maritess M. Bedona, Gail Franka C.
Beligrado, and Christelle Jolie O. Bulala*

Nurses play an important role in a patient's healing process. Complicating the ability to care is the increasing workload of nurses brought about by the increasing nurse to patient ratio. According to the international standard, the ideal ratio of nurses to patients in hospitals is 1:4. However in the Philippines, the ideal is often overlooked and nurses may have up to nine patients each. Clinical nurses have been drilled in the importance of completing their assignments before the end of the shift (Iyer, 2006). Hence, the disproportional ratio, the medical management that is needed to be implemented accurately and timely, and the demands of the patient incline the nurses to accomplish all tasks first, then "care" later.

PURPOSE OF THE STUDY

This study sought to understand the extent of the utilization of the Clinical Caritas Process as perceived by the staff nurses and the unit managers in standard units and critical care units.

METHODS

This study was conducted on standard and critical care units in a private, 570-bed, tertiary hospital in Makati City, the Philippines. The five standard units included the 9th floor (Suite), 8th floor (Medical-Surgical, Communicable Diseases), 7th floor (Medical-Surgical), 6th floor

(Medical Surgical, Pediatric), 5th floor (OB-GYN, Medical Surgical) nursing units, and the Carlos P. Manahan (CPM Ward). Critical care units included a medical intensive care unit, a surgical intensive care unit, neuroscience, telemetry, newborn services, a pediatric intensive care unit, and nurses of the cardio rehab and pain (CATLAP) department. Data were collected from September 15 to September 20, 2009. The researchers focused on the staff nurses working in the said areas that are rendering direct patient care and are regular employees of the hospital, and the unit managers in charge of planning, organizing, coordinating, and directing activities of one unit.

Staff nurses were given survey forms for them to answer that focused on their own perception of up to what extent they utilize the Clinical Caritas Process as proposed by Watson (2005). The unit managers were also given survey forms that will show their perceptions of the extent of utilization of the Clinical Caritas Process of the staff nurses in the said unit as a whole.

The survey was developed by the researchers of this study, using the 10 concepts of caring within Watson's theory of Caritas. There were 53 items within the new instrument. Items 1–5 describe the first clinical Caritas, which is the practice of loving kindness within the context of caring consciousness; 6–10 describe being authentically present and enabling the beliefs of the one being cared for and the one giving care; 11–15 denote cultivation of one's own spiritual practices, going beyond self, opening to others with compassion and sensitivity; 16–21 denote developing and maintaining a trusting, authentic, caring relationship; 22–27 denote being present to and supporting the positive and negative feelings with a connection to a deeper spirit; numbers 28–32 refer to clinical Caritas no. 6, which is the creative use of self; 33–37 stand for Caritas no. 7, which is engaging in a genuine teaching and learning experience; numbers 38–42 are for creating a healing environment at all levels; 43–48 are for assisting with patients' needs with a caring consciousness to align mind-body-spirit; and numbers 49–53 represent Caritas no. 10, which is soul care for the one being cared for.

The instrument was designed to inquire about how frequently the concept of Caritas was used within practice. The survey used a Likert scale that gave the respondent five choices: 5 = always (10 out of 10 situations); 4 = often (7 out of 10 situations); 3 = sometimes (4 out of 10 situations); 2 = rarely (1 out of 10 situations); and 1 = never (0 out of 10 situations). Responses were then sorted by mean scores for each concept in relationship to the extent the concept was used in practice (see Table C.1).

A t-test would be used to compare the difference between staff nurses and managers, using an alpha of .05. A t-test would also be used to compare the differences of response between staff nurses and managers.

TABLE C.1 Qualitative Interpretation of Mean Scores

MEAN SCORE	QUALITATIVE INTERPRETATION
4.21–5.00	Very great extent
3.41–4.20	Great extent
2.61–3.40	Moderate extent
1.81–2.60	Minimal extent
1.00–1.80	No extent

RESULTS

There were 138 nurses who responded from standard units, 48 from critical care, and 10 unit managers. Upon examination of the responses from the nurses, loving kindness was ranked first, and authentic presence was ranked last. All 10 concepts of Caritas were reported to be used to a very great extent (see Table C.2).

TABLE C.2 Responses of All Staff Nurses (From Both Standard and Critical Care Units)

CLINICAL CARITAS PROCESS	WEIGHTED MEAN	QUALITATIVE INTERPRETATION
Practice of loving kindness within the context of caring consciousness	4.65	Very great extent
Being authentically present and enabling the beliefs of the one being cared for and the one giving care	4.25	Very great extent
Cultivation of one's spiritual practices, going beyond self, opening to others with compassion and sensitivity	4.55	Very great extent
Developing and maintaining a trusting, authentic, caring relationship	4.49	Very great extent
Being present for and supporting the positive and negative feelings with a connection to a deeper spirit	4.48	Very great extent
Creative use of self	4.45	Very great extent
Engaging in a genuine teaching and learning experience	4.51	Very great extent
Creating a healing environment at all levels	4.42	Very great extent
Assisting with basic needs with a caring consciousness to align mind, body, spirit	4.46	Very great extent
Soul-care for the one being cared for	4.46	Very great extent

TABLE C.3   Responses of All Managers

CLINICAL CARITAS PROCESS	WEIGHTED MEAN	VERBAL INTERPRETATION
Practice of loving kindness within the context of caring consciousness	4.44	Very great extent
Being authentically present and enabling the beliefs of the one being cared for and the one giving care	3.92	Great extent
Cultivation of one's spiritual practices, going beyond self, opening to others with compassion and sensitivity.	4.42	Very ereat extent
Developing and maintaining a trusting, authentic, caring relationship	4.1	Great extent
Being present for and supporting the positive and negative feelings with a connection to a deeper spirit	4.47	Very great extent
Creative use of self	4.46	Very great extent
Engaging in a genuine teaching and learning experience	4.36	Very great extent
Creating a healing environment at all levels	4.25	Very great extent
Assisting with basic needs with a caring consciousness to align mind, body, spirit	4.50	Very great extent
Soul-care for the one being cared for	4.16	Great extent

When looking at the manager responses, it was noted that meeting the patients' basic needs was ranked first. Being authentically present was ranked last (see Table C.3).

When combining the total score for all Caritas processes as reported by staff nurses, it was noted that the standard units were 4.44 and the critical care units were 4.42. Both these scores were in the "very great extent" range. The t-test revealed the difference between these two scores was not statistically significant.

When combining the total score for all Caritas processes as reported by managers, it was noted that the standard units were 4.33 and the critical care units were 4.25. Both these scores were in the "very great extent" range. The t-test revealed the difference between these two scores was not statistically significant.

Comparison of the staff nurses' and managers' total scores did not reveal any difference that was statistically significant. This was true for both the standard and critical care units.

CONCLUSION

Based on the analysis and interpretation of the findings, it is therefore concluded that nurses are caring, and utilization of the Clinical Caritas Processes is evident in work performance in the selected tertiary hospital in the Philippines.

RECOMMENDATIONS

Based on the summary of findings and the conclusion, the researchers recommend the following:

To the *Nursing Service Division:*
- Use this study as a basis for planning and developing trainings and programs that will improve caring behaviors and the staff nurses' competencies.
- Use this study in putting emphasis on the value of providing genuine, caring behavior toward patients.

To the *Faculty:*
- Use the results of this study to put emphasis on the importance of a patient-centered, genuine kind of care in their curriculum. For Theoretical Foundation in the first year of Bachelor of Science Nursing, hold in-depth discussions on Jean Watson's Clinical Caritas Process because it is the core of being a nurse. For Personal, Moral, Social Development, V and VI, wherein the discussions revolve around "me, as a caring nurse" and "me, as a spiritual nurse," the faculty could put greater emphasis on the value of caring behavior.
- Use the results of this study and its questionnaire in evaluating the students' caring behavior.
- Use the results of this study to teach the students that, apart from the general nursing care that they will apply in their future workplaces, applying the clinical Caritas Process also plays a major role in the provision of holistic care for patients.
- Use the results of this study to instill the value of caring as the core of nursing and to show that it can help in the healing process of their patients.

To the *future researchers:*
- Use this study and its results as reference for further similar studies in different settings such as public hospitals, community settings, and specialized hospitals.
- Make a qualitative study about the way the nurses perceive their caring behavior.

Appendix D

The Presence of Caring Among Long-Term Care Nurses in the United States

Melinda M. Phillips and Linda S. Rieg

A s a profession, nursing has had caring as its foundation and central focus. In early centuries the motive for caring was understood as following Christ's example and living out His command to love and care for others. Nursing grew out of this call to fulfill God's command—to love one another and minister to the needy and outcasts of society (Mt. 25:31–46; Heb. 13:1–3; Jas. 1:27). In more recent history, nursing as a call to serve God was demonstrated when Catholics formed the Sisters of Charity and Sisters of Mercy; Protestants established the Kaiserwerth Institute, the training organization of Florence Nightingale (Trafecanty, 2006).

Influenced by modern-era thinking, nursing made an effort to become more "scientific" and thus earn respect as a true profession. As a result, these caring roots were often ignored and at times even shunned. In recent years the nursing profession has witnessed a movement to reestablish caring as the heart of nursing. However, the roots of caring in postmodern thinking have not been embedded in Christianity and the transcendent God, but are often based on humanism and a spirituality of being one with the universe (Watson, 2007).

CARING AS A NURSING PHENOMENON

The study of human caring as an essential characteristic of nursing practice has gradually expanded from early definitional, philosophical, and cultural writing on the meaning of caring (Boykin & Schoenhofer, 2001). Caring has been analyzed extensively, and comprehensively discussed in the nursing literature. Cook and Cullen (2003) described caring as the essential component of nursing. Caring has been described as the central core of all that is nursing (Bassett, 2002) and the major construct of contemporary nursing (Rawnsley, 1990). Leininger (1991, p. 44) recognized caring as the "essence of nursing and a distinct, dominant, central and unifying focus" for nursing practice.

Watson (2007) acknowledged Erikson's work, including the term *caritas* as reflecting love. The theory of human caring evolved as Watson's perspective of the caring process and the science of caring expanded. She translated her original Carative Factors into clinical Caritas Processes. According to Watson, the major differentiation between the Carative Factors and her more recent clinical Caritas framework focuses on the element of spirituality.

Although the term *caritas* is used to connote love, the source of *caritas* is not similarly described. Within Watson's clinical Caritas Processes, "This relationship between love and caring connotes inner healing for self and others, extending to nature, and the larger universe, unfolding and evolving within a cosmology that is both metaphysical and transcendent with the coevolving human in the universe" (Watson, 2007). In other words, it stems from within and extends out. Within the Judeo-Christian perspective, the source of Caritas is God, because God is love. Because of a loving relationship with God, we are compelled to love others, including providing culturally based care for all. It is this source of love that motivates caring.

PURPOSE OF THE STUDY

The purpose of this study was to evaluate the presence of caring by long-term care (LTC) nurses, administrative personnel, and nursing students and its effect on healing. Caring, as perceived by the residents, was also explored.

RESEARCH ITEMS

Based on the principal researcher's experience in LTC, and an extensive review of the literature, the study included the following areas:

1. How do LTC nurses view caring and caring behaviors?
2. Do facility residents sense the presence of caring among the nursing staff?
3. Do administrative personnel and nursing students perceive caring as an important component to healing?

Responses to the items were determined through the data analysis and interpretation process. Additional information was gleaned through analysis of the findings.

METHODOLOGY

This exploratory, descriptive, correlational study used a purposive sample of 20 alert and oriented LTC residents (10 from each of two facilities, identified as CE and ME), 10 nurses (5 from CE and 5 from ME), 3 members of administration (2 from CE and 1 from ME), and 9 nursing students; the total sample size was 42 participants. Permission to use Jean Watson's Caring Factor Survey (CFS) and Caring Factor Survey–Care Provider Version (CFS-CPV) as instruments for this study was granted.

There was a total of 44 participants in the sample from two different facilities, CE and ME. The residents were chosen on a voluntary basis, and for those who volunteered the unit managers and the principal researcher decided together which residents met the criteria for subjects in this study. Participants were chosen strictly on the basis of mental capacity, and each resident had to be his or her own power of attorney.

The CFS consisted of 10 items regarding the residents' perceptions of the caring behaviors provided by the nurses in their facility. The remainder of the participants were given the CFS-CPV (comprising 20 items with response ranges identical to the CFS), which they completed during the time that the data were being collected from the residents.

RESULTS

The makeup of each group was as follows: there were 5 nurses in each group for CE and ME, 10 patients in each group, and 2 administrators in CE and 1 administrator in ME. The remaining 9 of the 42 were students and were not divided by CE and ME. They were thus not included in this analysis. The t test included 17 in the CE group and 16 in the ME group.

A power analysis using an alpha of .05 and an effect size of .30 revealed low power of .21; thus an alpha of .15 was used to decrease the likelihood of committing a type II error of falsely accepting the null hypothesis. A significance of $p < .15$ was chosen because levels of significance less than .05 were judged to be too stringent, causing more type II errors. It was recognized that .15 was a liberal p level to use; but considering this was an exploratory study, relationships that may exist within the study's theoretical framework might have been missed if a more strict p level of .05 had been used.

When comparing the grouping of CE and ME, the only differences at the 0.15 level were for loving kindness (mean difference of .678, p of .123) and for helping/trusting relationship (mean difference of .998, p of .012). The ME group perceived more caring for 8 of 10 caring factors, plus more caring for the total caring score, derived from all factors combined (Figure D.1).

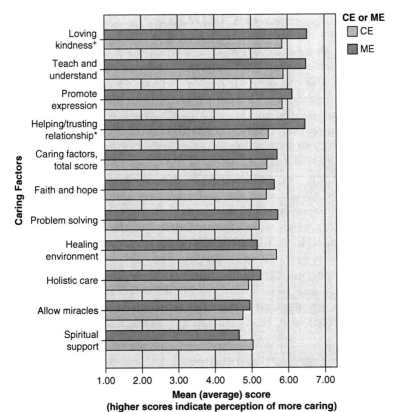

*Statistically significant using an alpha of .05; +statistically significant using an alpha of .15.

FIGURE D.1   Caring factors, comparing CE and ME groupings.

Differences Comparing Roles

The four groups of roles were compared using a one-way ANOVA. Groups included students ($n = 9$), nurses ($n = 10$), administrators ($n = 3$), and patients ($n = 20$). Results revealed statistically significant differences at the .15 level, including: instilling faith/hope (F 3.22, p .033); spiritual support (F 9.45, p .00009); holistic care (F 6.73, p .001); promotions of expression (F 3.63, p .021); allow miracles (F 14.35, p .000002); healing environment (F 2.13, p .112); and the total CFS score (F 5.41, p .003). The most interesting overall pattern noted was that the only caring factor that patients were more satisfied with than nurses was the perception of a helping/trusting relationship (Figure D.2).

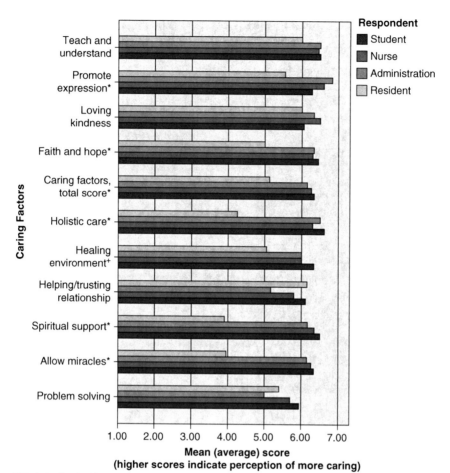

*Statistically significant using an alpha of .05; +statistically significant using an alpha of .15.

FIGURE D.2 Comparing four roles.

IMPLICATIONS AND RECOMMENDATIONS

As the findings of this study suggest, the only caring factor that residents in both facilities found more satisfactory than did the nurses was the perception of the helping/trusting relationship. Based on this finding alone, it is clear that these nurses perceive that they are demonstrating caring behaviors with residents, but the residents' perceptions do not reflect the same level of caring.

There could be many reasons for some of these differences. Perhaps the most important factor would be not having a clear understanding of what the residents identify as caring behaviors. Future qualitative studies should be conducted to identify how residents individually and as a group define caring behaviors. It may be that nurses are doing many things they perceive as caring, without clearly understanding the meaning as defined by the residents.

Additional research needs to be conducted to determine the "source" of caring. Some have identified the source of caring as coming from human transcendence, professional ethics, or personal experiences. Christian nurses have identified the source of caring as their relationship with Christ. They quote Christ's teaching: "I tell you the truth, whatever you did for one of the least of these brothers of mine, you did for me" (Matthew 25:40 NIV). They believe they must care for others as if they were caring for Christ. This meaning is reflective of Nightingale's writings that describe nursing as a calling or vocation. This Caritas is the motivation for purposeful service to others: "For we are God's masterpiece. He has created us anew in Christ Jesus, so we can do the good things He planned for us long ago" (Ephesians 2:10, NLT).

It is important to evaluate if caring is something that can be learned through education, or if it is deeper—the personal values derived from our worldview that guide caring behaviors. In order to provide meaningful care to residents, it is essential for nurses to become more self-aware of the cultural perspectives they bring into the relationship.

CONCLUSION

The problem of nurses and nursing assistants who do not seem to care is urgent and must be addressed. Policies should be designed to help ensure the social, financial, physical, and psychological safety of the elderly and their caregivers. This would include: investing in attracting and retaining high-quality caregivers; implementing consistent assignments; and providing continuing education specific to the geriatric population. It would also include delivery-care environments and systems that promote caring—rather than task-oriented, cure-focused care. A renewed respect for the value of the elderly must be fostered by nurses who will advocate for reforms that will provide protection and dignity for those in their final years. In addition, resources need to be available for gerontology nurses to achieve their professional goals and to strengthen their knowledge and skills, so they can give the elderly the best care to meet their needs.

REFERENCES

Bassett, C. (2002). Nurses' perceptions of care and caring. *International Journal of Nursing Practice, 8*, 8–15.

Boykin, A., & Schoenhofer, S. (2001). *Nursing as caring: A model for transforming practice.* Sudbury, MA: Jones and Bartlett.

Cook, P. R., & Cullen, J. A. (2003). Caring as an imperative for nursing education. *Nursing Education Perspectives, 24*, 192–197.

Leininger, M. (1991). *Culture care diversity and universality: A theory of nursing.* New York, NY: National League for Nursing.

Rawnsley, M. (1990). Of human bonding: The context of nursing as caring. *Advances in Nursing Science, 13*(1), 41–48.

Trafecanty, L. (2006). Biblical caring comes full circle: Identifying what constitutes caring in the 21st century remains imperative to defining nursing. *Journal of Christian Nursing, 23*(3), 6–13.

Watson, J. (2007). Theory of human caring: Caring theory defined. Retrieved from http://www.ucdenver.edu/academics/colleges/nursing/caring/humancaring/Pages/CaringTheoryDefined.aspx

Appendix E

Caring Attitudes of Nurses From the United States Toward Medical-Surgical Patients Who Have a Diagnosis of Drug Addiction

Gerri Clubb

*D*rug addiction is a chronic disease of the brain that develops into more complicated diseases. Drug addiction affects spiritual, mental, physical, and emotional components of human life. According to the Substance Abuse and Mental Health Services Administration (Substance Abuse and Mental Health Services Administration [SAMHSA], 2010), an estimated 22.6 million people (9.2% of the population of the United States) suffered from substance abuse that resulted in 1.7 million emergency department visits in 2006. With the risk of drug addiction to physical and mental health, nurses increasingly have contact with hospitalized patients who have illnesses associated with drug addiction.

Nurses' perceptions about drug addiction often reflect the negative stigma of the general population and become part of a subculture of nursing (Sleeper, 2008). Throughout much of the last century, people addicted to drugs were thought to be morally defective and deficient in willpower. As a result, society responded to drug addiction as being a moral flaw versus being a chronic disease (National Institute on Drug Abuse [NIDA], 2009). Unfortunately, the negative stigma society placed on addiction as a choice rather than a disease may interfere with the appropriate caring behavior that medical-surgical patients with a diagnosis of drug addiction need. It is important that all nurses increase their knowledge related to the disease of addiction to provide a caring attitude to medical-surgical patients who have a diagnosis of drug addiction.

PURPOSE OF THE STUDY

The purpose of the current study was to assess nurses' caring practices toward medical-surgical patients with and without a diagnosis of drug addiction.

THEORETICAL FRAMEWORK

Watson's theory of human caring (2008) was the theoretical framework for this study. According to Watson, the nurse must develop and maintain a helping, trusting, genuine caring relationship with the patient in order to promote healing and health. The theory's well-developed framework incorporates 10 concepts of caring, which Dr. Jean Watson terms "Carative Factors" (Watson, 1988) and more recently referred to as "Caritas Processes" (Watson, 2008).

Research Items

Using the Caring Factor Survey–Care Provider Version (CFS-CPV), which measures the nurses' perceptions of delivering the 10 Caritas Processes, the items addressed in the research study were as follows:

1. What caring behaviors of the nurse are perceived by the nurse as being most and least important?
2. Do medical-surgical registered nurses feel differently regarding the care of medical-surgical patients without a diagnosis of drug addiction versus the care of medical-surgical patients with a drug addiction diagnosis?
3. Do medical-surgical registered nurses with a higher educational level in nursing have a more caring attitude toward medical-surgical patients with a history of drug addiction?

METHODS

The current study is a quasi-experimental study that used a paired t test to examine the difference of scores for the CFS-CPV questionnaire when comparing the nurses' responses to care for medical-surgical patients with a diagnosis of drug addiction and medical-surgical patients without a diagnosis of drug addiction. The paired t test is appropriate to understand, within subject differences, when each respondent has supplied responses for two different populations (Leedy & Ormrod, 2005). The paired t test is more sensitive than the independent t test due to comparing differences of the same individual rather than different individuals.

The third research question suggested that registered nurses with higher educational levels would affect responses of caring because higher education levels allow for broader and more in-depth education about cultural differences. These differences could impact the approach taken for the culture of patients with a diagnosis of drug addiction versus patients without a diagnosis of drug addiction. To examine the difference, a general linear was used to examine the interaction effect of education of nurse and drug addiction of patients on report of Caritas.

The CFS-CPV was used to examine the nurses' perceptions of Caritas. The CFS-CPV has been tested previously and shown to have good reliability. The CFS-CPV has been described in more detail in Chapter 11 by Herbst, Chapter 4 by Johnson, and Chapter 13 by Julian and Bott.

Nurses worked on a medical-surgical nursing unit in a small Catholic hospital in Louisville, Kentucky. Patients had to have had an established diagnosis of drug addiction. The subjects were chosen randomly and on a volunteer basis. A sample size of 50 participants was the goal for the current study because only approximately 100 registered nurses work on the medical-surgical units in the small Catholic hospital, and 50 was a reasonable number due to the availability of medical-surgical registered nurses at this facility. A letter of recruitment was sent to all staff on the medical-surgical unit and the first 50 who responded were accepted to participate in the study.

The participants were then asked to complete two versions of CFS-CPV. They were asked to respond to the CFS-CPV related to a patient with a known diagnosis of drug addiction, and were asked to respond to a second CFS-CPV in relation to a patient who did not have a diagnosis of drug addiction.

A paired t test was performed using a G-power of 2.0., an effect size of 0.5, an alpha of .05, and power of .79.

RESULTS

For the nonaddict group, all 50 surveys (100%) were returned. For the addict group, 49 of 50 surveys (98%) were returned. All items for the returned surveys were completed. No questionnaires were discarded because of incomplete information.

Psychometrics of the CFS-CPV revealed a reliability of 0.94 for the nonaddict group, using Cronbach's alpha. The addict group revealed a reliability of 0.96. No item, if deleted, would have resulted in an increased alpha.

Upon examining the rank-order mean scores for the nonaddict group, it was noted that the caring behavior to instill faith and hope was number one with a mean score of 6.84 (SD, .36). This had a small range, with 6.0 being the minimum score and 7.0 the maximum score. The lowest-scoring variable, in contrast, was perception of problem solving with a mean score of 6.1. The perception of problem solving had a wide range, with 2.5 being the minimum score and 7.0 being the maximum score. The full range of rank-order mean scores are noted in descending order in Table E.1.

TABLE E.1 Descriptive Statistics for Nonaddict Group

	n	MINIMUM	MAXIMUM	MEAN	STD DEVIATION
Faith and hope	50	6.00	7.00	6.8400	.35628
Loving kindness	50	4.50	7.00	6.8100	.46170
Spiritual support	50	5.50	7.00	6.7800	.41845
Allow miracles	50	4.50	7.00	6.7500	.49744
Holistic care	50	5.00	7.00	6.7200	.49652
Healing environment	50	5.50	7.00	6.6800	.47121
Teach and understand	50	5.00	7.00	6.6800	.49239
Promote expression	50	5.00	7.00	6.6800	.50265
CFS-CPV total	49	5.15	7.00	6.6071	.42044
Helping/trusting relationship	50	4.50	7.00	6.0800	.76505
Problem solving	49	3.00	7.00	6.0612	.91077

TABLE E.2 Descriptive Statistics for Addict Group

	n	MINIMUM	MAXIMUM	MEAN	STD DEVIATION
Allow miracles	49	5.00	7.00	6.3163	.65902
Spiritual support	49	4.00	7.00	6.1020	.76362
Faith and hope	49	4.50	7.00	5.9898	.71800
Loving kindness	48	4.00	7.00	5.9792	.84399
Teach and understand	49	4.50	7.00	5.8265	.76751
Promote expression	49	3.00	7.00	5.7653	.99531
CFS-CPV total score	47	4.65	7.00	5.7585	.67117
Holistic care	49	3.00	7.00	5.7245	.89011
Healing environment	49	4.00	7.00	5.6122	.79232
Problem solving	48	3.00	7.00	5.1042	1.07663
Helping/trusting relationship	49	2.50	7.00	5.0918	1.01383

The mean scores for the addict group revealed that the top-ranked caring behavior was allowing the patient to believe in a miracle, with a mean score of 6.32 (SD, .66) and a range of 2.0 with minimum of 5.0 and maximum of 7.0. The lowest-ranked caring behavior was perception of creating a helping and trusting relationship, with a mean score of 5.09 and a range of 4.5 (minimum of 2.5, maximum of 7.0). These data are noted in descending order in Table E.2.

When comparing the interaction effect for the medical-surgical patient without a diagnosis of drug addiction and the level of education of the registered nurse, the descriptive statistics revealed that the mean

TABLE E.3 Descriptive Statistics for Nonaddict and Addict Groups, by Education Level

ADDICTION OR NONADDICTION	EDUCATION LEVEL (ASSOCIATE'S DEGREE, NURSE: ADN; BACCALAURE-ATE OF SCIENCE IN NURSING: BSN)	MEAN	STD DEVIATION	n
Not addicted	ADN	6.5531	.53959	16
	BSN	6.6893	.33978	14
	Total	6.6167	.45511	30
Addicted	ADN	5.9321	.92832	14
	BSN	5.6727	.50565	11
	Total	5.8180	.76851	25
Total	ADN	6.2633	.79762	30
	BSN	6.2420	.65902	25
	Total	6.2536	.73130	55

TABLE E.4 Results of Paired *t* Test

CARITAS PROCESS		MEAN	SD	t	DF	p
Pair 1	Loving kindness	−.77083	.92804	−5.755	47	.0000006
Pair 2	Problem solving	−.84043	1.26880	−4.541	46	.00004
Pair 3	Faith and hope	−.81633	.76167	−7.502	48	.000000001
Pair 4	Teach and understand	−.83673	.84402	−6.940	48	.000000009
Pair 5	Spiritual support	−.63265	.77578	−5.709	48	.0000007
Pair 6	Healing environment	−1.02041	.84754	−8.428	48	.00000000005
Pair 7	Helping/trusting relationship	−.92857	1.13652	−5.719	48	.0000007
Pair 8	Holistic care	−.95918	1.04501	−6.425	48	.00000006
Pair 9	Promote expression	−.88776	1.03715	−5.992	48	.0000003
Pair 10	Allow miracles	−.38776	.72360	−3.751	48	.0005
Pair 11	CFS-CPV total	−.78804	.73320	−7.290	45	.000000004

score for the nurses who had a BSN was higher at 6.68 (SD of .34). The mean score for the nurses who had an ADN and who completed the same survey was 6.55 (SD of .54). For the patients with drug addiction, the score for ADNs was higher at 6.26 (SD of .93) and the mean score for the BSNs was decreased at 5.67 (SD of .50). These data are noted in Table E.3.

The final analysis was a paired *t* test to compare if there was a statistically significant difference between groups of addicts and nonaddicts. All 10 caring behaviors were found to have differences that were statistically significant using an alpha of .05. These findings are noted in Table E.4 and Figure E.1.

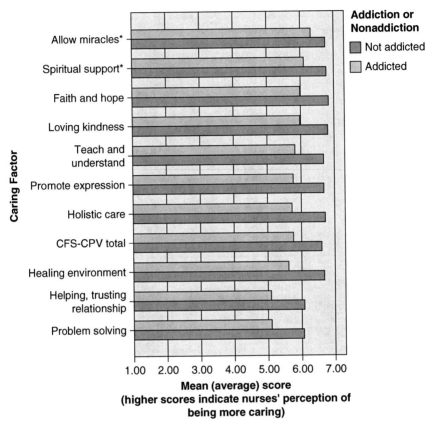

*Statistically significant using alpha of .05.

FIGURE E.1 Differences between addict and nonaddict groupings.

Results warrant careful interpretation due to the small sample size, which makes the sample vulnerable to bias. This should be considered a potential limitation of the study. The histogram of the comparison that had the largest sample difference (healing environment) reveals that the sample of the medical-surgical patient with a diagnosis of drug addiction is normally distributed. The sample of the medical-surgical patient without a known diagnosis of drug addiction has a left skew, because many scored very high. A study with a larger sample size would help determine the true distribution and eliminate the biased histogram to something that approaches a more central distribution.

CONCLUSION

The current study revealed that medical-surgical nurses at the small Catholic hospital in Louisville, Kentucky, determined faith and hope to be the highest-scoring caring factor and problem solving to be the lowest-scoring caring factor toward the patient without a diagnosis of drug addiction. The faith and hope caring factor ranked third highest toward the medical-surgical patient with a diagnosis of drug addiction. The study revealed the highest-scoring caring factor to be allowing for miracles toward the patient with a diagnosis of drug addiction. The lowest-scoring subscale was found to be helping/trusting toward the group with a diagnosis of drug addiction.

In comparison to the current study, Johnson's study which is described in Chapter 4 of this book, using the same CFS-CPV questionnaire on 76 nurses after a class of caring behaviors at Binghamton University, resulted in the same highest subscale (allowing for miracles) as the nurses' caring practice toward medical-surgical patients with a diagnosis of drug addiction. Allowing for miracles ranked fourth highest toward medical-surgical patients without a diagnosis of drug addiction in the current study.

A quasi-experimental study using the CFS-CPV with labor and delivery nurses (Herbst, in press) found the lowest-scoring caring factor to be problem solving, as did the medical-surgical nurses' caring practice toward medical-surgical patients without a diagnosis of drug addiction. Problem solving was the second-to-last-scoring caring factor toward the medical-surgical patient with a diagnosis of drug addiction. Ironically, problem solving was rated the second-to-last-scoring caring factor with the 76 nurses at Binghamton University after a class on caring behaviors (Johnson, in press).

Power analysis for a paired *t* test using a G-Power of 2.0 revealed higher caring factor scores relating to the medical-surgical patient without a diagnosis of drug addiction versus the caring factor scores relating to the medical-surgical patient with a diagnosis of drug addiction. It was found that the difference for all 10 caring factors, plus the total CFS-CPV score (all caring factors combined), were statistically significant using an alpha of .05. The comparison of responses between the two groups was quite large. The key finding in the study was that nurses connect far less with medical-surgical patients who also have a diagnosis of drug addiction.

Helping and trusting was found to be the lowest caring factor toward the patient who also had a diagnosis of drug addiction. According to Watson (1988), a helping/trusting relationship is imperative to promote healing and health. The findings were consistent with other studies that found health care providers often stereotype patients with a diagnosis of drug addiction and perceive them as untrustworthy.

A quantitative and qualitative study by Persky, Nelson, Watson, and Bent (2008) revealed that the profile of a nurse in caring may also be the nurse's individual biases/stereotypes. A study by Sleeper (2008) continually mentions themes of mistrust felt by substance abusers toward their health care providers. The patients did not feel that health care providers saw them as human beings with needs.

Results of the study did not reveal that a higher educational level was more significant with improved caring behaviors. Caring is a different construct than formal knowledge and this analysis may be showing that caring goes beyond education.

Implications

The purpose of the current study was to explore registered nurses' caring behaviors toward medical-surgical patients with and without a diagnosis of drug addiction. The study's findings revealed that problem solving was the lowest-scoring care factor toward the medical-surgical patient without a drug addiction diagnosis.

According to Watson (1988), the scientific problem-solving method is the only method that allows for control and prediction that will promote self-correction. The Caritas Process of problem solving is to promote problem-solving methods by engaging in creative practices with patients. This is done by using a holistic approach to understand and know the patient. Problem solving at the small, Catholic hospital being the lowest caring factor could be due to nursing time constraints and decreased resources.

Unfortunately, the key finding in the study revealed that medical-surgical registered nurses were less caring to patients who also have a diagnosis of drug addiction. Registered nurses perceive the patients who also have a diagnosis of drug addiction as untrustworthy. Perceiving patients as being untrustworthy is a negative factor that can influence the quality of care.

Because the population with a diagnosis of drug addiction will continue to be part of hospitalized patients, it will benefit registered nurses to develop an improved understanding of the etiology of drug addiction. Until nurses are more educated about the disease of addiction, the relationship between the nurse and patient with a diagnosis of drug addiction will be not as caring.

Recommendations

The relationship between medical patients with a drug addiction diagnosis and registered nurses will continue to be an important concern. Nurse caring behaviors should also remain a vital issue for enhanced physical and psychosocial healing of the patient.

Based on the current study's findings, it is recommended that a similar study be conducted with a larger sample size and in a different geographic area to validate the findings. Future research should investigate caring behaviors and perceptions of both nurses and medical-surgical patients with a diagnosis of drug addiction. Finally, future research should consider examining hospitals with formal caring programs versus those without formal caring programs, to understand how formal caring programs impact the perception of enacting caring behaviors.

Summary

The final results of the research study highlighted perceptions of registered nurses' caring behaviors toward medical-surgical patients with and without a diagnosis of drug addiction. The expanded knowledge gained insight that registered nurses have a negative perception of hospital patients who have a diagnosis of drug addiction. The study demonstrated that more education is needed for registered nurses about the chronic disease of drug addiction and the science of caring.

REFERENCES

Leedy, P., & Ormrod, J. (2005). *Practical research: Planning and design* (8th ed.). Upper Saddle River, NJ: Merril Prentice Hall.

National Institute on Drug Abuse. (2009). *Drugs, brains, and behavior—The science of addiction.* Retrieved May 1, 2010, from http://www.nida.nih.gov/scienceofaddiction

Persky, G., Nelson, J., Watson, J., & Bent, K. (2008). Creating a profile of a nurse effective in caring. *Nursing Administration, 32*(1), 15–20.

Sleeper, J. A. (2008). *Stigmatization by nurses as perceived by substance abuse patients: A phenomenological study.* MS dissertation, Southern Connecticut State University, Connecticut.

Substance Abuse and Mental Health Services Administration. (2010). Drug Abuse Warning Network. Retrieved May, 2010, from http://dawninfo.samhsa.gov/pubs/edpubs/default.asp

Watson, J. (1988). *Nursing: Human science and human care. A theory of nursing* (Vol. 15-2236, pp. 1–111). New York: National League for Nursing Publications.

Watson, J. (2008). *Nursing: The philosophy and science of caring.* Denver, CO: University Press of Colorado.

Appendix F

Caring for Patients With Breast Cancer in the Philippines

Jeff Vasquez

BACKGROUND AND RATIONALE

*I*t has been consistently affirmed that breast cancer is a major disease affecting women all over the world. Next to skin cancer, it is the most common cancer in women (Giuliano, 2009). The American Cancer Society (2008) states that breast cancer is the leading cancer among Asian women. In a study of 100,000 women, 55% of the Chinese; 73.1% of the Filipinos; 82.3% of the Japanese; and 28.5% of the Koreans are affected by breast cancer. In a report by the *Manila Times* (2008), the Philippines has the highest incidence rate of breast cancer in Asia and is considered to have the ninth-highest incidence rate in the world today. It was a report obtained from the International Agency for Research on Cancer by the World Health Organization. It further showed that approximately 70% of breast cancer cases occur in women with none of the known risk factors.

The late Rosa Francia Meneses, the founding president of the Philippine Breast Cancer Network, once said, "The greatest risk of getting breast cancer tomorrow is being born today in a developing country. The greatest risk of not surviving breast cancer today is being a woman in the Philippines." With this in mind, it is important that this study was conducted to investigate the lived experience of a patient with breast cancer using Jean Watson's clinical Caritas Processes. This broadens the understanding of the phenomenon surrounding the disease and contributes to the improvement of nursing care to patients with breast cancer. Most importantly, the previous experience of the researcher with a close family member afflicted with breast cancer who perished, gave the researcher the encouragement to conduct this study. The researcher's participation in "Silver Linings 2008," a homecoming for breast cancer survivors, made him realize the nurse's critical role in the recovery of a patient with breast cancer.

THEORETICAL FRAMEWORK

Patients with cancer need a special type of care that caters not only to the physical needs, but also to other needs of mankind. The adoption of Jean Watson's clinical Caritas Processes entails the holistic care that these patients need. This theory provides nurses the opportunity to practice altruism while attending to the dependent and independent nursing functions. It gives meaning to the actions of the nurse and gives value to the person being cared for. Hence, this study was anchored on Jean Watson's clinical Caritas Processes. The 10 processes are as follows:

1. Embracing altruistic values and practicing loving kindness with self and others
2. Instilling faith and hope and honoring others
3. Being sensitive to self and others by nurturing individual beliefs and practices
4. Developing helping, trusting, caring relationships
5. Promoting and accepting positive and negative feelings as you authentically listen to another's story
6. Using creative, scientific, problem-solving methods for caring decision making
7. Sharing teaching and learning that address the individual needs and comprehension styles
8. Creating a healing environment for the physical and spiritual self that respects human dignity
9. Assisting with basic physical, emotional, and spiritual human needs
10. Opening to mystery and allowing miracles to enter

The clinical Caritas framework exhibits an intense spiritual focus and a covert expression of love and caring. This perspective highlights the evolving face of nursing within a caring–healing theory. With the inclusion of love and caring in the work and in the nurse's life, there is discovery and affirmation that nursing is more than just a job but both life-giving and life-receiving that offers a lifetime of growth and learning (Parker, 2001).

Breast cancer is one disease that greatly affects women in the world. Its effects may be devastating if found at its malignant stage, or it may be manageable if discovered at a stage when medical management shows promise for a good prognosis. The management of breast cancer should not be limited only to the conventional care the patient receives from the hospital, but it should also cover areas not addressed by conventional therapy. The role of the nurse in the holistic care of the patient furnishes the patient the environment conducive for mind-body-spirit healing. These are the areas that are greatly affected by the multiple stressors to which a patient with breast cancer is subjected.

However, this is not a problem that concerns women alone. Inevitably, the social, psychological, and economic impact of the disease concerns both sexes. Patients with breast cancer and their families are compelled to make many difficult decisions pertaining to disease management (Black, Hawks, & Keene, 2008). This makes the whole experience not an easy one to bear. The male population becomes affected by the effects of the disease because a male would always be affiliated with a female person—be she a mother, wife, sister, cousin, niece, or a friend.

STATEMENT OF THE PROBLEM

This study aimed to investigate the lived experience of a patient with breast cancer, adopting Jean Watson's clinical Caritas Processes as a basis of improved nursing care. Specifically, it sought to determine the health experiences of the patient's phenomenal field that contributed to her current condition, psychopathophysiological changes observed, the nursing diagnoses and caring outcome criteria derived, caring–healing interventions and clinical Caritas Processes implemented, and the client's perception of care given.

METHODOLOGY

The researcher used qualitative design using the case-study research method. Through this design, the researcher was given the opportunity of acquiring intimate knowledge of the patient's condition, thoughts, feelings, past and present actions, and the environment, with the end result of a healing–caring modality designed especially for the patient. This study was conducted at Ward VI, the female surgical ward of the Vicente Sotto Memorial Medical Center.

The researcher made use of a researcher-made assessment tool based on Jean Watson's theory and guided by the Doenges, Moorhouse, and Murr's Adult Medical/Surgical Assessment Tool; in-depth interviews; and the Caring Factor Survey to validate the experiences of the patient. Direct nursing care was rendered to the patient while simultaneously gathering data through use of the assessment tool, interview responses, the patient's chart, and the Caring Factor Survey.

Quantitative data obtained from the Caring Factor Survey completed by the patient was used to triangulate the qualitative data obtained.

RESULTS AND DISCUSSION
Accessing the Phenomenal Field

Patient RGP is a 56-year-old Filipina. She is a Roman Catholic and married with two children. She sought health care upon complaining of a lump on her breast.

Two months prior to her confinement, she felt a relatively small lump on her right breast. Weeks passed by and the lump had increased in size. Although the presence of the mass did not interfere with her daily activities, she decided to submit for consultation at the Vicente Sotto Memorial Medical Center Breast Cancer Clinic. A month later, she underwent a biopsy, which showed Stage 2 CA. Thus, she was admitted for a planned mastectomy on her right breast.

Current Health Experiences

She was diagnosed with hypertension in 2005. She had no religious/cultural affiliations that dictated her diet. However, she preferred to eat fish rather than pork. She was placed on non per orem (NPO) the night before the scheduled mastectomy and was put back on a regular diet hours after the operation. Postoperatively, the incision made on her right breast covered with gauze made her feel a bit uncomfortable, but she was still happy that it did not interfere with her breathing. As a homemaker and part-time businesswoman, she was satisfied with how her business was going and claimed that the little income that her business could bring in was helping her family a lot. Because of the world financial crisis, a lot of wives like her were managing to help ease the financial burden.

The venoclysis affected her grooming activities, which gave her husband the opportunity to assist her with hygiene and grooming. This became a moment for the couple to bond together. The wife preferred to bathe in the morning as she was used to. She reported difficulty in abducting her affected arm, which was verified by the researcher. She reported a pain score of 6–7, on a scale of 1–10, on her incision, especially after she was brought to the ward from the recovery room. It gradually subsided.

She learned about breast self-examination when her neighbor showed her how. This was when she was made more aware of the breast mass she had.

After the operation, the patient verbalized the loss of her right breast and the changes that it brought to her appearance. She was a bit uncomfortable looking at the incision. Her husband also was very concerned, but with the disease rather than the loss of his wife's breast.

She had been married for 25 years and had been very happy. Her husband was with her throughout her stay in the hospital. While the patient was in the operating room, the husband patiently waited for his wife. His anxiety made him skip breakfast. When the patient had a hard time providing self-hygiene measures after the surgery, the husband did that for her without complaining.

The whole illness experience had made her closer to her husband. She was able to appreciate her husband's love for her because he always stayed with her. Despite what had happened, she was still grateful to

God for a successful surgery. She added that people would always encounter problems but that they would always overcome them by believing in God and His power.

The numerous expenditures consequential to her hospitalization had hurt their family's finances; however, she believed that money could be replenished. As a Roman Catholic, her faith had always helped her be optimistic about all obstacles that came along the way. She was generally calm during her hospital stay, although she was a bit anxious waiting for her biopsy result.

Nursing Diagnoses

Nursing problems are categorized mainly into: psychophysical, which includes acute pain, self-care deficit, disturbed sensory perception, risk for infection, and risk for sexual dysfunction; psychosocial, which includes disturbed body image; and intrapersonal-interpersonal, which comprises deficient knowledge, readiness for enhanced hope, and readiness for enhanced spiritual well-being.

Patient's Perception of Care Given

The patient "slightly agreed" in terms of the provision of the researcher of clinical Caritas Processes 2, 3, 5, 8, 9, and 10, whereas she "agreed" on clinical Caritas Processes 1, 4, 6, and 7. With a mean score of 5.4, the patient's general perception of care fell under "agree." This means that the patient agreed that the clinical Caritas Processes were practiced by the researcher, together with the rest of the health care team, throughout her hospital stay. This strengthens the researcher's caring–healing interventions that had become tangible to the patient. The duration of her hospital stay could have an effect on her perception of the care. Time is an important element in enabling the patient to experience fully the clinical Caritas Processes employed by the nurse.

Proposed Clinical Caritas Home-Based Care Program

A patient who has been diagnosed with breast cancer and who has submitted for a mastectomy will need the continuity of the provision of love and care, which are necessary to ensure physical, emotional, and spiritual healing. This considers the family members who also need healing. DUGHAN, a Filipino term for breast, also stands for Dakong Ulay nga Gugma, Hatagan ug Amuma Namo, which means, "With great and pure love, we will care." The objectives of the program DUGHAN are: to demonstrate correctly arm and hand exercises; to identify essential lifestyle changes that contribute to the mind-body-spirit healing; to participate in group sharing with fellow breast-cancer survivors and their families; and to advocate for the strengthening of breast-cancer awareness programs.

CONCLUSION AND RECOMMENDATIONS

The clinical Caritas Processes by Dr. Jean Watson are a useful means of providing a unique caring experience to a patient with breast cancer. The Caritas Processes provided a rich cultivation of the patient's life experiences, which was important to understand her better. The fight against cancer needs a strong spirit integral to the lifelong survival of the patient. True, the researcher was able to take care of the spiritual aspect of the person by first entering into her immediate physical needs. The practice of clinical Caritas Processes surmounts the conventional therapy that a patient with breast cancer receives. It is imperative that these patients receive this type of care, because the illness phenomenon cuts across all aspects of life—physical, social, mental, financial, and spiritual. It addresses the holistic care that a patient with breast cancer would need. Being hospitalized is not easy, but with the caring–healing nursing interventions distinguished by the clinical Caritas Processes, the whole experience is made lighter, inspiring, and empowering for the patient with breast cancer and her family.

It is also recommended that the clinical Caritas be adopted when taking care of patients with breast cancer, those with other types of cancers, and those with chronic conditions; that DUGHAN be incorporated into the home-care management of patients with breast cancer; that nurses strive hard to practice the clinical Caritas during a patient's entire stay at the hospital regardless of patient load because caring is irreducible; that Philippine academic institutions adopt Jean Watson's theory of human caring in their curriculum to support and promote the country's pride of producing the best and most caring nurses in the world; that various health care institutions use the clinical Caritas Processes in the care of their patients to fully cater to the multidimensional needs of the human person; and that government health agencies addressing cancer care adopt clinical Caritas-based programs to provide a life-changing experience through acceptable and effective caring–healing modalities.

REFERENCES

American Cancer Society (2008). *Breast Cancer Statistics.* Retrieved May 7, 2009, from http://www.gloriagemma.org/facts-statistics.html

Black, J., Hawks, J. H., & Keene, A. (2008). *Medical-surgical nursing: Clinical management for positive outcomes* (8th ed.). Philadelphia, PA: W. B. Saunders.

Giuliano, A. (2009). Breast Disorders. In S. J. McPhee & M.A. Papadakis (Eds.), *Current medical diagnosis and treatment.* Columbus, OH, USA: The McGraw-Hill companies

Jean Watson's philosophy of nursing. (2009). Retrieved April 27, 2009, from http://currentnursing.com/nursing_theory/Watson.htm

Parker, M. (2001). *Nursing theories and nursing practice* (1st ed.). Philadelphia, PA: F. A. Davis Company.

Philippines Breast Cancer Incidence Rate Asia's Highest (2008). *Manila Times.* Retrieved May 7, 2009, from http://www.manilatimes.net/national/2008/oct/05/yehey/metro/20081005met6.html

Appendix G

A U.S. Study of Nurses' Self-Care and Compassion Fatigue Using Watson's Concepts of Caritas

Sandra Johnson

*T*here is a cost to caring. Compassion fatigue (CF) describes the emotional, physical, social, and spiritual exhaustion that overtakes a person and causes a pervasive decline in his or her desire, ability, and energy to feel and care for others. The literature reflects that the health care field is becoming more aware of the cost of caring, of the significant stress that occurs in health care providers when they witness and/or learn of the suffering and pain of their patients. This notion is not a new one. Although the costs of caring vary, anyone who has sat at the bedside of a patient struggling to hang on to life, or talked with the family experiencing their anticipatory grief, or attempted to resuscitate a 4-year-old who fell into the pool, knows the heavy toll that is paid as a result of extending compassion and competence when life hangs in the balance. Not only is the toll on the hearts and lives of the caregivers, but organizations acutely experience the negative impact of a weary and worn workforce.

Anna Baranowsky, executive director of the Trauma Institute in Canada who has researched CF extensively, discussed the fact that the direct costs of workplace stress and health care challenges translated into 70 million workdays missed by Canadian employees for personal reasons in 2000 (Baronowsky, 2005). CF takes a toll with costs to not only the health care provider, but also on the workplace, causing high turnover, more sick days, and decreased productivity. The soul of health care—its heart that beats with its values of healing and service—is enabled to the degree of wholeness of its providers. What model of leadership aligns most closely with the leader characteristics needed to enhance and support "whole" providers of care?

CF is a relatively recent term, first coined by Johnson in 1992 while studying burnout in nurses working in emergency departments (Sabo, 2005). The majority of the emerging literature regarding CF leads with Charles Figley's body of work. Figley (1995) defined CF as "the natural

413

consequent behaviors and emotions resulting from knowing about a traumatizing event experienced by a significant other—the stress resulting from helping or wanting to help a traumatized or suffering person" (p. 7). CF differs from post-traumatic stress disorder (PTSD) in that the caregiver is exposed to the suffering person rather than the traumatic event itself (Sabo, 2005). This author points out that although CF came to be recognized as a feature of secondary trauma in therapists as they heard and empathized with their traumatized clients, in fact, nurses and other acute and emergency health care providers do bear primary witness to catastrophic and traumatic events while caring for their patients. Gentry (2002) discussed the result of the work of Gentry and Baronowsky in which they have expanded the definition of CF to include preexisting or concomitant primary post-traumatic stress and its symptoms when he wrote, "Many caregivers, especially those providing on-site services, will have had first-hand exposure to the traumatic events to which they are responding" (p. 73).

Figley (1995) expanded the concept of CF and described it as a stress response that occurs suddenly and without warning following repeated exposure to the trauma of others. Baranowsky (2005) identified the syndrome of CF as having a trajectory of phases: Phase 1—the Zealot Phase—when caregivers are committed, involved, and available; Phase 2—the Irritability Phase—when caregivers begin to cut corners and avoid patient contact and when lapses of concentration may cause mistakes; Phase 3—the Withdrawal Phase—when caregivers are tired all the time and begin to neglect family and coworkers, and others may complain about their behaviors; Phase 4—the Zombie Phase—when caregivers function on automatic pilot, not connected to their thoughts or feelings, having an apathy and loss of capacity to care, losing the sense of meaning and purpose in their work. This leaves them vulnerable to the silencing response—a reaction based on a series of assumptions that cause the caregiver to shutdown and to minimize or neglect the information coming from the patient. Along the trajectory, many stress symptoms are experienced physically, mentally, emotionally, and spiritually, and various stress behaviors are observed by others. The severity of CF and secondary traumatic stress (STS) is compounded by the caregiver's past, personal traumatic events. Those who are most vulnerable to CF are health care providers who work most closely with traumatized persons.

Figley's (1995) trauma transmission model suggests that in an effort to generate an understanding of the sufferer, caregivers require identification with the sufferer and his or her suffering, the condition he describes as compassion stress. His model of compassion stress begins with caregiver empathy, defined as the ability to notice the pain of others, and the motivation to want to act. "Both empathic ability and emotional contagion—one's susceptibility to the feelings of the sufferer—account for the extent to which the helper is exposed to the suffering of the sufferer"

(p. 262). The extent to which a helper is satisfied with his or her efforts (sense of achievement) and the extent to which the helper can distance himself or herself from the ongoing lived misery of the sufferer, accounts for how much the helper experiences compassion stress.

Gentry (2002), an internationally recognized educator in the study and treatment of CF, in a web-based CF education module, promoted his belief that, unaddressed, CF always gets worse, leads to caregiver self-destruction, and that it is possible for caregivers to be 100% resilient. He used a quote by Victor Frankl, Holocaust survivor, who said, "That which is to give light must endure burning." Gentry builds the pathophysiological understanding of CF, identifying the central nervous system and brain responses to actual or perceived threat. The sympathetic nervous system activation is meant for acute, perceived threat and to ready us for fright or flight; yet when we are exposed to its effects chronically, it diminishes our cognitive, frontal lobe function and our immune system capacity. His studies have shown that when we use personal practices that activate the parasympathetic nervous system, especially during times of caring for sufferers, we remain calm and capable and can provide compassionate and competent care without the deleterious effects of CF.

RECOMMENDED SELF-CARE FOR AMELIORATION OF COMPASSION FATIGUE

We are most vulnerable to CF and vicarious traumatization when we are unaware of the state of our own body, mind, and spirit (Rothschild, 2006). Many sources could be discussed here in relation to recommending self-care for CF. Three are discussed briefly for the purposes of this appendix. Gentry (2009) identified five "antibodies" that serve to "vaccinate" the caregiver against CF: (1) self-regulation—the ability to switch from the sympathetic to the parasympathetic nervous system; this requires relaxation of the pelvic muscles; (2) intentionality—the ability to follow one's life mission and purpose; (3) self-validating care giving—the ability to give self-acknowledgment and validation for one's work; the ability to monitor and provide self with physical, emotional, and spiritual needs; (4) connection/support—the employment of three or more "safe" peers to serve as support, who can listen without judgment and provide encouragement; and (5) self-care—developing practices that "re-fuel."

Yassin (as found in Figley, 1995) stated, "Unless we prepare, plan, and attend to the effects of STS, we can cause harm to ourselves, to those who are close to us, or to those who are in our professional care" (p. 179). She discussed, at length, components of STS/CF that address the personal, professional, and environmental dimensions of STS: (1) personal—self-care practices such as aerobic exercise, adequate sleep, and therapeutic body work; for example, massage, good nutrition, life balance, relaxation, contact with nature, creative expression, skill building, meditation/spiritual practice that includes group fellowship, self-awareness, humor, social supports, and social activism; (2) professional—work/life balance, setting boundaries such as time boundaries, personal boundaries, therapeutic boundaries with client/patient, knowing one's own limits, asking for help, peer support, relationship with supervisor, mentors, and training; and (3) environmental—societal and work-setting factors.

Watson (2005) wrote, "As a beginning, we have to impose our own will to care and love upon our own behavior and not onto others. We have to treat ourselves with gentleness, loving kindness, equanimity, and dignity before we can respect and care for others with gentleness, kindness, equanimity and dignity" (p. 19). Watson identified four heart-centered self-care tasks as necessary to sustain one's own healing work for self and others: forgiveness, gratitude, surrender, and compassionate human service.

One final, yet significant note regarding caregiver self-care, which is worthy of another article in itself, is the place of caregiver spirituality and faith as an enhancer of compassion resiliency.

As a note of background, San Joaquin Community Hospital (SJCH), where the study for this appendix was conducted, is venturing on an organizational culture transformation called "Sacred Work." Sacred Work for SJCH is messaged as "the expression of God's love in the work we do every day. It is experienced whenever need is met with love" (Johnson & Phillips, 2008, p. 4). SJCH believes that caregivers create the healing environment to the extent of personal wholeness they bring to each caregiving moment, and that their intention imperative is to bring a healing presence to every interaction. Healing presence is defined by Miller (2001) as, "The condition of being consciously and compassionately in the present moment with another, believing in and affirming their potential for wholeness wherever they are in life" (p. 12). SJCH's commitment is to "Take care of the people who take care of people" (Johnson & Phillips, 2008, p. 5), and to develop strategies that examine and support the well-being of the caregivers who are often wounded healers.

METHODOLOGY

The primary objective of this quantitative, cross-sectional study was to determine the relationship between nurse self-care and nurse CF. The research items included the following: (1) What is the relationship of nurse self-care with nurse CF? and (2) What is the relationship of nurse self-care with risk for burnout? The method of measurement (data collection) was nurse surveys with two instruments: Caring Factor Survey–Caring for Self (CFS-CS), a 10-item, 7-point Likert scale; and Compassion Fatigue Self-Assessment, a 40-item, 5-point Likert scale assessment. Both instruments have been psychometrically tested.

The two subscales of the CF survey inquired about the perceptions of nurses related to CF and burnout. Responses secured the nurses' responses to the frequency of events consistent with the construct of CF. Responses ranged from 1, *rarely/never*, to 5, *very often*. Approximately half of the items were then added to obtain a CF score and the remaining half were added to obtain a burnout score.

The CFS-CS inquired about self-care using a 1–7 Likert scale. Responses ranged from 1, *strongly disagree*, to 7, *strongly agree*. Pearson's correlation was used to examine if a relationship exists between variables. A power analysis was also conducted by a colleague, John Nelson, to examine the sample size needed for adequate power. Software G-Power 2.0 was used and revealed that a sample of 65 nurses would be needed using an alpha of .05, power of 0.80, and an effect size of 0.30. The effect size reveals the magnitude of effect and 0.30 was considered appropriate for the dynamic and complex environment like health care. Prior to the analysis being run, an ANOVA procedure was conducted to ensure that there were no differences between nursing units.

The unit of analysis was acute hospital staff nurses. Six hundred nurses from SJCH were invited to participate. This was a convenience sample of nurses from 15 departments where nurses work in patient care.

RESULTS

Sixty-five nurses responded to both the CF and CFS-CS, a 10.8% response rate. The data from these 65 nurses were used for analysis for this study. The psychometrics revealed significant reliability with Cronbach's alpha of .94 for the CFS-CS and .91 for the CF subscale component of the CF survey, and .92 for the burnout subscale component of the CF survey.

Pearson's correlation, using an alpha of .05, revealed a statistically significant negative relationship between self-care and CF ($r = -.597$) and self-care and burnout ($r = -.604$).

Figure G.1 displays the mean scores for the self-perception of the caring concepts. Note that the lowest-perceived self-care concept was "practice loving kindness for myself."

Some of the narrative comments by the responders who reported scores less than 4.0, on the 1–7 scale, are noted as follows:

- "I'm already burnt out."
- "I am always taking care of others; it is often difficult to remember to take care of one's self."
- "I have a hard time expressing emotions or allowing myself to heal. I feel selfish to take care of my needs before others."

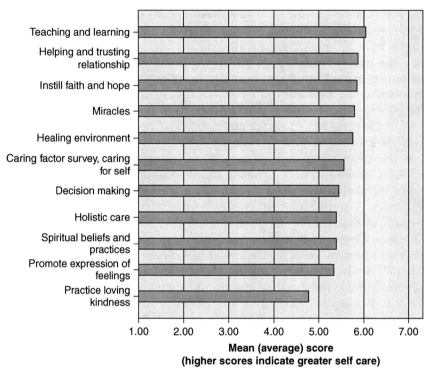

FIGURE G.1   Rank order of self-care scores.

■ "I feel I do not get enough time to appreciate and take care of myself."
■ "I have just never really believed in my own self. I believe in the Lord and the Spirit and they are important to me and life. I just wish I could believe in me."

CONCLUSION

This significant study joins a growing body of research and an emerging awareness in the health care community related to CF about the resulting potential for the effects of CF on caregivers and their families, those they serve, and their organizations. Health care organizations must invest in and support the emerging evidence showing that the quality of the healing environment is created by direct caregivers who, for the most part, came into health care to make a difference and answer a "call to care."

One nurse at SJCH stated one day, "If I didn't have all of these patients, I could get my work done!" This author, in hearing that remark, reflected on a caregiver's true work. Where have we come in health care today if the caregiver's "work" is everything else but the whole person care of the patient who is experiencing life at its most vulnerable? This study has shown that the nurse who made that statement was likely experiencing CF. More research is needed that will link caregiver CF with patients' perceptions of caring.

In her discussion of the words of Christ, Jones (1995) wrote, "If you love this people, and serve them, and speak kind words to them, they will love you and follow you forever" (II Chronicles 10:7, New International Version). The call to the leaders of today and tomorrow is to take care of the people who take care of people—to serve the servers—and to help the growth of their capacity to work compassionately and resiliently from their hearts.

REFERENCES

Baranowsky, A. (2005). *Compassion fatigue: Resiliency and recovery, a presentation for care providers manual* (7th ed.). Toronto, Canada: Traumatology Institute.

Figley, C. (1995). *Compassion fatigue: Secondary traumatic stress in those who treat the traumatized.* New York, NY: Brunner-Routledge.

Gentry, E. (2002). Compassion fatigue: A crucible of transformation. *Journal of Trauma Practice, 1*(3), 37–61.

Johnson, S., & Phillips, J. (2008). *The sacred work manual.* Retrieved from https//www.sjch.us

Jones, L. B. (1995). *Jesus, CEO.* New York, NY: Hyperion.

Miller, J. (2001). *The art of being a healing presence.* Fort Wayne, IN: Willowgreen Publishing

Rothschild, B. (2006). *Help for the helper: Self-care strategies for managing burnout and stress.* New York, NY: Norton.

Sabo, B. (2005). Compassion fatigue and nursing work: Can we accurately capture the consequences of caring work. *International Journal of Nursing Practice, 12*, 136–142.

Watson, J. (2005). *Caring science as sacred science.* Philadelphia, PA: F. A. Davis.

Appendix H

Caring in the Context of Curing: What Are Patients' Perceptions of Nurse Caring When Receiving ECT in the PACU?

Cheryl McDavitt and Penelope Glynn

According to Gass (2006), nurses have a long history of practice in the area of electroconvulsive therapy (ECT), and opinions on their involvement in the treatment reflect the wider professional and media debate on the appropriateness of its use. Among patients undergoing ECT, there is little debate. Although the literature is sparse regarding patients' experiences and satisfaction with ECT, especially as related to satisfaction with nursing care, patients report it as causing anxiety and fear, particularly related to the fear of anesthesia, brain damage, dying, personality changes, memory loss, and loss of control (Beyer, Weiner, & Glenn, 1998; Dowman, Patel, & Rajput, 2005; Sienaert, Becker, Vansteel-andt, Demyttenaere, & Peuskens, 2005). They reported feeling safe during its administration, and the majority would be willing to have it again, whereas the minority would not (Rose, Wykes, Bindman, & Fleischmann, 2003). Most recently, Sienaert, Vansteelandt, Demyttenaere, and Peuskens (2010) studied predictors of patient satisfaction with ECT but the factors related to patient attributes and patients' perceived outcomes, and not to the care received. More recent studies do indicate that patients and families continue to want more information about ECT as a procedure and that they value being treated respectfully and with dignity (Harrison & Kaarsemaker, 2000; Malekian, Amini, Maracy, & Barekatain, 2008; Myers, 2007; Sienaert et al., 2005; Smith, Vogler, Zarrouf, Sheaves, & Jesse, 2009).

Kavanagh and McLaughlin (2010) report the functions of the ECT nurse today as including ensuring that the environment, equipment, and medications used in ECT are in accordance with the best practice guidelines and that the psychological needs of the patient, including fully informing the patient about his or her illness, why ECT has been recommended, describing the process, and allaying the patients' and families' fears regarding ECT, have been addressed. The need for the ECT nurse to address the educational and psychological needs of the patient is also described in a study of the effectiveness of an ECT training program for nurses conducted by Munday, Deans, and Little (2003). They describe the role as increasingly multifaceted and, among other things, as including the provision of education to patients and families; ensuring patients' physical well-being before, during, and after ECT; and ensuring that patients' psychological needs are met.

Although the role and functions of the ECT nurse are clear, the extent to which they are implemented is less clear, especially as ECT treatment is being moved to the postanesthesia care unit (PACU) setting in some hospitals. Gass (2006) suggests that what is missing in the literature is research on what ECT nurses actually do when providing care to ECT patients. This question was of particular interest to the researchers, given the multifaceted role of the ECT nurse, and the recent move of their hospital's designated ECT setting to the PACU. The PACU nurses, given the challenge of rendering ECT care in a PACU setting, had raised their concern as to whether or not their patients could perceive them as "caring" given the high-tech, fast-paced environment of the PACU, and the need to move ECT patients efficiently through the prephase, the ECT, and postphase of ECT in a span of two to three hours.

In attempting to answer the question, a review of the literature revealed one report on the successful implementation of an ECT program in the PACU (Petty, 2000), a study of the effect on education about ECT on patient satisfaction (Arkan & Ustun, 2008), and one study by Gass (2006) that focused specifically on the work of mental health nurses and ECT, including the concept of caring. This grounded-theory study, conducted in Scotland with a sample of 20 mental health nurses and 4 students, revealed two roles for nurses in ECT: relational roles and treatment roles. The nurses described: the role of information giver, persuader, and supporter with the patients, a relational role of "being there," being present and engaged with the patient; and a treatment role with the medical staff, which was sometimes in direct contradiction to the relational role. Conducting a study to explore the PACU nurses' "caring" for ECT patients was determined to be an important performance-improvement project, given the need to address the nurses' concerns regarding the role of ECT nurses in providing so many caring interventions, and their own commitment to evidence-based practice. Exploring the issue from the patients' perspective was deemed most appropriate in view of the Institute of Medicine's charge that care be patient centered.

Thus, a descriptive study using survey methodology was implemented to assess patients' perceptions of caring while undergoing ECT therapy. The Caring Factor Survey by Watson and Nelson was used to measure the perceptions of patients, who received ECT in a small community hospital in New England from May through October 2010. The Caring Factor Survey was chosen because it is short (factor analysis conducted on data from a sample of 600 surveys, permitting the reduction of the original 20 items down to 10), it addresses the caring behaviors about which the PACU nurses were concerned, and its reliability and validity have been established (DiNapoli, Nelson, Turkel, & Watson, 2010). Items are measured on a Likert scale, from 1 = *strongly disagree*, to 7 = *strongly agree*, and a total score is calculated for each survey. To participate in the survey, the patient had to be 18, had to have completed at least 8 weeks of therapy, and be capable of reading English. After gaining approval by the hospital's institutional review board (IRB), the survey was mailed to all 73 patients who were eligible, with a response rate of 37%, and $N = 27$. The mean age of the 73 eligible patients was 53, including 47 females and 26 males. In order to achieve the best possible response rate, anonymity was guaranteed, all surveys were hand-addressed, and a stamped, return envelope was included. Minimal demographic data were collected because of the need for anonymity, the vulnerable nature of the population, and the need to obtain patients' honest perceptions. Completion of the survey was an indication of their willingness to participate and surveys were re-sent to patients a second time in order to achieve an acceptable response rate.

RESULTS

It may be the contradiction in roles reported by Gass (2006), the less familiar role of the ECT nurse, and the high-tech PACU environment that precipitated the PACU nurses' concerns regarding their provision of "caring," but the results did not corroborate their concerns. The patients' total mean score for perception of caring was 6.24 out of 7, suggesting that this sample of patients, in fact, do perceive themselves as recipients of caring. Table H.1 presents the caring factors in descending order with the factor perceived by patients as most present at the top. It is important that patients perceived the nurses as having established helping and trusting relationships with them, given the fear and anxiety patients experience with ECT treatment. The fact that the patients' mean score for "caregivers addressing all their needs and concerns" was 6.67 is also noteworthy, but must be viewed in the context of the last three caring factors (caregivers recognized the connection between mind, body, and spirit; caregivers' acceptance and support of beliefs regarding a higher power; and caregivers encouraged practice of patients' health beliefs), given that these factors received the lowest mean scores (<6), and were significantly correlated with the total perceived caring mean score at .672, .832, .697, respectively, and ($p = .000$).

It would be important to examine these factors again after attempts are made to better address them.

The qualitative data provided by the patients also were analyzed, using qualitative descriptive analysis. The data provided additional support for the patients' perceptions of the PACU nurses as caring, and the

TABLE H.1   CFS Scores Reported by ECT Patients, Descending Order

CARITAS PROCESS/FACTOR	n	MEAN	STD DEVIATION
Caregiver addressed all needs and concerns	27	6.67	.734
Caregiver established a helping and trusting relationship with patient	26	6.65	.689
Care provided with loving kindness	26	6.62	.752
Creative problem solving to meet patient's needs	26	6.54	.761
Caregiver's teaching is understandable	24	6.46	.779
Care provided instilled faith and hope	25	6.32	.988
Caregiver's embracement of patient's thoughts and feelings	24	6.17	.963
Caregiver recognized connection between mind, body, and spirit	25	5.96	1.428
Caregiver's acceptance and support of beliefs regarding a higher power	21	5.43	1.777
Caregivers encouraged practice of patient's health beliefs	25	5.28	1.768

achievement of Watson's four components of caring: caring, competence, communication, and commitment.

Each and every PACU ECT nurse has the ultimate respect and treats depression as an illness beyond my control, leaving me feeling that I am not singularized as nonsensical and insane. Each and every nurse is authentic and demonstrates genuine kindness, respect, concern, and devotion to their patients.

We are all [the patients] treated with true respect and dignity as we are spoken to and treated with a level of kindness and love that seems as though it would ordinarily be reserved for the staff members' own family members. I have never come away from a "treatment" experience with anything other than a feeling of having received the best care imaginable!

So, yes, caring can be provided in a PACU setting, as evidenced by the findings of this study. These quotes, and the quantitative data, provided sufficient evidence for the PACU nurses. However, as with any study, the generalizability of the findings and the conclusions drawn must be tempered by any limitations inherent in the study's design and conduct—in this case, the small sample size, the conduct of the study in one hospital, and the inability to collect demographic data. The effect of these limitations was tempered by the use of a reliable and valid tool to measure perceptions of caring (the reliability and transferability of which were further demonstrated in this study), but use of this tool to measure patients' perceptions of caring provided by another group of nurses may not yield the same positive results.

REFERENCES

Arkan, B., & Ustun, B. (2008). Examination of the effect of education about electroconvulsive therapy on nursing practice and patient satisfaction. *Journal of ECT, 24*, 254–259.

Beyer, J. L., Weiner, R. D., & Glenn, M. D. (1998). *Electroconvulsive therapy: A programmed text.* Washington, DC: American Psychiatric Press.

DiNapoli, P., Nelson, J., Turkel, M., & Watson, J. (2010). Measuring the Caritas processes: Caring factor survey. *International Journal of Human Caring, 14*(3), 16–21.

Dowman, J., Patel, A., & Rajput, K. (2005). Electroconvulsive therapy: Attitudes and misconceptions. *Journal of ECT, 21*, 84–87.

Gass, J. (2006). Electroconvulsive therapy and the work of mental health nurses: A grounded theory study. *International Journal of Nursing Studies, 45*, 191–202. doi:10.1016/j.ijnurstu.2006.08.011

Harrison, B., & Kaarsemaker, B. (2000). Continuous quality improvement to an electroconvulsive therapy delivery system. *Journal of Psychosocial Nursing and Mental Health Services, 38*, 27–35.

Kavanagh, A., & McLaughlin, D. (2010). Electroconvulsive therapy and nursing care. *British Journal of Nursing, 18*(22), 1370, 1372, 1374–1377.

Malekian, A., Amini, Z., Maracy, M. R., & Barekatain, M. (2008). Knowledge of attitude toward experience and satisfaction with electroconvulsive therapy in a sample of Iranian patients, *Journal of ECT, 25*(2), 106–112.

Munday, J., Deans, C., & Little, J. (2003). Effectiveness of a training program for ECT nurses. *Journal of Psychosocial Nursing and Mental Health Services, 41*(11), 20–26.

Myers, D. H. (2007). A questionnaire study of patients' experience of electroconvulsive therapy. *Journal of ECT, 23*, 169–174.

Petty, D. (2000). ECT in the PACU? It's possible. *Nursing Management, 31*(11), 42, 44.

Rose, D., Wykes, T., Bindman, J., & Fleischmann, O. (2003). Patients' perspectives on electroconvulsive therapy: Systematic review. *British Medical Journal, 326* (7403), 1363–1365.

Sienaert, P., Becker, T., Vansteelandt, K., Demyttenaere, K., & Peuskens, J. (2005). Patient satisfaction after electroconvulsive therapy. *Journal of ECT, 21*(4), 227–231.

Sienaert, P., Vansteelandt, K., Demyttenaere, K., & Peuskens, J. (2010). Predictors of patient satisfaction after ultrabrief, bifrontal and unilateral electroconvulsive therapies for major depression. *Journal of ECT, 26*, 55–59.

Smith, M., Vogler, J., Zarrouf, F., Sheaves, C., & Jesse, J. (2009). Electroconvulsive therapy: Struggles in the decision-making process and the aftermath of treatment. *Issues in Mental Health Nursing, 30*, 554–559.

Index

RBC. *See* Relationship-Based
Care (RBC)
Reception of patients/clients in health
care, in Italy, 291–295
Reflection, importance of
definition of, 307
as learning tool, 306
practical support for, 316
self-care, 306
structured, 308, 310
Reflection-in-action, 307–308
Reflective practice, 306–307
Registered Nurse-Bachelor
of Science in Nursing
(RN-BSN), 251
Registered nurses (RNs), 66, 93, 153,
166–167, 196, 398, 404
Relationship-Based Care (RBC), 40–41,
97, 195
background, 125–126
components of, 126, 128
education, 134–135
educational programming
RBC introduction, 130
RBC leader practicum, 130
UPC orientation, 130
elements of, 41
evaluation, 135–137
guiding principles of, 127
Healthcare Environment Survey
(HES), 137, 138
and human caring, 40–41
implementation, 147
inspiration and infrastructure,
131–134
integrated outcomes dashboard,
139, 141–142
journey, 145
baseline assessment of caring
factors, 146, 148, 149
beginning at unit level, 146
BHS adult unit, 151
implementation strategies,
147, 148
nurse case management, 150–151
rehabilitation nursing unit,
148–150
model, 127
ongoing journey, 143

Press Ganey patient satisfaction,
137, 139, 140
shared governance, infrastructure of
committee structure, 128–129
coordination council, 127–128
department councils, 129
unit practice councils, 127
and strategy, 126–127
structure of, 98
Relationship-Based Care (RBC)
in England
clinical supervision, 312–313
implementation of, 303, 304
community setting, challenges, 305
outcomes of, 304
interprofessional working,
310–311
reflection
definitions of, 307
importance of, 307–309
as learning tool, 306
practical support for, 316
self-care, 306
structured, 308, 310
reflective practice, 306–307
in community environment,
309–310
results used within, 313–315
transformational change, 305–306
as world pilot, 303–307
Religiosity, concept of, 9
Roots of nursing (caring), 30–31
Rotherham Community Health
Services (RCHS), 304

Sacred Work, definition of, 416
San Joaquin Community Hospital
(SJCH), 416
Self-authoring mind, xvii, xviii
Self-care, 357, 358
lack of, 39
for professional nurse, 108, 114
questionnaire, 303, 306
Self-transforming mind, xviii
"Silver Linings 2008," 407
Social and cognitive skills, 11
Sound validation in critical care, 12
Spirituality, concept of, 9